Recent Advances in Understanding Systemic Sclerosis

Recent Advances in Understanding Systemic Sclerosis

Guest Editor

Joerg Henes

MDPI

Basel • Beijing • Wuhan • Barcelona • Belgrade • Novi Sad • Cluj • Manchester

Guest Editor
Joerg Henes
Center for Interdisciplinary
Clinical Immunology,
Rheumatology and Autoimmune Diseases
(INDIRA) and Internal Medicine II
University Hospital Tübingen
Tübingen
Germany

Editorial Office
MDPI AG
Grosspeteranlage 5
4052 Basel, Switzerland

This is a reprint of the Special Issue, published open access by the journal *Sclerosis* (ISSN 2813-3064), freely accessible at: https://www.mdpi.com/journal/sclerosis/special_issues/systemic_sclerosis.

For citation purposes, cite each article independently as indicated on the article page online and as indicated below:

Lastname, A.A.; Lastname, B.B. Article Title. *Journal Name* **Year**, *Volume Number*, Page Range.

ISBN 978-3-7258-5803-3 (Hbk)
ISBN 978-3-7258-5804-0 (PDF)
https://doi.org/10.3390/books978-3-7258-5804-0

Cover image courtesy of Joerg Henes

Contents

About the Editor

Joerg Henes

Joerg Henes is a Professor of rheumatology at the University Hospital Tuebingen, one of the oldest universities in Germany. Prof. Henes started early on in his career to take care of patients with systemic sclerosis and other connective tissue diseases, with a special focus on new cellular therapies to enhance the therapeutic options for these patients. He plays a key role in the development and recommendations for autologous stem cell transplantation in autoimmune diseases in Europe. Very recently, he and several colleagues established the first German guidelines for the diagnosis and treatment of systemic sclerosis.

Another focus of his is on topics such as sexuality, fertility, and pregnancy in autoimmune diseases.

sclerosis

MDPI

Article

Uncovering Subclinical Cardiac Involvement in VEDOSS: An Echocardiographic Driven Study

Eugenio Capparelli [1,2,*], Eleonora Zaccara [1], Ilaria Suardi [3,4], Antonella Laria [3], Laura Castelnovo [1], Eleonora Mauric [3], Daniela Bompane [1], Antonio Tamburello [1], Maria Iacovantuono [2], Maria Sole Chimenti [2], Antonino Mazzone [1] and Paola Faggioli [1,3]

[1] Internal Medicine Unit, ASST Ovest Milanese, Legnano Hospital, 20025 Milan, Italy; eleonora.zaccara@asst-ovestmi.it (E.Z.); laura.castelnovo@asst-ovestmi.it (L.C.); daniela.bompane@asst-ovestmi.it (D.B.); antonio.tamburello@asst-ovestmi.it (A.T.); antonino.mazzone@asst-ovestmi.it (A.M.); paola.faggioli@asst-ovestmi.it (P.F.)

[2] Rheumatology, Allergology and Clinical Immunology, Departement of Medicine of Systems, University of Rome Tor Vergata, 00133 Rome, Italy; mariaiacovantuono@gmail.com (M.I.); maria.sole.chimenti@uniroma2.it (M.S.C.)

[3] Rheumatology Unit, ASST Ovest Milanese, Magenta Hospital, 20123 Milan, Italy; ilaria.suardi@asst-ovestmi.it (I.S.); antonella.laria@asst-ovestmi.it (A.L.); eleonora.mauric@asst-ovestmi.it (E.M.)

[4] Department of Clinical Sciences and Community Health, Università degli Studi di Milano, 20122 Milan, Italy

* Correspondence: capparelli.eugenio@yahoo.it

Abstract: Background: The 2011 Very Early Diagnosis of Systemic Sclerosis (VEDOSS) criteria include both patients at risk of progression and those with mild non-progressive forms of SSc. Early diastolic and systolic dysfunction can indicate myocardial fibrosis in SSc patients, yet data on myocardial impairment in the VEDOSS population are limited. **Objectives:** This study aimed to identify subclinical echocardiographic changes and predictive markers of cardiac dysfunction in both very early and mild-longstanding forms of VEDOSS. **Methods:** We conducted a cross-sectional observational study involving 61 patients meeting VEDOSS criteria followed up regularly within our Scleroderma referral center. Patients were categorized as early VEDOSS (e-VEDOSS) or mild-longstanding VEDOSS (ml-VEDOSS) based on disease duration ($\geq$10 years). We analyzed clinical and demographic data, focusing on echocardiographic parameters such as the E/A ratio and left ventricular (LV) thickness. Statistical analyses included chi-square, Fischer exact, and student's t tests, with a significance threshold of $p < 0.05$. **Results:** ml-VEDOSS patients were older and reported a higher burden of comorbidities. Autoantibody-positive patients exhibited lower E/A ratios and increased left atrial size. Late nailfold videocapillaroscopic pattern patients exhibited increased PWED thickening and aortic valve insufficiency. Notably, patients undergoing vasodilators experienced larger right atrial volume, while patients receiving Renin-Angiotensin-Aldosterone System (RAAS) inhibitors reported reduced E/A ratio. Multivariable analysis confirmed DLCO% as the sole predictor of both diastolic and systolic impairment in VEDOSS population. **Conclusions:** Careful monitoring of cardiac function in VEDOSS patients is crucial as subclinical alterations may occur even in the absence of symptoms. DLCO% emerged as an important predictor of LV diastolic dysfunction.

Keywords: VEDOSS; systemic sclerosis; early diagnosis; cardiac involvement; diastolic dysfunction; echocardiography

1. Introduction

Systemic sclerosis (SSc) is a rare autoimmune disease characterized by the classical triad of microvascular damage, autoimmune dysregulation, and fibrosis of the skin and internal organs [1]. The extensive fibrotic process of vital organs, including the lungs and heart, is significantly associated with a high burden of morbidity and mortality [2]. In this context, it is essential to perform a prompt diagnosis to shape the trajectories of potentially progressive disease [3]. Currently, SSc diagnosis can be oriented by consolidated classification criteria such as those proposed by LeRoy and Medsger in 2001 [4], together with the 2013 ACR/EULAR guidelines [5]. However, it is well recognized that these classifications do not encompass all patients within the broader scleroderma spectrum, particularly in the earlier stages of the disease [6]. The 2011 criteria for a Very Early Diagnosis of Systemic Sclerosis (the VEDOSS criteria) and their validation in 2021, have enhanced clinicians' ability to identify the disease in its initial phase [7,8].

Thus, while VEDOSS may represent the early stage of SSc, it could also reflect a milder form that remains stable over time and does not progress to clinically established disease. Currently, despite the lack of validated criteria that allow clinicians to differentiate between these two forms, VEDOSS represents a critical stage in the scleroderma continuum, in which it is crucial to identify early organ involvement [9,10].

Moreover, while some organs, such as the gastrointestinal tract, have been investigated in VEDOSS [11], cardiac involvement remains a neglected area. All layers of the heart—endocardium, myocardium, and pericardium—can be affected by the pathogenic processes of SSc, with myocardial fibrosis being the predominant pathological finding in postmortem studies [12]. Subclinical left ventricular (LV) diastolic and systolic impairments represent the initial expression of myocardial fibrosis, which may often be asymptomatic [13]. However, several echocardiographic parameters, such as mitral early diastolic inflow velocity (E wave), mitral late filling peak velocity (A wave), early diastolic annular velocity (E′), and the E/A and E/E′ ratios may enable the detection of early myocardial involvement in asymptomatic SSc patients. For instance, an E/A ratio less than 1.0 and E/E′ ratio ≥ 15 indicate elevated filling pressure and predict the development of diastolic heart failure [14]. Moreover, given that cardiac involvement in SSc is highly predictive of poor prognosis and mortality [15], detecting subclinical echocardiographic signs of systolic and diastolic dysfunction seems to be fundamental even in the VEDOSS population.

The aim of the present study is to identify subclinical echocardiographic alterations in VEDOSS patients by analyzing certain clinical, serological, and functional predictive markers of systolic and diastolic dysfunction in both mild-longstanding cases and the very early form of SSc, offering insights into the progression and early detection of cardiac involvement in this patient group.

2. Materials and Methods

2.1. Sample Definition

We conducted a cross-sectional observational study involving a cohort of VEDOSS patients attending the Scleroderma Unit of ASST Ovest Milanese (Italy). Participants were selected if they fulfilled the 2011 preliminary VEDOSS criteria [7] while not meeting the 2013 ACR/EULAR and/or 2001 LeRoy and Medsger criteria for a definitive diagnosis of SSc [4,5]. Patients with severe heart failure, a positive history of congenital heart disease, severe chronic obstructive pulmonary disease, pulmonary thromboembolism, and individuals who underwent cardiac surgery, percutaneous coronary intervention (PCI) and pacemaker implant were excluded from the study. The presence of other autoimmune disease-related antibodies and/or the fulfillment of additional classification criteria for any systemic autoimmune disease served as further exclusion criteria.

Written informed consent was obtained from each participant, and the study was conducted in accordance with the ethical guidelines of the Declaration of Helsinki, with the ethic protocol number S00125/2023 obtained from the Ethic Committee of Milan Area 3 on 29th of May 2023.

2.2. Data Collection

Data collection was conducted by experienced rheumatologists and spanned between June and December 2024. Demographic data including sex, age at enrollment, alcohol consumption or smoking habit, age at the first appearance of Raynaud's Phenomenon (RP), and age at VEDOSS diagnosis were extracted from medical records. Diagnostic delay was calculated as the time interval between the onset of the first VEDOSS symptom and the confirmation of a definitive VEDOSS diagnosis.

Key clinical and anthropometric parameters were recorded at last follow up visit, including height, weight, body mass index (BMI) and body surface area (BSA). The presence of RP and puffy hands was noted, along with the presence of any gastrointestinal complaints that could be attributed to VEDOSS. Additionally, for the main purpose of the study, the absence of skin fibrosis, sclerodactyly, digital ulcers, pitting scars, calcinosis, and telangiectasias was documented. Therefore, clinical evaluation involved a comprehensive physical, functional, and radiological assessment for dyspnea and other heart-related symptoms. Data from pulmonary function tests (PFTs), including predicted forced vital capacity (FVC%), predicted diffusing capacity for carbon monoxide (DLCO%), and the FVC/DLCO% ratio, were obtained from the most recent available assessments, and along with chest X-ray, were allowed to exclude suspected or established interstitial lung disease (ILD) and pulmonary arterial hypertension (PAH) as compelling causes of unexplained dyspnea. Analogously, all patients underwent nailfold Videocapillaroscopy (NVC) at the last follow-up visit, with the NVC results reported according to Cutolo classification [16].

Laboratory detection of antinuclear antibodies (ANA), anticentromere antibodies (ACA), and anti-topoisomerase I antibodies (ATA) were performed using standardized methods during the initial clinical evaluation.

Data on current comorbidities were collected, including cardiovascular conditions such as chronic systemic arterial hypertension and atrial fibrillation, as well as thyroid disorders, pulmonary diseases, gastrointestinal disorders, renal diseases, malignancies, hematological conditions, and psychiatric and neurological issues.

Data concerning treatment modalities were registered, encompassing the administration of Iloprost infusions, the use of calcium channel blockers (CCBs), and low-dose aspirin (LDA). Additionally, treatments employed for managing cardiovascular comorbidities with a known influence on microvascular system were documented, such as angiotensin-converting enzyme inhibitors (ACE-Is), angiotensin receptor blockers (ARBs), beta-blockers, and diuretics. Immunosuppressive therapies and the use of hydroxychloroquine were also recorded.

2.3. Echocardiography Procedure

Echocardiographic parameters were collected at the last follow-up visit. All selected patients were imaged by transthoracic echocardiography (TTE) in the left lateral decubitus position by experienced cardiologists at the same hospital in accordance with the guidelines of the American Society of Echocardiography (ASE) [17]. All images and measurements were obtained from the standard views with stable electrocardiograph (EKG). The following parameters were measured: interventricular septum (IVS) thickness (mm), posterior wall at end diastole (PWED) thickness (mm), left ventricular (LV) volumes and diameters in both end systole and end diastole, aorta diameter at sinuses, along with right and left atrial (RA and LA) volumes at the end systole in monoplane apical 4 chamber (4CH) view through both Simpson and indexed methods. RA and LA end systolic diameters were measured via monoplane 4CH view in the longitudinal side (superior-inferior) direction, and the RA and LA end systolic area was assessed in cm^2. Left ventricular (LV) ejection fraction (EF) was measured with the modified biplane Simpson's method from the apical 4CH view [18].

Left ventricular (LV) mass was calculated according to the Devereux formula [19]. Pathological thickening of both IVS and PWED was defined as more than 10 mm and more than 9 mm, respectively. Additionally, the systolic pulmonary artery pressure (sPAP) was estimated using modified Bernoulli's formula [20]. The tricuspid annular plane systolic excursion (TAPSE) was measured by placing the M-mode line at the junction of the tricuspid valve annulus and the RV free wall [21]. Tricuspid regurgitation and the tricuspid maximum regurgitation pressure gradient were also assessed. Doppler echocardiographic measurements included: Trans-mitral early diastolic inflow velocity (E), trans-mitral late filling peak velocity (A), and E/A ratio measured in the apical 4-CH view [22]. Tissue Doppler imaging was used to measure the early diastolic annular velocity (E′). Left ventricular dysfunction was defined as mitral E/A ratio < 1.0 and E/E′ ratio ≥ 15 [23]. Additionally, the presence of mitral, aortic, and tricuspid valve insufficiencies was evaluated by the color Doppler method, along with any noted sclerosis of the aortic and mitral valve leaflets and then reported according to the 2020 ACC/AHA guideline for the management of patients with valvular heart disease [24]. Lastly, the presence of pericardial effusion was identified by the appearance of an echo-free space between the two layers of the pericardium.

2.4. Statistical Analysis

Patients' data were summarized as mean and standard deviation for normally distributed variables or as median and interquartile range (IQR) for skewed ones. Discrete or qualitative variables were summarized as counts and percentages. Mean differences of continuous variables were assessed using student's *t*-test or Mann–Whitney U-test, depending on whether the data followed a parametric or non-parametric distribution. Chi-squared and Fisher's exact tests were used to compare categorical variables based on sample size. ANOVA test served for multiple comparison analysis.

Based on their established relevance on SSc progression and heart involvement, several clinical determinants, such as BMI, age at VEDOSS diagnosis, DLCO% predicted, ACA/ATA positivity, late NVC patterns, and puffy hands were included in the multiple general regression model to assess their independent contribution on left ventricular diastolic and systolic dysfunction. E/A ratio, IVS thickness, and PWED thickness served as dependent variables in the multiple general regression model.

A *p*-value of ≤ 0.05 or a 95% confidence interval not crossing zero were considered statistically significant. All statistical analyses were performed using IBM SPSS Statistics version 27 (IBM SPSS Software, Armonk, NY, USA).

3. Results

3.1. Overall Patients' Characteristics

The study cohort consisted of 61 participants, with a female predominance (58 out of 61—95.1%). Based on VEDOSS disease duration, patients were distributed into two subgroups: mild longstanding VEDOSS with a disease duration $\geq$10 years (ml-VEDOSS, 24/61—39.3%) and early VEDOSS group with a disease duration <10 years (e-VEDOSS, 37/61—60.7%) (Table 1).

Table 1. Patient's main characteristics according to VEDOSS disease duration.

	TOTAL $n = 61$	e-VEDOSS $n = 37$	ml-VEDOSS $n = 24$	p-Value
Female, n(%)	58 (95.1)	36 (97.3)	22 (91.7)	0.56
Male, n(%)	3 (4.9)	1 (2.7)	2 (8.3)	0.56
Age at enrollment, mean ± SD	58.7 ± 14.5	55.2 ± 14.6	64.0 ± 12.8	0.01
Age at VEDOSS diagnosis, mean ± SD	49.8 ± 14.7	51.7 ± 15.1	47.3 ±14.1	0.27
Age at RP onset, mean ± SD	43.2 ±17.1	44.2 ± 17.4	41.8 ± 16.9	0.62
Disease duration of VEDOSS, mean ± SD	9.9 ± 7.9	4.9 ± 2.7	16.8 ± 7.7	<0.001
Disease duration of RP, mean ± SD	16.1 ± 11.6	12.3 ± 10.9	21.6 ± 10.4	0.002
Diagnostic delay, mean ± SD	6.4 ± 9.5	7.5 ± 10.6	4.7 ± 7.4	0.28
Body mass index (Kg/m^2), mean ± SD	23.5 ± 5.9	22.4 ± 5.7	25.2 ± 5.9	0.07
Smoking habits, n(%)	10 (16.4)	8 (21.6)	2 (8.3)	0.29
Alcohol consumption, n(%)	13 (21.3)	2 (5.3)	1 (4.2)	1.0
Puffy hands, n(%)	18 (29.5)	10 (27.0)	8 (33.3)	1.0
ANA (positive) only, n(%)	21 (34.4)	16 (43.2)	5 (20.8)	0.09
Anticentromere (positive), n(%)	21 (34.4)	9 (24.3)	12 (50)	0.05
Anti-topoisomerase I (positive), n(%)	3 (4.9)	2 (5.3)	1 (4.2)	1.0
Gastrointestinal tract symptoms, n(%)	30 (49.2)	15 (40.5)	15 (62.5)	0.12
COMORBIDITIES, n(%)				
Cardiovascular diseases,	29 (47.5)	13 (35.1)	16 (66.7)	0.02
Dyslipidemia	17 (27.9)	9 (24.3)	8 (33.3)	0.56
Hyperuricemia	2 (3.3)	0 (0)	2 (8.3)	0.15
Type 2 diabetes mellitus	4 (6.6)	2 (5.3)	2 (8.3)	0.64
Thyroid disorders	13 (21.3)	7 (18.9)	6 (25.0)	0.75
Lung diseases	12 (19.6)	6 (16.2)	6 (25.0)	0.51
Kidney diseases	8 (13.1)	4 (10.8)	4 (16.7)	0.7
Gastrointestinal diseases	35 (57.4)	17 (45.9)	18 (75.0)	0.03
Hematological disorders	8 (13.1)	2 (5.3)	6 (25.0)	0.04
Malignancies	10 (16.4)	5 (13.5)	5 (20.8)	0.49
Psychiatric disorders	3 (4.9)	2 (5.3)	1 (4.2)	1.0
Neurological disorders	11 (18.0)	5 (13.5)	6 (25.0)	0.32
Comorbidities count, mean ± SD	2.7 ± 2.1	2.1 ± 1.9	3.6 ± 2.0	0.005
Comorbidities count ≥ 3, n(%)	31 (50.8)	15 (40.5)	16 (66.7)	0.01
NVC PATTERN, n(%)				
Aspecific alterations	7 (11.5)	5 (13.5)	2 (8.3)	0.69
Early pattern	34 (55.7)	23 (62.2)	11 (45.8)	0.29
Active pattern	14 (23.0)	9 (24.3)	5 (20.8)	1.0
Late pattern	6 (9.8)	0 (0)	6 (25.0)	0.002
TREATMENT, n(%)				
Iloprost	44 (72.1)	23 (62.2)	21 (87.5)	0.04
Calcium channel blockers	20 (32.7)	8 (21.6)	12 (50.0)	0.03
Low-dose aspirin	39 (63.9)	23 (62.2)	16 (66.7)	0.78
ACE-I/ARBs	16 (26.2)	6 (16.2)	10 (41.7)	0.04
Beta-blockers	4 (6.6)	2 (5.3)	2 (8.3)	0.64
Diuretics	1 (1.6)	1 (2.7)	0	1.0
Hydroxychloroquine	20 (32.7)	9 (24.3)	11 (45.8)	0.09
Immunosuppressants	3 (4.9)	1 (2.7)	2 (8.3)	0.56

Acronyms: n = number; % = percentage; SD = standard deviation; e-VEDOSS = early very early diagnosis of systemic sclerosis; ml-VEDOSS = mild longstanding very early diagnosis of systemic sclerosis; RP = Raynaud's phenomenon; ANA = antinuclear antibodies; ACE-I = angiotensin converting enzyme inhibitors; Angiotensin receptor blockers; ns = not significant; Kg = Kilograms; m^2 = square meters, NVC = Nailfold videocapillaroscopy.

The mean age at enrollment was significantly higher in the ml-VEDOSS group compared to the e-VEDOSS group (64.0 ± 12.8 vs. 55.2 ± 14.6 years; $p = 0.01$). As expected, the disease durations for VEDOSS and RP were substantially longer in the ml-VEDOSS group

(16.8 ± 7.7 vs. 4.9 ± 2.7 years; $p < 0.001$ and 21.6 ± 10.4 vs. 12.3 ± 10.9; $p = 0.002$, respectively). Regarding autoimmunity profile, ACA+ patients were more frequently present in the ml-VEDOSS group (50% vs. 24.3%, $p = 0.05$).

A greater mean comorbidity count was observed in the ml-VEDOSS group compared to the e-VEDOSS group (3.6 ± 2.0 vs. 2.1 ± 1.9; $p = 0.005$), with higher prevalence of patients exhibiting more than three comorbidities (66.7% vs. 40.5%, $p = 0.01$). Within the same group, there was a higher prevalence of cardiovascular and gastrointestinal diseases (66.7% vs. 35.1%; $p = 0.02$ and 75% vs. 45.9%; $p = 0.03$, respectively), along with hematological disorders (25% vs. 5.3%, $p = 0.04$). Furthermore, the late NVC pattern was significantly more common within the ml-VEDOSS group (six out of 24, 25%; $p = 0.002$).

Similarly, treatment modalities displayed notable variations between the two groups. The administration of vasodilators, such as Iloprost infusion and CCBs, were prescribed significantly more often in the ml-VEDOSS group (87.5% vs. 62.2%, $p = 0.04$ and 50% vs. 21.6%, $p = 0.03$, respectively). The use of ACE-Is or ARBs was more common in the ml-VEDOSS group compared to the e-VEDOSS group (41.7% vs. 16.2%, $p = 0.04$). Immunosuppressants were prescribed in only three out of 61 patients, two of whom were receiving methotrexate due to musculoskeletal symptoms, while one patient received azathioprine for a concurrent diagnosis of autoimmune hepatitis.

3.2. Subclinical Echocardiographic Findings

Main echocardiographic findings of the entire population are reported in Table 2. Specifically, mean E/A ratio was 0.99 ± 0.39 and 37/61 (60.7%) patients exhibited an E/A ratio less than 1, mean PWED thickness was 8.4 ± 1.6 mm and 19 out of 61 (31.1%) presented with a PWED thickening more than 9 mm, while the pathological IVS thickening (>10 mm) was documented in 17/61 participants (27.9%). A reduced EF% (less than 55%) was reported only in 3/61 patients (4.9%) while the mean value of EF% was 64.5 ± 4.8%. A reduced TAPSE (<22 mmHg) was reported in 36/61 patients (59%) while only one patient exhibited a TAPSE less than 16 mmHg. Mean sPAP of the entire population was 27.2 ± 5.3 mmHg.

Since the comparison between e-VEDOSS and ml-VEDOSS group did not reveal any statistical difference on echocardiographic parameters (Supplementary Table S1), we further focused on assessing these findings within three intergroups by selecting the late NVC pattern, SSc specific autoantibodies positivity, and puffy hands as compelling variables (Table 3).

Notably, the prevalence of patients exhibiting PWED thickness > 9 mm was significantly greater in the late NVC pattern group (66.7% vs. 23.6 %, $p = 0.04$). Furthermore, the presence of aortic valve insufficiency (66.7% vs. 18.2%, $p = 0.02$) and sclerosis (66.7% vs. 16.4%, $p = 0.01$) were significantly more prevalent in the same group. Moreover, the E/A ratio was significantly lower in the ACA/ATA+ group (0.84 ± 0.27 vs. 1.08 ± 0.42, $p = 0.02$) by exhibiting a longer A wave measurement (0.84 ± 0.20 vs. 0.70 ± 0.15 m/s, $p = 0.006$). Additionally, IVS thickness was greater in the same group (9.9 ± 1.3 vs. 8.9 ± 1.9 mm, $p = 0.03$). Further significant differences were noted in the LA end systolic (LAES) volume, even indexed for BSA, which were significantly higher in the ACA/ATA+ group ($p = 0.01$ for both). Likewise, the LAES diameter (49.7 ± 5.9 vs. 45.0 ± 8.4 mm/m^2, $p = 0.04$) and the relative wall thickness (0.48 ± 0.09 vs. 0.42 ± 0.10, $p = 0.04$) were significantly larger in the ACA/ATA+ group. Additionally, the ACA/ATA+ group revealed a greater proportion of both aortic and mitral valve insufficiency and sclerosis of valve leaflets. Lastly, in the puffy hands group, E deceleration time was significantly longer compared to the non-puffy hands group (194.4 ± 47.9 vs. 230.5 ± 52.8 m/s, $p = 0.02$). Any differences in RV and RA function parameters emerged from the intergroup comparisons of TAPSE, sPAP, and the tricuspid maximum regurgitation gradient, along with RAES volumes and diameters.

Table 2. Echocardiographic findings across the entire population.

Echocardiographic Parameters	TOTAL $n = 61$
E deceleration time (m/s), mean ± SD	244.3 ± 281.7
E/E′ ratio, mean ± SD	6.9 ± 1.9
E wave, (m/s), mean ± SD	0.69 ± 0.17
A wave, (m/s), mean ± SD	0.75 ± 0.19
E/A ratio, mean ± SD	0.99 ± 0.39
E/A ratio < 1.0, *n* (%)	37 (60.7)
LVED diameter, (mm), mean ± SD	40.3 ± 4.8
PWED thickness, (mm), mean ± SD	8.4 ± 1.6
PWED > 9 mm, *n* (%)	19 (31.1)
IVS thckness, (mm), mean ± SD	9.3 ± 1.8
IVS > 10 mm, *n* (%)	17 (27.9)
LVED volume 4CH Simpson, (mL), mean ± SD	67.7 ± 16.6
LVES volume 4CH Simpson, (mL), mean ± SD	25.5 ± 11.8
LVED volume 4CH AL, (mL/m^2), mean ± SD	43.4 ± 8.8
LVES volume 4CH AL, (mL/m^2), mean ± SD	14.7 ± 4.3
EF%, mean ± SD	64.5 ± 4.8
EF% < 55%	3 (4.9)
Mass ASE, (g), mean ± SD	123.2 ± 123.9
Mass/BSA, (g/m^2), mean ± SD	66.3 ± 17.3
Relative wall thickness, mean ± SD	0.44 ± 0.10
Mass/height, (g/m), mean ± SD	65.8 ± 18.2
Aortic diameter, (mm^2), mean ± SD	29.7 ± 3.9
LAES area, (cm^2), mean ± SD	15.6 ± 3.6
LAES 4CH Simpson, (mL), mean ± SD	40.4 ± 13.7
LAES 4CH ind, (mL/m^2), mean ± SD	24.4 ± 7.5
LAES diameter sup-inf 4CH, (mm/m^2), mean ± SD	46.5 ± 7.6
RAES diameter AL, (mm), mean ± SD	46.1 ± 5.8
RAES 4CH Simpson, (mL), mean ± SD	30.3 ± 8.9
RAES 4CH ind, (mL/m^2), mean ± SD	18.5 ± 5.0
RAES area, (cm^2), mean ± SD	13.5 ± 3.1
TAPSE, (mmHg), mean ± SD	21.5 ± 3.0
TAPSE < 22 mmHg, *n* (%)	36 (59.0)
TAPSE < 16 mmHg, *n* (%)	1 (1.6)
TAPSE/sPAP, mean ± SD	0.72 ± 0.32
TAPSE/sPAP < 0.55, *n* (%)	1 (1.6)
sPAP, (mmHg), mean ± SD	27.2 ± 5.3
Tricuspid maximum regurgitation gradient, (mmHg), mean ± SD	22.2 ± 6.5
Mitral Valve Insufficiency, *n* (%)	42 (68.9)
Mitral Valve Sclerosis, *n* (%)	25 (40.9)
Tricuspid Valve Insufficiency, *n* (%)	33 (54.1)
Aortic Valve Insufficiency, *n* (%)	13 (21.3)
Aortic Valve Sclerosis, *n* (%)	11 (18.0)
Pericardial Effusion, *n* (%)	4 (6.6)

Acronyms: SD = Standard deviation. ACA = Anti-centromere autoantibodies; ATA = Anti Topoisomerase I autoantibodies; E wave = early diastolic filling velocity of the left ventricle; E′ = early diastolic tissue velocity of the mitral annulus; A = late diastolic filling velocity; LVED = left ventricular end diastolic; LVES = left ventricular end systolic; PWED = posterior wall end diastolic; IVS = interventricular septum; LAES = left atrial end systolic; RAES = right atrial end systolic; TAPSE = tricuspid annular plane systolic excursion; sPAP = systolic pulmonary artery pressure; 4CH = 4 chamber; AL = anterolateral; EF = ejection fraction; % = percentage; BSA = body surface area; ASE = American Society of echocardiography; ind = indexed; sup-inf = superior–inferior; m/s = meter/seconds; mm = millimeters; g = grams; g/m^2 = grams/square meters; cm^2 = square centimeters; mmHg = millimeters of mercury.

Table 3. Echocardiographic findings among intergroups analysis.

	Late Pattern $n = 6$	No Late Pattern $n = 55$	p-Value	ACA/ATA+ $n = 24$	ACA/ATA− $n = 37$	p-Value	Puffy Hands $n = 18$	No Puffy Hands $n = 43$	p-Value
E deceleration time (m/s), mean ± SD	225.2 ± 46.1	246.7 ± 298.9	0.86	213.4 ± 56.2	261.6 ± 349.9	0.55	230.5 ± 52.8	194.4 ± 47.9	0.02
E/E′ ratio, mean ± SD	7.55 ± 1.37	6.92 ± 1.90	0.52	7.6 ± 1.8	6.7 ± 1.8	0.12	7.0 ± 1.3	6.8 ± 1.9	0.77
E wave, (m/s), mean ± SD	0.70 ± 0.22	0.68 ± 0.16	0.86	0.71 ± 0.17	0.65 ± 0.17	0.27	0.68 ± 0.19	0.69 ± 0.16	0.78
A wave, (m/s), mean ± SD	0.81 ± 0.17	0.75 ± 0.19	0.46	0.84 ± 0.20	0.70 ± 0.15	0.006	0.79 ± 0.20	0.74 ± 0.18	0.38
E/A ratio, mean ± SD	0.92 ± 0.40	1.0 ± 0.39	0.61	0.84 ± 0.27	1.08 ± 042	0.02	0.92 ± 0.4	1.02 ± 0.39	0.39
E/A ratio < 1.0, n (%)	3 (50)	34 (61.8)	0.12	18 (75)	19 (51.4)	0.11	10 (55.6)	27 (62.8)	0.77
LVED diameter, (mm), mean ± SD	38.5 ± 3.6	40.5 ± 4.9	0.34	39.4 ± 5.6	40.8 ± 4.4	0.45	40.2 ± 6.2	40.4 ± 4.07	0.86
PWED thickness, (mm), mean ± SD	8.4 ± 1.5	8.3 ± 1.6	0.89	8.6 ± 1.2	8.2 ± 1.8	0.31	8.5 ± 1.5	8.3 ± 1.7	0.63
PWED > 9 mm, n(%)	4 (66.7)	13 (23.6)	0.04	9 (37.5)	8 (21.6)	0.24	8 (44.4)	9 (20.9)	0.11
IVS thckness, (mm), mean ± SD	9.9 ± 1.6	9.3 ± 1.8	0.37	9.9 ± 1.3	8.9 ± 1.9	0.03	9.4 ± 1.6	9.4 ± 2.0	0.90
IVS > 10 mm, n (%)	2 (33.3)	20 (36.4)	0.39	10 (41.7)	12 (32.4)	0.58	6 (33.3)	16 (37.2)	1.0
LVED volume 4CH Simpson, (mL), mean ± SD	69.7 ± 22.2	67.5 ± 16.1	0.76	66.9 ± 17.3	68.3 ± 16.4	0.75	24.8 ± 3.5	85.3 ± 363.2	0.49
LVES volume 4CH Simpson, (mL), mean ± SD	24.8 ± 9.7	25.6 ± 12.1	0.88	24.0 ± 9.9	26.4 ± 12.8	0.46	68.3 ± 17.8	68.7 ± 16.3	0.93
LVED volume 4CH AL, (mL/m²), mean ± SD	41.3 ± 12.4	43.6 ± 8.4	0.88	41.7 ± 10.3	44.3 ± 7.8	0.29	25.7 ± 10.9	26.0 ± 12.7	0.92
LVES volume 4CH AL, (mL/m²), mean ± SD	14.8 ± 5.6	14.7 ± 4.2	0.54	14.7 ± 6.2	14.7 ± 2.9	0.92	43.1 ± 10.5	44.3 ± 8.2	0.64
EF%, mean ± SD	64.5 ± 6.8	64.6 ± 4.6	0.92	64.9 ± 5.7	64.4 ± 4.3	0.64	15.6 ± 6.2	14.6 ± 3.2	0.42
EF% < 55%	1 (16.7)	2 (3.6)	0.27	2 (8.3)	1 (2.7)	0.55	2 (11.1)	1 (2.3)	0.21
Mass ASE, (g), mean ± SD	108.3 ± 30.9	124.9 ± 130.8	0.96	129.1 ± 153.4	112 ± 30.3	0.63	63.5 ± 5.7	65.1 ± 4.5	0.26
Mass/BSA, (g/m²), mean ± SD	65.5 ± 17.0	66.4 ± 17.0	0.90	68.8 ± 17.4	64.9 ± 17.4	0.42	163.3 ± 217.5	107.3 ± 36.9	0.14
Relative wall thickness, mean ± SD	0.48 ± 0.08	0.44 ± 0.1	0.35	0.48 ± 0.09	0.42 ± 0.10	0.04	68.3 ± 19.5	66.5 ± 17.0	0.73
Mass/height, (g/m), mean ± SD	69.2 ± 21.8	65.5 ± 17.9	0.64	68.1 ± 20.3	64.7 ± 17.2	0.51	0.45 ± 0.12	0.44 ± 0.09	0.65
Aortic diameter, (mm²), mean ± SD	29.7 ± 2.4	29.6 ± 4.1	0.96	29.7 ± 3.7	29.6 ± 4.1	0.94	65.3 + 20.6	67.5 ± 17.8	0.68
LAES area, (cm²), mean ± SD	16.1 ± 2.7	15.6 ± 3.7	0.75	16.7 ± 4.1	15.1 ± 3.2	0.11	28.5 ± 2.5	30.0 ± 4.3	0.19
LAES 4CH Simpson, (mL), mean ± SD	41.6 ± 10.5	40.3 ± 14.3	0.83	46.7 ± 18.7	37.2 ± 8.9	0.01	15.4 ± 3.3	16.1 ± 3.8	0.52
LAES 4CH ind, (mL/m²), mean ± SD	24.6 ± 5.7	24.4 ± 7.8	0.95	27.7 ± 10.2	22.6 ± 5.1	0.01	42.3 ± 13.2	40.8 ± 14.2	0.73
LAES diameter 4CH, (mm/m²), mean ± SD	50.3 ± 5.8	46.1 ± 8.1	0.27	49.7 ± 5.9	45.0 ± 8.4	0.04	25.6 ± 8.3	24.6 ± 7.3	0.68
RAES diameter AL, (mm), mean ± SD	47.2 ± 1.7	46.0 ± 6.1	0.74	47.8 ± 45.4	45.4 ± 5.8	0.22	46.9 ± 6.0	46.7 ± 9.1	0.91
RAES 4CH Simpson, (mL), mean ± SD	32.9 ± 9.6	30.0 ± 8.9	0.55	30.1 ± 8.1	30.5 ± 9.5	0.91	44.8 ± 4.5	47.0 ± 6.2	0.27
RAES 4CH ind, (mL/m²), mean ± SD	19.1 ± 5.4	18.4 ± 5.1	0.78	18.5 ± 3.6	18.5 ± 5.6	0.98	28.4 ± 7.9	31.7 ± 9.5	0.33
RAES area, (cm²), mean ± SD	13.8 ± 2.5	13.5 ± 3.2	0.83	14.4 ± 2.9	13.0 ± 3.2	0.12	17.9 ± 4.8	18.9 ± 5.4	0.59
TAPSE, (mmHg), mean ± SD	22.0 ± 4.9	21.5 ± 2.9	0.70	21.9 ± 3.7	21.4 ± 2.7	0.61	13.1 ± 2.2	13.8 ± 3.6	0.43
TAPSE < 22 mmHg, n (%)	4 (66.7)	32 (58.2)	1.0	14 (58.3)	22 (59.4)	1.0	12 (66.7)	23 (53.5)	0.40
TAPSE < 16 mmHg, n (%)	0 (0)	1 (1.8)	1.0	1 (4.2)	0 (0)	0.39	0 (0)	1 (2.3)	1.0
TAPSE/sPAP, mean ± SD	0.98 ± 0.31	0.69 ± 0.32	0.24	0.71 ± 0.38	0.72 ± 0.29	0.92	21.8 ± 3.3	21.3 ± 2.8	0.59
TAPSE/sPAP < 0.55, n (%)	1 (16.7)	3 (5.5)	0.35	1 (4.2)	3 (8.1)	1.0	1 (5.6)	3 (7.0)	1.0
sPAP, (mmHg), mean ± SD	28.0 ± 4.2	27.1 ± 5.5	0.83	26.7 ± 4.4	27.7 ± 6.2	0.63	0.7 ± 0.36	0.69 ± 0.33	0.29
Tricuspid maximum regurgitation gradient, (mmHg), mean ± SD	21.9 ± 3.4	22.2 ± 6.7	0.93	22.4 ± 4.8	22.1 ± 7.4	0.88	27.7 ± 3.9	26.8 ± 6.3	0.75
Mitral valve insufficiency, n (%)	5 (83.3)	37 (67.3)	0.66	21 (87.5)	21 (56.8)	0.01	12 (66.7)	30 (69.8)	1.0
Mitral valve sclerosis, n (%)	3 (50)	22 (40)	0.68	17 (70.8)	8 (21.6)	<0.001	9 (50)	16 (37.2)	0.40
Tricuspid valve insufficiency, n (%)	3 (50)	30 (54.5)	1.0	15 (62.5)	18 (48.6)	0.31	10 (55.6)	23 (53.5)	1.0
Aortic valve insufficiency, n (%)	4 (66.7)	10 (18.2)	0.02	10 (41.7)	4 (10.8)	0.01	5 (27.8)	9 (20.9)	0.74
Aortic valve sclerosis, n (%)	4 (66.7)	9 (16.4)	0.01	9 (37.5)	4 (10.8)	0.02	5 (27.8)	8 (18.6)	0.49
Pericardial effusion, n (%)	0 (0)	4 (7.3)	1.0	1 (4.2)	3 (8.1)	1.0	2 (11.1)	2 (4.7)	0.57

Acronyms: SD = standard deviation. ACA = anti-centromere autoantibodies; ATA = anti Topoisomerase I autoantibodies; E wave = early diastolic filling velocity of the left ventricle; E′ = early diastolic tissue velocity of the mitral annulus; A = late diastolic filling velocity; LVED = left ventricular end diastolic; LVES = left ventricular end systolic; PWED = posterior wall end diastolic; IVS = interventricular septum; LAES = left atrial end systolic; RAES = right atrial end systolic; TAPSE = tricuspid annular plane systolic excursion; sPAP = systolic pulmonary artery pressure; 4CH = 4 chamber; AL = anterolateral; EF = ejection fraction; % = percentage; BSA = body surface area; ASE = American Society of echocardiography; ind = indexed; sup-inf = superior–inferior; m/s = meter/seconds; mm = millimeters; g = grams; g/m² = grams/square meters; cm² = square centimeters; mmHg = millimeters of mercury.

Additionally, patients receiving ACE-Is/ARBs showed a statistically significant reduction in the E/A ratio compared to those who did not receive these treatments (0.81 ± 0.28 vs. 1.06 ± 0.4, p = 0.01). This treatment group also exhibited a statistically larger LA diameter measured in the superior-inferior direction at end-systole (49.5 ± 5.8 vs. 45.3 ± 8.4 mm/m²,

$p = 0.04$) and a greater prevalence of aortic valve leaflets sclerosis (35.3% vs. 11.6%, $p = 0.03$) (Figure 1).

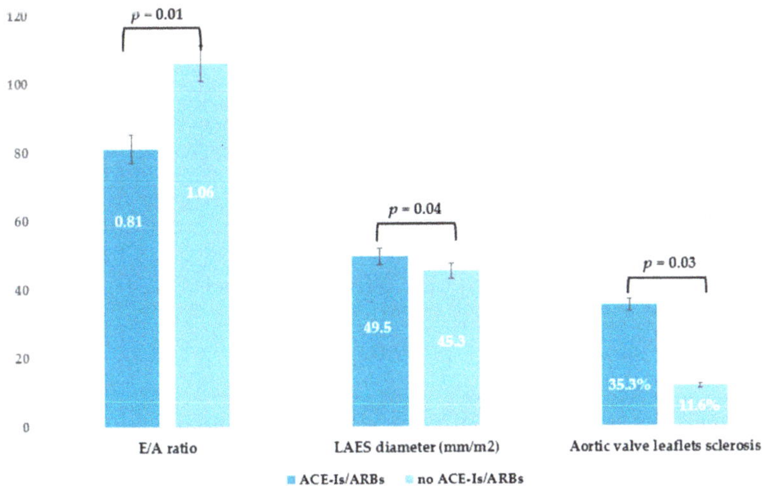

Figure 1. Bar chart showing main echocardiographic findings differences between patients undergoing ACE-Is/ARBs treatment versus patients not receiving ACE-Is/ARBs therapy. Acronyms: ACE-Is/ARBs = angiotensin converting enzyme inhibitors; ARBs = angiotensin receptor blockers; E/A ratio = early diastolic tissue velocity of the mitral annulus/late diastolic filling velocity ratio; LAES = left atrial end systolic; m^2 = square meters.

3.3. Subclinical Echocardiographic Findings by Comparing Patients Receiving Current Therapy with Vasodilators

Subclinical echocardiographic alterations in patients receiving vasodilators were further assessed. We exclusively selected Iloprost iv administration and/or calcium channel blockers, as no other vasodilator was administered to our patients. Accordingly, patients were divided into four groups: Group 1 encompassing patients receiving Iloprost intravenously only ($n = 25$), Group 2 comprised patients receiving CCBs orally only ($n = 8$), while Group 3 included patients undergoing both monthly Iloprost infusion and daily oral CCB ($n = 18$), and Group 4 encompassed patients receiving no vasodilators ($n = 13$). Our analysis revealed that patients receiving CCBs only exhibited a greater LVES volume measured by the Simpson method ($p = 0.001$), while reporting a reduced RAES volume compared to each group ($p = 0.005$). Moreover, patients undergoing the combination therapy with Iloprost and CCBs exhibited a greater RAES volume measured via the indexed method compared to the other groups ($p = 0.01$) (Table 4).

Table 4. Echocardiographic findings across patients undergoing vasodilators compared to those not receiving vasodilators.

Echocardiographic Parameters	Iloprost Iv $n = 25$	CCBs $n = 8$	Iloprost + CCBs $n = 18$	No Vasodilators $n = 13$	p-Value
E deceleration time (m/s), mean ± SD	295.0 ± 422.8	176.7 ± 40.7	203.6 ± 62.8	220.9 ± 49.7	0.74
E/E′ ratio, mean ± SD	7.3 ± 2.1	7.8 ± 2.8	6.8 ± 1.8	6.6 ± 1.1	0.71
E wave, (m/s), mean ± SD	0.67 ± 0.18	0.68 ± 0.22	0.68 ± 0.15	0.77 ± 0.23	0.59
E/A ratio, mean ± SD	1.08 ± 0.44	0.92 ± 0.35	0.85 ± 0.21	1.0 ± 0.46	0.32
LVED diameter, (mm), mean ± SD	40.6 ± 5.1	42.5 ± 7.4	39.6 ± 4.4	40.4 ± 5.0	0.72
PWED thickness, (mm), mean ± SD	8.2 ± 1.9	8.7 ± 0.8	8.2 ± 0.9	8.7 ± 2.1	0.75
IVS thckness, (mm), mean ± SD	9.3 ± 1.8	8.9 ± 1.4	9.5 ± 1.4	9.3 ± 2.6	0.93

Table 4. *Cont.*

Echocardiographic Parameters	Iloprost Iv $n = 25$	CCBs $n = 8$	Iloprost + CCBs $n = 18$	No Vasodilators $n = 13$	p-Value
LVED volume 4CH Simpson, (mL), mean ± SD	67.5 ± 13.8	54.1 ± 31.5	67.8 ± 15.3	73.8 ± 14.6	0.17
LVES volume 4CH Simpson, (mL), mean ± SD	23.7 ± 6.5	47.2 ± 35.1	23.8 ± 6.0	24.6 ± 7.4	0.001
LVED volume 4CH AL, (mL/m^2), mean ± SD	42.8 ± 9.8	41.4 ± 8.4	42.1 ± 8.7	46.9 ± 7.1	0.46
LVES volume 4CH AL, (mL/m^2), mean ± SD	14.5 ± 3.6	16.5 ± 12.9	14.4 ± 3.5	15.3 ± 4.0	0.84
EF%, mean ± SD	64.9 ± 4.4	59.6 ± 6.7	65.1 ± 5.0	65.2 ± 4.2	0.12
Mass ASE, (g), mean ± SD	109.3 ± 33.5	95.9 ± 60.3	160.1 ± 217.4	109.1 ± 42.2	0.56
Mass/BSA, (g/m^2), mean ± SD	66.1 ± 16.8	71.9 ± 21.4	65.0 ± 13.5	68.1 ± 23.4	0.89
Relative wall thickness, mean ± SD	0.44 ± 0.11	0.45 ± 0.10	0.46 ± 0.08	0.44 ± 0.13	0.93
Mass/height, (g/m), mean ± SD	67.4 ± 20.8	57.0 ± 21.1	66.9 ± 14.4	66.7 ± 18.9	0.78
Aortic diameter, (mm^2), mean ± SD	30.8 ± 2.9	26.9 ± 4.8	28.9 ± 4.7	29.3 ± 4.1	0.27
LAES area, (cm^2), mean ± SD	14.4 ± 2.4	15.5 ± 4.1	16.3 ± 3.8	17.0 ± 4.7	0.16
LAES 4CH Simpson, (mL), mean ± SD	36.1 ± 8.1	41.0 ± 19.8	44.7 ± 16.3	42.1 ± 16.3	0.26
LAES 4CH ind, (mL/m^2), mean ± SD	21.6 ± 4.3	25.5 ± 11.4	26.9 ± 8.3	26.0 ± 9.8	0.14
LAES diameter 4CH, (mm/m^2), mean ± SD	45.8 ± 5.9	46.9 ± 5.8	48.5 ± 6.2	44.0 ± 13.7	0.54
RAES diameter AL, (mm), mean ± SD	45.1 ± 5.9	40.5 ± 6.1	48.7 ± 5.3	46.2 ± 5.4	0.12
RAES 4CH Simpson, (mL), mean ± SD	31.2 ± 8.4	14.1 ± 6.5	26.5 ± 5.4	30.2 ± 9.1	0.005
RAES 4CH ind, (mL/m^2), mean ± SD	18.1 ± 5.1	12.4 ± 6.7	21.7 ± 4.5	16.6 ± 2.1	0.01
RAES area, (cm^2), mean ± SD	13.4 ± 3.6	12.1 ± 3.0	14.8 ± 3.1	12.6 ± 1.9	0.24
TAPSE, (mmHg), mean ± SD	20.8 ± 2.9	20.9 ± 3.1	21.3 ± 2.7	22.9 ± 3.3	0.29
TAPSE/sPAP, mean ± SD	0.79 ± 0.33	0.31 ± 0.44	0.76 ± 0.10	0.65 ± 0.39	0.28
sPAP, (mmHg), mean ± SD	25.1 ± 4.8	24.5 ± 6.4	29.5 ± 6.1	29.4 ± 3.6	0.21
Tricuspid maximum regurgitation gradient, (mmHg), mean ± SD	21.0 ± 4.6	20.4 ± 6.2	24.5 ± 4.9	21.6 ± 11.3	0.23

Acronyms: iv = intravenous; CCB = calcium channel blockers; SD = standard deviation. E wave = early diastolic filling velocity of the left ventricle; E′ = early diastolic tissue velocity of the mitral annulus; A = late diastolic filling velocity; LVED = left ventricular end diastolic; LVES = left ventricular end systolic; PWED = posterior wall end diastolic; IVS = interventricular septum; LAES = left atrial end systolic; RAES = right atrial end systolic; TAPSE = tricuspid annular plane systolic excursion; sPAP = systolic pulmonary artery pressure; 4CH = 4 chamber; AL = anterolateral; EF = ejection fraction; % = percentage; BSA = body surface area; ASE = American Society of echocardiography; ind = indexed; sup-inf = superior–inferior; m/s = meter/seconds; mm = millimeters; g = grams; g/m^2 = grams/square meters; cm^2 = square centimeters; mmHg = millimeters of mercury.

3.4. General Multivariable Regression Model

Furthermore, E/A ratio, IVS thickness, and PWED thickness were identified as key descriptors of diastolic and systolic LV dysfunction. A general multivariable regression model incorporating BMI, age at VEDOSS diagnosis, DLCO% predicted, ACA/ATA positivity, late NVC patterns, and puffy hands as relevant clinical determinants, revealed that only DLCO% emerged as a significant predictor of both IVS thickening ($p = 0.034$) and PWED thickening ($p = 0.002$). Additionally, ACA positivity was significantly associated with PWED thickening ($p = 0.004$). These findings persisted even when the model was applied exclusively to the e-VEDOSS group.

4. Discussion

The present study provides relevant insights into subclinical echocardiographic abnormalities of patients meeting the VEDOSS criteria. The occurrence of cardiac involvement at the early stage of SSc was previously reported by researchers Gotschy A et al. and De Luca G et al. The former conducted a cardiac magnetic resonance-driven study which proved the presence of myocardial fibrosis in a cohort of 24 VEDOSS patients [25], while the latter described three cases of myocardial involvement, emphasizing the role of vasculopathy, inflammation and fibrosis as major SSc-related pathogenic mechanisms [26].

Our cohort was initially divided into mild longstanding VEDOSS (ml-VEDOSS) and early VEDOSS (e-VEDOSS) groups based on disease duration, as suggested by Blaja et al. [9]. The authors stated that subjects fulfilling the criteria for VEDOSS encompass a heterogeneous mixture of patients with both early disease who are potentially at risk of progression and long-standing, very mild diseases. This observation has important implications, as these two subgroups cannot be easily differentiated based on clinical phenotype at first presentation, and since patients with mild long-standing disease need different frequencies of follow up and therapeutic considerations [9].

The ml-VEDOSS group exhibited a greater comorbidity count compared to the e-VEDOSS group, reflecting the cumulative burden of disease. This observation is consistent with previous research indicating that prolonged disease duration is correlated with prolonged chronic inflammation and prolonged exposure to altered vasoreactivity, ultimately increasing cardiovascular comorbidity [27,28]. These findings are particularly relevant given that SSc patients account for a five–fold increased mortality rate due to cardiac causes, and sudden cardiac death occurring in 21–54% of cases [15,29].

The intergroup comparisons showed several differences in LV diastolic function parameters. In fact, as demonstrated by Giunta A et al., LV function can reflect heart involvement of SSc more sensitively than RV function [30]. Firstly, VEDOSS patients with late NVC patterns had significantly greater PWED thickness and a higher prevalence of aortic valve insufficiency. This aligns with findings of Markusse IM et al., who confirmed the independent association between advanced NVC pattern and heart/lung involvement [31]. The relationship between macrovascular and microvascular damage in SSc has been largely investigated. Pagkopoulou et al. demonstrated that reduced capillary density was inversely correlated with arterial stiffness. The authors reported also that the Framingham Risk Score, QRISK3, and ASCVD (atherosclerotic cardiovascular disease) were inversely correlated with capillary density [32]. Conversely, Szucs et al. showed that the flow-mediated endothelium-dependent dilation was substantially reduced in SSc patients compared to healthy controls, indicating that impaired endothelium-dependent vasodilation is also present in pre-atherosclerotic stages [33]. Nevertheless, accurately quantifying the roles of intrinsic microangiopathy versus more common atherosclerotic processes in shaping the cardiovascular risk of SSc patients remains challenging.

Our results support these findings, providing additional evidence for the VEDOSS population, revealing that more advanced microarchitectural changes in NVC are related to greater echocardiographic alterations.

Additionally, it is worth mentioning that the ongoing process of endothelial dysfunction also affects coronary microvasculature [34]. Due to abnormal vasoreactivity, patients with SSc may experience repeated cycles of myocardial ischemia-reperfusion, potentially contributing to the development of myocardial fibrosis, even in the absence of significant heart-related symptoms.

Furthermore, we observed that VEDOSS patients with specific SSc autoantibody positivity exhibited a reduced E/A ratio, greater modifications in LAES area, valve dysfunction, and an increased PWED thickness, positioning this study along with previous research that has shown a relationship between specific autoantibodies and cardiac involvement [35]. Even though the causal relationship between autoantibodies and myocardial fibrosis is not yet fully understood, Henault et al. demonstrated that ATA can directly bind to fibroblast surfaces, inducing their activation and proliferation in endothelial tissue [36]. Moreover, Shen et al. found that ACA and ATA antibodies could induce vascular endothelial cell senescence via mechanisms distinct from the classic p53-p21 pathway in vitro, as observed in the sera of patients with Raynaud's phenomenon [37].

Moreover, Bellando-Randone et al. stated that autoimmunity plays a crucial role in shaping the progressive trajectories of VEDOSS patients, highlighting that SSc-specific antibodies are the most significant isolated predictor of progression from VEDOSS to definitive SSc, whereas negativity for antinuclear antibodies (ANA) at baseline has a strong negative predictive value [7].

Interestingly, by comparing patients undergoing vasodilators to patients not receiving such treatment, the former reported a greater percentage of enlarged RA, potentially reflecting an increased pressure or volume load on the RV. However, our echocardiographic findings did not show any discrepancies in RV functionality, as reported by the similar values of TAPSE, sPAP, and Tricuspid maximum regurgitation gradient.

Our intriguing data did not allow easy interpretation. On one hand, our observation suggests that vasodilators may exert detrimental effects on right atrial enlargement without causing detectable changes in RV measurements. On the other hand, patients in the VEDOSS cohort could be characterized by an overall greater disease severity due to more severe microvascular involvement, which encompasses RA abnormalities, and vasodilators may simply be insufficient to detain the damage progression.

As demonstrated by Guedón et al., in a prospective three-years survival analysis, Iloprost administration did not show any effect on either reducing or increasing the occurrence of diastolic dysfunction and PAH, while Sildenafil demonstrated a potential protective role in preventing the progression toward diastolic dysfunction and heart failure with altered EF [38]. The authors also emphasized the need for a comprehensive analysis of the potential benefits of sodium-glucose cotransporter 2 (SGLT2) inhibitors, such as empagliflozin and dapagliflozin, on diastolic dysfunction in patients with SSc. These medications have demonstrated beneficial effects in patients with heart failure and preserved EF [39]. However, we have no evidence regarding their efficacy in the VEDOSS population, as the present study focused on detecting subclinical echocardiographic changes in patients without heart-related symptoms.

Nevertheless, the increased use of both ACE-Is and ARBs in ml-VEDOSS points to a proactive approach in mitigating cardiovascular risk in patients experiencing a longer disease duration. This strategy is supported by evidence implying that these medications can improve cardiovascular and renal outcomes in the general population. In fact, ACE-Is and ARBs encompass the same Renin-Angiotensin-Aldosterone System (RAAS) inhibitors group, although they exert different mechanisms of action, including increased bradykinin levels, potentiated bradykinin response, and stimulated nitric oxide production with ACE-Is [40]. Moreover, the reduced E/A ratio in RAAS inhibitors group could reinforce the theory of their usage in more at-risk individuals, potentially mitigating the occurrence of major cardiac events and mortality. However, the preventive role of RAAS inhibitors in the early stages of SSc is still debated, and their usage should be practiced with caution. In fact, as reported by Bütikofer L. et al. in an EUSTAR cohort analysis, ACE-Is in SSc patients with concomitant arterial hypertension display an independent risk factor for the development of scleroderma renal crisis (SRC) but they still represent the first choice in SRC treatment. This study advocates that ARBs might be a safer alternative than ACE-Is, yet the overall safety of alternative antihypertensive drugs needs to be further investigated [41].

Furthermore, the multivariable analysis, indicating that DLCO% was the only significant predictor of IVS and PWED thickening, supported the role of pulmonary function in uncovering subclinical cardiac changes within our population. As recently described by He H. et al. in a magnetic resonance guided study, the DLCO% values are inversely correlated with myocardial native T1 values in SSc patients, suggesting that DLCO might be a potential indicator for subclinical myocardial fibrosis [42].

Although the present study adds new evidence on the underexplored occurrence of subclinical cardiac involvement in VEDOSS, it is limited by several factors. The relatively limited sample size of 61 participants may impact on the robustness of our conclusions. However, this small sample size primarily stems from the low prevalence of systemic sclerosis, as well as the even lower prevalence of VEDOSS. Therefore, multicenter studies involving larger cohorts are necessary to enhance the validity of these findings. Furthermore, inter-operator variability in the echocardiographic technique should be considered, although standardized protocols in accordance with the 2020 ACC/AHA guidelines were implemented to minimize its impact, as detailed in the methods section. Additionally, since the study was conducted at a single center in Italy, the generalizability of these findings may be limited. Due to the cross-sectional nature of the study, causal inferences cannot be made. To address this limitation, we strongly recommend conducting further multicenter prospective studies.

In conclusion, we demonstrated that various subclinical echocardiographic alterations occur in both early and mild-longstanding form of VEDOSS, however, we excluded patients initially classified as VEDOSS who further developed an established SSc. Future research is warranted to detect early differences in echocardiographic parameters between progressive and stable forms.

5. Conclusions

This study highlighted critical echocardiographic changes among patients fulfilling VEDOSS criteria. The associations between pulmonary function, cardiac structure, specific autoantibodies profile, and microvascular damage underscored the complexity of VEDOSS and the need for comprehensive management strategies. Timely detection of heart involvement, especially in patients with advanced microangiopathy and features of SSc-related autoimmunity, is crucial for predicting disease progression and mortality.

Supplementary Materials: The following supporting information can be downloaded at: https://www.mdpi.com/article/10.3390/sclerosis3010007/s1, Table S1: Echocardiographic findings comparison between e-VEDOSS and ml-VEDOSS.

Author Contributions: E.C.: Conceptualization, Software, Methodology, Validation, Formal analysis, Investigation, Resources, Data curation, Writing—original draft, Writing—review & editing. E.Z.: Conceptualization, Methodology, Software, Validation, Formal analysis, Investigation, Resources, Data curation, Writing—review & editing. I.S.: Resources, Data curation. A.L.: Resources, Data curation, L.C.: Resources, Data curation. E.M. Resources, Data curation. D.B.: Resources, Data curation. A.T.: Resources, Data curation. M.I.: Methodology, Supervision. M.S.C.: Methodology, Supervision A.M.: Conceptualization, Validation, Resources, Supervision. Project administration. P.F.: Conceptualization, Validation, Resources, Writing—review & editing, Supervision, Project administration. All authors have read and agreed to the published version of the manuscript.

Funding: This research received no external funding.

Institutional Review Board Statement: The study was conducted in accordance with the Declaration of Helsinki and approved by the Ethics Committee of Milan Area 3 under protocol number S00125/2023 (29 May 2023).

Informed Consent Statement: Informed consent was obtained from all participants involved in the study.

Data Availability Statement: The data supporting this study's findings are available from the corresponding author upon reasonable request. The data is not publicly available due to ethical restrictions.

Conflicts of Interest: The authors declare no conflicts of interest.

References

1. Ko, J.; Noviani, M.; Chellamuthu, V.R.; Albani, S.; Low, A.H.L. The Pathogenesis of Systemic Sclerosis: The Origin of Fibrosis and Interlink with Vasculopathy and Autoimmunity. *Int. J. Mol. Sci.* **2023**, *24*, 14287. [CrossRef]
2. Rosa, I.; Romano, E.; Fioretto, B.S.; Manetti, M. The contribution of mesenchymal transitions to the pathogenesis of systemic sclerosis. *Eur. J. Rheumatol.* **2020**, *7* (Suppl. 3), S157–S164. [CrossRef]
3. Herrick, A.L.; Assassi, S.; Denton, C.P. Skin involvement in early diffuse cutaneous systemic sclerosis: An unmet clinical need. *Nat. Rev. Rheumatol.* **2022**, *18*, 276–285. [CrossRef] [PubMed]
4. LeRoy, E.C.; Medsger, T.A., Jr. Criteria for the classification of early systemic sclerosis. *J. Rheumatol.* **2001**, *28*, 1573–1576.
5. van den Hoogen, F.; Khanna, D.; Fransen, J.; Johnson, S.R.; Baron, M.; Tyndall, A.; Matucci-Cerinic, M.; Naden, R.P.; Medsger, T.A., Jr.; Carreira, P.E.; et al. 2013 classification criteria for systemic sclerosis: An American College of Rheumatology/European League against Rheumatism collaborative initiative. *Arthritis Rheum.* **2013**, *65*, 2737–2747. [CrossRef]
6. Yang, M.; Goh, V.; Lee, J.; Espinoza, M.; Yuan, Y.; Carns, M.; Aren, K.; Chung, L.; Khanna, D.; McMahan, Z.H.; et al. Clinical Phenotypes of Patients with Systemic Sclerosis with Distinct Molecular Signatures in Skin. *Arthritis Care Res.* **2023**, *75*, 1469–1480. [CrossRef] [PubMed]
7. Bellando-Randone, S.; Del Galdo, F.; Lepri, G.; Minier, T.; Huscher, D.; Furst, D.E.; Allanore, Y.; Distler, O.; Czirják, L.; Bruni, C.; et al. Progression of patients with Raynaud's phenomenon to systemic sclerosis: A five-year analysis of the European Scleroderma Trial and Research group multicentre, longitudinal registry study for Very Early Diagnosis of Systemic Sclerosis (VEDOSS). *Lancet Rheumatol.* **2021**, *3*, e834–e843. [CrossRef]
8. Avouac, J.; Fransen, J.; Walker, U.; Riccieri, V.; Smith, V.; Muller, C.; Miniati, I.; Tarner, I.; Randone, S.B.; Cutolo, M.; et al. Preliminary criteria for the very early diagnosis of systemic sclerosis: Results of a Delphi Consensus Study from EULAR Scleroderma Trials and Research Group. *Ann. Rheum. Dis.* **2011**, *70*, 476–481. [CrossRef]
9. Blaja, E.; Jordan, S.; Mihai, C.M.; Dobrota, R.; Becker, M.O.; Maurer, B.; Matucci-Cerinic, M.; Distler, O. The Challenge of Very Early Systemic Sclerosis: A Combination of Mild and Early Disease? *J. Rheumatol.* **2021**, *48*, 82–86. [CrossRef]
10. Ross, R.L.; Caballero-Ruiz, B.; Clarke, E.L.; Kakkar, V.; Wasson, C.W.; Mulipa, P.; De Lorenzis, E.; Merchant, W.; Di Donato, S.; Rindone, A.; et al. Biological hallmarks of systemic sclerosis are present in the skin and serum of patients with Very Early Diagnosis of Systemic Sclerosis (VEDOSS). *Rheumatology* **2024**, keae698, *Epub ahead of print*. [CrossRef]
11. El Aoufy, K.; Melis, M.R.; Bandini, G.; Ghezzi, G.; Russo, E.; Fioretto, B.S.; Romano, E.; Amedei, A.; Rosa, I.; Manetti, M.; et al. POS1593-HPR Gastrointestinal involvement is already reported in an Italian VEDOSS cohort: Results from a rheumatological nurse assessment. *Ann. Rheum. Dis.* **2023**, *82*, 1172–1173. [CrossRef]
12. Zhu, L.; Wang, Y.; Zhao, S.; Lu, M. Detection of myocardial fibrosis: Where we stand. *Front. Cardiovasc. Med.* **2022**, *9*, 926378. [CrossRef] [PubMed]
13. Piccione, M.C.; Zito, C.; Oreto, G.; Di Bella, G.; Bagnato, G.; Carerj, S. Role of 2D strain in the early identification of left ventricular dysfunction and in the risk stratification of systemic sclerosis patients. *Cardiovasc. Ultrasound* **2013**, *11*, 6. [CrossRef] [PubMed]
14. Lee, S.-W.; Choi, E.-Y.; Jung, S.Y.; Choi, S.T.; Lee, S.-K.; Park, Y.-B. E/E′ ratio is more sensitive than E/A ratio for detection of left ventricular diastolic dysfunction in patients with systemic sclerosis. *Clin. Exp. Rheumatol.* **2010**, *28* (Suppl. 58), S12–S17. [PubMed]
15. Pokeerbux, M.R.; Giovannelli, J.; Dauchet, L.; Mouthon, L.; Agard, C.; Lega, J.C.; Allanore, Y.; Jego, P.; Bienvenu, B.; Berthier, S.; et al. Survival and prognosis factors in systemic sclerosis: Data of a French multicenter cohort, systematic review, and meta-analysis of the literature. *Arthritis Res. Ther.* **2019**, *21*, 86. [CrossRef]
16. Ruaro, B.; Smith, V.; Sulli, A.; Decuman, S.; Pizzorni, C.; Cutolo, M. Methods for the morphological and functional evaluation of microvascular damage in systemic sclerosis. *Korean J. Intern. Med.* **2015**, *30*, 1–5. [CrossRef] [PubMed]
17. Mitchell, C.; Rahko, P.S.; Blauwet, L.A.; Canaday, B.; Finstuen, J.A.; Foster, M.C.; Horton, K.; Ogunyankin, K.O.; Palma, R.A.; Velazquez, E.J. Guidelines for Performing a Comprehensive Transthoracic Echocardiographic Examination in Adults: Recommendations from the American Society of Echocardiography. *J. Am. Soc. Echocardiogr.* **2019**, *32*, 1–64. [CrossRef]
18. Lang, R.M.; Bierig, M.; Devereux, R.B.; Flachskampf, F.A.; Foster, E.; Pellikka, P.A.; Picard, M.H.; Roman, M.J.; Seward, J.; Shanewise, J.S.; et al. Recommendations for Chamber Quantification: A Report from the American Society of Echocardiography's Guidelines and Standards Committee and the Chamber Quantification Writing Group, Developed in Conjunction with the European Association of Echocardiography, a Branch of the European Society of Cardiology. *J. Am. Soc. Echocardiogr.* **2015**, *18*, 1440–1463.
19. Devereux, R.B.; Alonso, D.R.; Lutas, E.M.; Gottlieb, G.J.; Campo, E.; Sachs, I.; Reichek, N. Echocardiographic assessment of left ventricular hypertrophy: Comparison to necropsy findings. *Am. J. Cardiol.* **1986**, *57*, 450–458. [CrossRef]
20. Pyxaras, S.A.; Pinamonti, B.; Barbati, G.; Santangelo, S.; Valentincic, M.; Cettolo, F.; Secoli, G.; Magnani, S.; Merlo, M.; Giudice, F.L.; et al. Echocardiographic evaluation of systolic and mean pulmonary artery pressure in the follow-up of patients with pulmonary hypertension. *Eur. J. Echocardiogr.* **2011**, *12*, 696–701. [CrossRef] [PubMed]

21. Skinner, H.; Kamaruddin, H.; Mathew, T. Tricuspid Annular Plane Systolic Excursion: Comparing Transthoracic to Transesophageal Echocardiography. *J. Cardiothorac. Vasc. Anesthesia* **2017**, *31*, 590–594. [CrossRef] [PubMed]
22. Nagueh, S.F.; Appleton, C.P.; Gillebert, T.C.; Marino, P.N.; Oh, J.K.; Smiseth, O.A.; Waggoner, A.D.; Flachskampf, F.A.; Pellikka, P.A., Evangelisa, A. Recommendations for the evaluation of left ventricular diastolic function by echocardiography. *Eur. J. Echocardiogr.* **2009**, *10*, 165–193. [CrossRef]
23. Schwarz, E.R.; Dashti, R. The clinical quandary of left and right ventricular diastolic dysfunction and diastolic heart failure. *Cardiovasc. J. Afr.* **2010**, *21*, 212–220.
24. Otto, C.M.; Nishimura, R.A.; Bonow, R.O.; Carabello, B.A.; Erwin, J.P., 3rd; Gentile, F.; Jneid, H.; Krieger, E.V.; Mack, M.; McLeod, C.; et al. 2020 ACC/AHA Guideline for the Management of Patients with Valvular Heart Disease: Executive Summary: A Report of the American College of Cardiology/American Heart Association Joint Committee on Clinical Practice Guidelines. *Circulation* **2021**, *143*, e35–e71; Erratum in *Circulation* **2021**, *143*, e228; Erratum in *Circulation* **2021**, *143*, e784. [CrossRef] [PubMed]
25. Gotschy, A.; Jordan, S.; Stoeck, C.T.; von Deuster, C.; Peer, T.; Gastl, M.; Vishnevskiy, V.; Wissmann, L.; Dobrota, R.; Mihai, C.; et al. Diffuse myocardial fibrosis precedes subclinical functional myocardial impairment and provides prognostic information in systemic sclerosis. *Eur. Heart J. Cardiovasc. Imaging* **2023**, *24*, 373–382. [CrossRef]
26. De Luca, G.; Campochiaro, C.; Peretto, G.; Busnardo, E.; Matucci-Cerinic, M.; Dagna, L. Cardiac involvement, a threatening very early manifestation of systemic sclerosis: Evidence from VEDOSS patients. *Clin. Exp. Rheumatol.* **2023**, *41*, 1723–1724. [CrossRef] [PubMed]
27. Volkmann, E.R.; Fischer, A. Update on Morbidity and Mortality in Systemic Sclerosis-Related Interstitial Lung Disease. *J. Scleroderma Relat. Disord.* **2021**, *6*, 11–20. [CrossRef] [PubMed]
28. Alfaddagh, A.; Martin, S.S.; Leucker, T.M.; Michos, E.D.; Blaha, M.J.; Lowenstein, C.J.; Jones, S.R.; Toth, P.P. Inflammation and cardiovascular disease: From mechanisms to therapeutics. *Am. J. Prev. Cardiol.* **2020**, *4*, 100130. [CrossRef] [PubMed]
29. Rangarajan, V.; Matiasz, R.; Freed, B.H. Cardiac complications of systemic sclerosis and management: Recent progress. *Curr. Opin. Rheumatol.* **2017**, *29*, 574–584. [CrossRef] [PubMed]
30. Giunta, A.; Tirri, E.; Maione, S.; Cangianiello, S.; Mele, A.; De Luca, A.; Valentini, G. Right ventricular diastolic abnormalities in systemic sclerosis. Relation to left ventricular involvement and pulmonary hypertension. *Ann. Rheum. Dis.* **2000**, *59*, 94–98. [CrossRef]
31. Markusse, I.M.; Meijs, J.; de Boer, B.; Bakker, J.A.; Schippers, H.P.C.; Schouffoer, A.A.; Ajmone Marsan, N.; Kroft, L.J.M.; Ninaber, M.K.; Huizinga, T.W.J.; et al. Predicting cardiopulmonary involvement in patients with systemic sclerosis: Complementary value of nailfold videocapillaroscopy patterns and disease-specific autoantibodies. *Rheumatology* **2017**, *56*, 1081–1088. [CrossRef] [PubMed]
32. Pagkopoulou, E.; Soulaidopoulos, S.; Triantafyllidou, E.; Arvanitaki, A.; Katsiki, N.; Loutradis, C.; Karagiannis, A.; Doumas, M.; Garyfallos, A.; Kitas, G.D.; et al. Peripheral microcirculatory abnormalities are associated with cardiovascular risk in systemic sclerosis: A nailfold video capillaroscopy study. *Clin. Rheumatol.* **2021**, *40*, 4957–4968. [CrossRef] [PubMed]
33. Szucs, G.; Tímár, O.; Szekanecz, Z.; Dér, H.; Kerekes, G.; Szamosi, S.; Shoenfeld, Y.; Szegedi, G.; Soltész, P. Endothelial Dysfunction Precedes Atherosclerosis in Systemic Sclerosis–Relevance for Prevention of Vascular Complications. *Rheumatology* **2007**, *46*, 759–762. [CrossRef]
34. Zanatta, E.; Famoso, G.; Boscain, F.; Montisci, R.; Pigatto, E.; Polito, P.; Schiavon, F.; Iliceto, S.; Cozzi, F.; Doria, A.; et al. Nailfold avascular score and coronary microvascular dysfunction in systemic sclerosis: A newsworthy association. *Autoimmun. Rev.* **2019**, *18*, 177–183. [CrossRef]
35. Tsai, C.-Y.; Hsieh, S.-C.; Wu, T.-H.; Li, K.-J.; Shen, C.-Y.; Liao, H.-T.; Wu, C.-H.; Kuo, Y.-M.; Lu, C.-S.; Yu, C.-L. Pathogenic Roles of Autoantibodies and Aberrant Epigenetic Regulation of Immune and Connective Tissue Cells in the Tissue Fibrosis of Patients with Systemic Sclerosis. *Int. J. Mol. Sci.* **2020**, *21*, 3069. [CrossRef] [PubMed]
36. Hénault, J.; Robitaille, G.; Senécal, J.; Raymond, Y. DNA topoisomerase I binding to fibroblasts induces monocyte adhesion and activation in the presence of anti–topoisomerase I autoantibodies from systemic sclerosis patients. *Arthritis Rheum.* **2006**, *54*, 963–973. [CrossRef]
37. Shen, C.Y.; Lu, C.H.; Wu, C.H.; Li, K.J.; Kuo, Y.M.; Hsieh, S.C.; Yu, C.L. Molecular Basis of Accelerated Aging with Immune Dysfunction-Mediated Inflammation (Inflamm-Aging) in Patients with Systemic Sclerosis. *Cells* **2021**, *10*, 3402. [CrossRef] [PubMed]
38. Guédon, A.F.; Carrat, F.; Mouthon, L.; Launay, D.; Chaigne, B.; Pugnet, G.; Lega, J.-C.; Hot, A.; Cottin, V.; Agard, C.; et al. Vasodilator drugs and heart-related outcomes in systemic sclerosis: An exploratory analysis. *RMD Open* **2024**, *10*, e004918. [CrossRef] [PubMed]
39. Lee, H.-C.; Shiou, Y.-L.; Jhuo, S.-J.; Chang, C.-Y.; Liu, P.-L.; Jhuang, W.-J.; Dai, Z.-K.; Chen, W.-Y.; Chen, Y.-F.; Lee, A.-S. The sodium–glucose co-transporter 2 inhibitor empagliflozin attenuates cardiac fibrosis and improves ventricular hemodynamics in hypertensive heart failure rats. *Cardiovasc. Diabetol.* **2019**, *18*, 45. [CrossRef] [PubMed] [PubMed Central]

40. Alcocer, L.A.; Bryce, A.; De Padua Brasil, D.; Lara, J.; Cortes, J.M.; Quesada, D.; Rodriguez, P. The Pivotal Role of Angiotensin-Converting Enzyme Inhibitors and Angiotensin II Receptor Blockers in Hypertension Management and Cardiovascular and Renal Protection: A Critical Appraisal and Comparison of International Guidelines. *Am. J. Cardiovasc. Drugs* **2023**, *23*, 663–682. [CrossRef]
41. Collaborators, O.B.O.E.; Bütikofer, L.; Varisco, P.A.; Distler, O.; Kowal-Bielecka, O.; Allanore, Y.; Riemekasten, G.; Villiger, P.M.; Adler, S. ACE inhibitors in SSc patients display a risk factor for scleroderma renal crisis—A EUSTAR analysis. *Arthritis Res. Ther.* **2020**, *22*, 59.
42. He, H.; Tong, X.; Ning, Z.; Zhou, J.; Du, C.; Wang, Y.; Wang, Q.; Xu, D.; Zeng, X.; He, Z.-X.; et al. Diffusing capacity of lungs for carbon monoxide associated with subclinical myocardial impairment in systemic sclerosis: A cardiac MR study. *RMD Open* **2023**, *9*, e003391. [CrossRef]

sclerosis MDPI

Review

Systemic Sclerosis in Women—Impact on Sexuality, Fertility, Pregnancy, and Menopause

Ann-Christin Pecher [1], Melanie Henes [2] and Joerg Henes [1,*]

[1] Center for Interdisciplinary Rheumatology, Immunology and Autoimmune Diseases (INDIRA) and Department for Internal Medicine II (Haematology, Oncology, Rheumatology and Clinical Immunology), University Hospital Tuebingen, 72076 Tuebingen, Germany; ann-christin.pecher@med.uni-tuebingen.de

[2] Department of Obstetrics and Gynaecology, University Hospital Tuebingen, Calwerstrasse 7, 72076 Tuebingen, Germany; melanie.henes@med.uni-tuebingen.de

* Correspondence: joerg.henes@med.uni-tuebingen.de; Tel.: +49-7071-2984095; Fax: +49-7071-292763

Abstract: Background: Systemic sclerosis is a systemic autoimmune disease that also impacts women's health in very different ways. Methods: This review summarises the most important data on sexuality, fertility, pregnancy, and menopause from the last 10 years. Findings: We identified nine articles with data on sexuality and a prevalence of sexual dysfunction varying between 46 and 90%. Fertility was examined in six studies, with evidence for a negative influence at least on ovarian reserve. With regard to menopause, only three studies are mentioned that show an increased risk for premature menopause in SSc women. Although pregnancies are rare in SSc women after disease onset, there is growing evidence that pregnancies are feasible but go along with a higher maternal and foetal risk compared to healthy controls. Interpretation: SSc is dominated by female gender, but aspects of women's health influenced by the disease are still often ignored. The treating physician should be aware of the mostly negative impact on sexuality, fertility, and pregnancy and address these topics with the patients to adapt treatment and follow-up examinations to the patients' complaints and life situation.

Keywords: women; systemic sclerosis; sexuality; fertility; pregnancy; menopause

1. Background

Systemic sclerosis (SSc) is a chronic autoimmune disease characterised by fibrosis of the skin and internal organs [1]. The estimated global prevalence of SSc is 17.6–18.9 per 100,000 individuals, with 28.0–31.2/100,000 females and 6.0–6.8/100,000 males [2]. The manifestations of the disease can vary significantly, often impacting the vascular system, lungs, kidneys, gastrointestinal tract, and musculoskeletal system. SSc in most cases starts with vasculopathy leading to Raynaud's phenomenon with trophical damage like digital ulcers that can lead to severe infections and the loss of parts of the fingers. The skin thickening usually starts at the fingers/hand and feet but can affect the whole body and especially the face, leading to a reduction in movement and changes in the patient's look. For organ manifestations, inflammatory changes in the lung and heart lead to deterioration of the organ function by progressive lung fibrosis or myocardial fibrosis, which is the most common reason for mortality in these patients [1,3]. The whole gastrointestinal tract can be affected, with motility disturbance of the oesophagus being the most frequent manifestation. One of the most severe complications in SSc is scleroderma renal crisis (SRC), which is associated with high morbidity and mortality. It is a rare manifestation and usually manifests in the first years after diagnosis [1]. The extent of the skin fibrosis defines the differentiation between limited (lc) and diffuse cutaneous (dc)SSc and thus their prognosis, although the autoantibody status plays an even more important role [1]. Patients with antibodies against centromes have more often an lcSSc and a better prognosis than patients with antibodies against topoisomerase I or RNA polymerase III [3].

Systemic sclerosis affects women's health in very different ways. Vaginal dryness and atrophy have a negative impact on sexuality and desire, fertility and pregnancy are negatively affected by systemic sclerosis, and patients appear to go into menopause earlier. However, although more women than men are affected by the disease, there is very little research on the topic of women's health. Here we tried to summarise the few data from the last 10 years.

2. Methods

A PubMed search over the last 10 years was carried out using the search terms "systemic sclerosis and sexuality", "systemic sclerosis and fertility", "systemic sclerosis and pregnancy", and "systemic sclerosis and menopause". Inclusion criteria were the diagnosis of SSc independent of lcSSc or dcSSc. Only data on adult women were taken into consideration. Case reports were excluded.

For the search term "systemic sclerosis and sexuality", 50 papers were identified, of which 9 were suitable. For "systemic sclerosis and fertility", 6 out of 25 publications, for "systemic sclerosis and pregnancy" 19/140, and for "systemic sclerosis and menopause", only 3/29 articles were considered.

3. Results

3.1. SSc and Sexuality

Sexual dysfunction (SDF) has been reported frequently among individuals diagnosed with SSc, largely due to physical and emotional factors. SSc is known to cause vascular abnormalities, which can also lead to reduced perfusion of the genitals [4]. This may contribute to erectile dysfunction in men and vaginal dryness or dyspareunia in women. Thickening of the skin can extend to the genital area, potentially causing discomfort or reduced sensation during sexual activity. Furthermore, fibrosis in vaginal tissue may result in vaginal atrophy, contributing to painful intercourse. Joint stiffness or pain due to musculoskeletal involvement may render sexual activity physically challenging or uncomfortable, especially when finger movement is reduced due to contractures. SSc has also been demonstrated to result in neuropathy, manifesting as a reduction in sensitivity or an alteration in sexual response in some patients. The chronic nature of SSc, in conjunction with its overt physical manifestations, has the potential to engender feelings of anxiety and body image concerns, all of which can significantly impact sexual desire and intimacy. Patients experience feelings of self-consciousness or fear regarding their ability to engage in sexual activity, or they may experience a lack of desire due to emotional distress. The impact of the disease on depression affects nearly half of SSc patients, exacerbating sexual dysfunction [5,6]. Furthermore, emotional distress associated with body image changes also plays a significant role in one's sense of identity, especially concerning femininity, and this can also affect sexual functioning. The presence of fatigue, a common complaint in SSc, can further impair sexuality.

There are a number of approaches to the investigation of SDF. The most commonly used is the validated Female Sexual Dysfunction Index (FSFI) [7]. The FSFI comprises a series of questions designed to assess various domains of sexual function, including desire, arousal, lubrication, orgasm, satisfaction, and pain. The scale consists of 19 items, some of which address particularly intimate subjects; consequently, the questionnaire is completed independently and without guidance from a physician. Other questionnaires, such as the shorter Qualisex questionnaire, which has been developed for rheumatoid arthritis (RA), have also been used in SSc [8]. In the context of measuring depression, the Beck Depression Inventory (BDI) is a frequently employed instrument, comprising 21 questions designed to assess symptoms of depression [9].

Several surveys of affected patients with SSc have been carried out, sometimes with comparisons to other connective tissue diseases, sometimes also with comparisons to healthy controls. In most cases, the cut-off of the FSFI questionnaire was <26.55 as recommended in the original publication [7], whereas some studies also used a stricter cut-off of <19, meaning that the data cannot be fully compared. Nevertheless, the prevalence of SDF is high and varies between 46.7% [4] and 90.7% [6] with differences in included patients. Age plays an important role when comparing these data, but also other differences in inclusion criteria influence sexual activity leading to large variety of SDF of 53% and 100%. The largest and latest study so far had the highest age and proportion of postmenopausal women but not the highest prevalence of SDF [10]. The highest prevalence of SDF, with around 90%, was found in two studies from Turkey and Italy, although the number of postmenopausal women was much lower, indicating the various influencing factors [6,11]. A study from Germany compared patients with SSc to an age-matched cohort of SLE patients and found no difference between the two groups with regard to SDF [5].

In summary, the prevalence of SDF in SSc women is high and significantly higher when compared to healthy controls [4,12,13]. Vaginal dryness is reported to be a major problem in these patients [5,11,13].

Table 1 provides an overview of recent publications on female sexual function in SSc.

Table 1. Most recent publications on female sexual function in SSc; abbreviations: BDI = Beck's depression inventory, SDF = sexual dysfunction; FSFI = female sexual function index; NK = not known.

Article	N	Mean or Median Age in Years	Mean or Median Disease Duration	% of Menopausal Women	Sexually Active	Prevalence of Vaginal Dryness	Prevalence of Dyspareunia	Prevalence of SDF FSFI	Prevalence of Depression According BDI
Lazzaroni M et al. [10]; 2025; Italy	168	58 (44–67)	9.0 (5–11)	70.2%	NK	NK	NK	66.2%	NK
Marcoccia A et al. [14]; 2024; Italy	65	44.71 (+/−11.96)	4.6 (+/−2.7)	NK	NK	NK	NK	Mean FSFI 15.85 not mentioning the %	NK
Dag A et al. [6]; 2024; Turkey	50	44.9 (+/−8.7)	10.1 (+/−5.8)	34%	NK	NK	NK	90%	60%
Ruffolo AF et al. [11]; 2023; Italy	107	53.47 (+/−13.27)	12.48 (+/−10.28)	54.2%	90.7%	83.2%	82.2%	89.7%	NK
Heřmánková B et al. [12]; 2022, Czech Republic	90	49.1 (+/−11.6)	4.0 (2–8)	56%	69%	NK	NK	73%	NK
Schmalzing M et al. [5]; 2020; Germany	83	48.5 (+/−11.07	9.85 (+/−8.4)	NK	62.6%	43.3	28.9%	49%	53%
Gigante A et al. [4]; 2019, Italy	15	41 (35–47)	9 (8–11)	0%	NK	NK	NK	46.7% (cut-off <19)	NK
Ucar I et al. [13]; 2018, Turkey	30	45.3 (+/−9.22)	NK	0%	100%	63.3%	23.3%	86.6%	NK
Sanchez K et al. [15]; 2016, France	60	55.9 (+/−14.0)	8.6 (+/−7.7)	NK	53.2%	NK	NK	62.5%	NK

3.2. SSc and Fertility

The impact of SSc on fertility may be influenced by both the disease itself and the therapeutic interventions employed to manage the condition. A significant proportion of women diagnosed with SSc report menstrual irregularities, including oligomenorrhea (infrequent menstrual cycles), amenorrhea (absence of menstruation), and preterm menopause. Several data on premature ovarian insufficiency (POI) and its correlation with immune cell dysfunction underline the link between autoimmune diseases and the female hormonal status as autoimmune diseases, especially thyroiditis, autoimmune polyglandular syndromes, hypophysitis, thrombocytopenia purpura, RA, systemic lupus erythematosus (SLE), primary biliary cholangitis, and diabetes are more common in patients with POI [16,17]. Differences in hormone levels during the female reproductive life, such as menarche, pregnancy, or menopause, may also influence disease activity [18,19].

Most of the studies on fertility are quite old and might reflect the concerns of both physicians and patients with regard to pregnancy and pregnancy complications after disease onset. Nevertheless, the trials suggest that infertility could be a feature of SSc [20,21]. Today there is some evidence that SSc can affect ovarian function, leading to premature ovarian failure or reduced ovarian reserve. This may result from the direct effects of the disease on the ovaries or the use of immunosuppressive drugs that may have a toxic effect on the ovaries. Two studies addressed this point but included different types of patients. The most recent paper included only patients younger than 40 years without cyclophosphamide (CYC) pretreatment and compared AMH and number of children to a healthy control group [22], whereas the paper from Thailand also allowed pretreatment with CYC [23]. Both groups found a high prevalence of low ovarian reserve, underlining the negative impact of SSc on ovarian reserve and thus fertility. The most recent studies found a very low number of pregnancies in India, with a rate of infertility of 8.3% [24], but no significant differences with regard to fertility in China when comparing 342 SSc women to 110 healthy controls [25].

The reason for AMH and thus fertility reduction is still a matter of debate. As reduced AMH levels are also found in other chronic autoimmune diseases, chronic inflammation seems to have an impact [26–28]. In addition, vascular problems and fibrosis of the ovaries can be discussed in SSc patients.

In summary, data on fertility in SSc women are still limited, but there is evidence for a negative influence at least on ovarian reserve. Like in sexual dysfunction, there are many confounders that interfere with a definite conclusion. Nevertheless, treating physicians should address family planning early, not to miss the ideal timepoint for fertility preservation, pregnancy, or artificial reproductive therapies.

3.3. *SSc and Pregnancy*

Pregnancy in women with SSc is a complex issue that requires careful management due to the potential risks to both maternal and foetal health.

3.3.1. Risks to Maternal Health

Skin: The hallmark of SSc is skin thickening; however, concerns regarding the progression of the condition appear to be negligible during pregnancy. A meta-analysis summarised reports on skin evolution during pregnancy, yielding rather favourable results. The analysis revealed that the deterioration of skin involvement (2.9% during pregnancy and 13.6% postpartum) appeared to be less prevalent than that of improvement (20% during pregnancy) [29].

Renal Involvement: Older works showed no elevated risk of SRC during pregnancy [30]. However, the progression of renal disease during pregnancy can result in complications, including preeclampsia, renal failure, or severe hypertension. There are documented cases of SRC in pregnancy, mostly occurring after the 20th week of gestation [31–34]. This may complicate the distinction between SRC and preeclampsia. ACE inhibitors have been used to treat SRC in pregnancy but are not recommended during pregnancy because of the associated risk of congenital anomalies. In view of the high frequency of SRC in patients with RNA Pol III antibodies, it may be advisable to postpone pregnancy in the first years following diagnosis.

Cardiopulmonary involvement: Women with SSc may have underlying lung or heart disease, which can exacerbate during pregnancy, increasing the risk of respiratory failure, pulmonary hypertension, or heart failure. Interstitial lung disease (ILD) is prevalent among patients suffering from SSc, affecting approximately 60% of the patient population, albeit with variable degrees of severity [35]. A retrospective analysis of women with ILD of different origins demonstrated that adverse pregnancy outcomes, including prematurity and preeclampsia, were prevalent (28% of women with CTD-ILD) and affected a greater number of individuals when severe ILD was present (60%) [36]. Similar data has been published by other groups [37,38]. However, the progression of ILD seems to not be common.

The prevalence of pulmonary artery hypertension (PAH) in SSc varies, but it has been demonstrated to worsen pregnancy outcomes in women with PAH of different aetiology. This is attributable to the fact that pregnancy-associated physiologic changes in cardiac output and plasma volume increase might negatively impact the maternal and, consequently, foetal cardiovascular system. It is evident that the occurrence of adverse outcomes is associated with this condition, including an elevated risk of preterm birth and intrauterine growth restriction (IUGR) [39,40]. Moreover, there is a paucity of knowledge regarding PAH-targeted drugs such as sildenafil, bosentan, macitentan, and riociguat and their impact on pregnancy. The most recent recommendations made by the European League Against Rheumatism (EULAR) include the potential use of sildenafil [41]. Furthermore, calcium channel blockers and prostacyclin have historically been utilised as therapeutic agents in this context [42].

Preeclampsia and SSc: Different groups demonstrated an elevated risk of preeclampsia in patients suffering from SSc [43,44]. Consequently, the utilisation of acetylsalicylic acid in these patients should be contemplated, despite the paucity of studies conducted on this particular entity. It is a noteworthy observation that women afflicted with preeclampsia exhibit a 69% elevated probability of subsequently manifesting SSc [45].

3.3.2. Foetal Risks

Foetal loss: The incidence of early pregnancy loss (first trimester miscarriage) appears to slightly exceed that of the general population, which is typically about 5–20% [25,29,43]. In contrast, a multicentre Italian study reported an abortion rate of only 4% [46]. Furthermore, a study conducted on a nationwide U.S. basis demonstrated a significant decrease in foetal mortality over the years, thereby indicating an enhancement in the management of pregnant patients suffering from SSc [47].

IUGR and low birth weight: IUGR has been consistently reported through numerous publications, with varying rates (5–30%) [25,43,46,47].

Preterm delivery is also a frequent complication (20–30%). A higher incidence of preterm delivery was observed in pregnancies in SSc patients compared with healthy individuals (OR 6.74, 95%CI 1.29–35.09) [43]. And as in the aforementioned U.S. study, an OR of 2.65 (95%CI 2.23–3.14) was calculated when comparing SSc and non-SSc delivery-related hospitalisations over the entire study period [47]. Some groups suggested a higher incidence in patients with dcSSc [25,43].

Congenital anomalies: Most reports did not reveal an increased rate of congenital malformations in children born to women with SSc. Indirectly, SS-A/SS-B antibodies, which are associated with neonatal Lupus [48], an immune-mediated disease caused by maternal antibodies, can lead to congenital anomalies, as SS-A antibodies are also frequently (approximately 25% of cases) detected in patients with SSc [49]. There is some evidence suggesting that autoimmune diseases, including SSc, may increase the risk of certain congenital anomalies, although this remains an area of ongoing research.

Table 2 summarises the most recent data on pregnancy outcomes in SSc patients.

Table 2. Pregnancy outcomes in patients after disease onset; abbreviations: IUGR = intrauterine growth restriction; NK = not known; SGA = small for gestational age; OR = odds ratio.

Article	N	Mean Age in Years 1. Pregnancy	Autoantibodies	Gestational Age	Prevalence or Risk of Foetal Loss or Miscarriage	Prevalence of Live Births	Prevalence or Risk of Sga or Iugr	Prevalence or Risk of Preterm Delivery	Prevalence or Risk of Preeclampsia
Chicharo et al. [50]	12 pregnancies in 9 women	35.9 +/− 4.9	6 ACA 3 Scl70 2 SSA/SSB	38.2 +/− 1.8	2 miscarriages	10/12 (83.3%)	SGA 33.3%	1/12 (8.3)	NK
Sieiro et al. [51]	88 pregnancies in 50 women	29.5 +/− 7.2	27 ACA 18 Scl70 18 SSA 4 RNP	NK	18% foetal loss	77%	NK	0	3%
Lazzaroni et al. [10]	48	32.0 (29–36)	NK	39.0 (37.0–40.0)	4/36 (11.1)	88.9%	NK	7/36 (19.4)	0/36 (0.0%)
Alrifai et al. [52]	1165	31.2 (5.2)	NK	NK	20 (1.72%)	98.3%	IUGR 80 (6.87%)	105 (9.01%)	NK
Crisafulli et al. [44] and Singh et al. [53]	1403 (meta-analysis from 16 studies)	NK	NK	NK	OR 1.6 (1.22–2.22)	NK	OR 3.2 (2.21–4.53)	OR 2.4 (1.14–4.86)	OR 2.20 (2.21–4.53)
Kawano et al. [47]	3740	30.2	NK	NK	28.9/1000	NK	IUGR 5.5%	21.9%	NK
Barilaro et al. [43]	33 pregnancies in 21 women	35.4 +/− 4.1	NK	31.6 +/− 11.7	21.2%	NK	IUGR 15.2% SGA 21.2%	24.2%	12.1%
Kharbanda et al. [24]	15 pregnancies	NK	NK	NK	40%	60%		26.7%	NK
Taraballi et al. [46]	99 pregnancies	31.8 +/− 5.3	20 ACA 59 Scl70	NK	6% 4% therapeutic abortion	90%	IUGR 6%	25%	0%

In conclusion, the data on maternal and foetal pregnancy outcomes are very heterogeneous due to the different ways of reporting and collecting the data and the included patients' medical health care in the different countries. Nevertheless, there are signs of a higher incidence of adverse pregnancy outcomes in SSc.

3.4. SSc and Menopause

Menopause is defined as cessation of the menstrual period and thus ability to get pregnant. As mentioned before, several influencing factors play a role, and the timepoint of menopause usually varies between the ages of 45 and 55 but can be much younger in patients with SSc [44].

The impact of SSc on the lives of those affected is profound, extending beyond the physical health dimension to encompass the psychological, social, and sexual aspects of life. As most of our patients are women, this paper aims to explore the impact of SSc on sexuality, fertility, pregnancy, and menopause, focusing on both the physiological and emotional challenges faced by women living with this condition.

In the Chinese population, the mean age at which menopause occurred in patients with SSc who had disease onset prior to menopause was found to be significantly younger than in the general population [25]. As stated in the preceding paper from Thailand, early menopause was observed in 35.7% of patients, a phenomenon that was found to be significantly associated with CYC. The study also identified a correlation between early menopause and both elevated cumulative doses of prednisone and a protracted disease duration [23]. A study conducted in Croatia also reported a reduction in androgen levels (i.e., testosterone, androstenedione, and DHEAS) in postmenopausal women with SSc when compared with a group of healthy, age-matched controls [54].

The reason for non-treatment-related early menopause in SSc is rooted in the reduction in female hormone levels triggered by chronic inflammation, vasculopathy, and fibrosis of hormone-producing organs.

In a recent review article, the authors also found evidence of the impact of hormonal status on the manifestation of diseases. Subsequent to the onset of menopause, there was an improvement in the condition of the skin. However, there is a concomitant increase in the risk of PAH. Moreover, the positive effects of hormone replacement therapy (HRT) on PAH have been delineated in the extant literature [55]. Conversely, Swedish researchers identified a heightened probability of developing new SSc in women undergoing HRT, with an OR of 1.4 (1.2–1.7) [56]. As patients with SSc have a higher risk for osteoporosis [57,58] and premature menopause has been demonstrated to increase this risk, it is recommended that bone density assessment be incorporated into the standard SSc workup [58,59].

4. Discussion

SSc significantly affects various aspects of a woman's life, including sexuality, fertility, pregnancy, and menopause. Figure 1 summarises the different manifestations/influences of SSc on female health. Comprehensive care addressing physical symptoms, emotional well-being, and interdisciplinary collaboration ensures that affected individuals can navigate these aspects of life effectively. The disease itself, coupled with the physical and psychological challenges it presents, can make sexual health and reproductive choices difficult for those living with it. Understanding these issues, along with appropriate medical management, is essential for improving quality of life and ensuring that individuals with systemic sclerosis receive comprehensive care. With advances in medical treatment, psychosocial support, and fertility preservation techniques, many individuals with SSc can lead fulfilling lives and make informed decisions about their sexual health and reproductive futures.

In the Italian and German surveys, patients were asked whether they discussed their sexual disorders with their physicians. The results indicated that 58% and 90.4% of SSc patients, respectively, had never addressed this topic [5,11]. Therefore, it is of utmost importance that medical professionals are open to addressing and finding a way to help our patients by frankly asking about complaints with regard to sexuality, or at least using questionnaires. This will improve the awareness and thus facilitate the identification of the necessity for assistance.

Although the issue of SDF in SSc has been addressed in several studies, there are no clear treatment options so far. It is generally known that physical exercise has a positive effect on the functional and mental health of all patients [60]. Targeted pelvic floor training and physiotherapy have been shown to improve sexuality in healthy individuals [60]. A recently published study from the Czech Republic also showed a significant improvement in a small group through targeted 8-week physiotherapy, including pelvic floor training, even in women with SSc [61]. In general, regular physical activity, including physiotherapy and occupational therapy, is recommended to maintain hand–finger function, which, of course, also plays a role in sexuality. Drug treatment options for SDF in women are limited. Vaseline-containing ointments as lubricants are definitely recommended for vaginal dryness. The data on reduced clitoral blood flow and its negative correlation with FSFI score [4] might indicate that vasoactive substances might improve female sexuality, but studies with phosphodiesterase-5-inhibitors, for example, are missing.

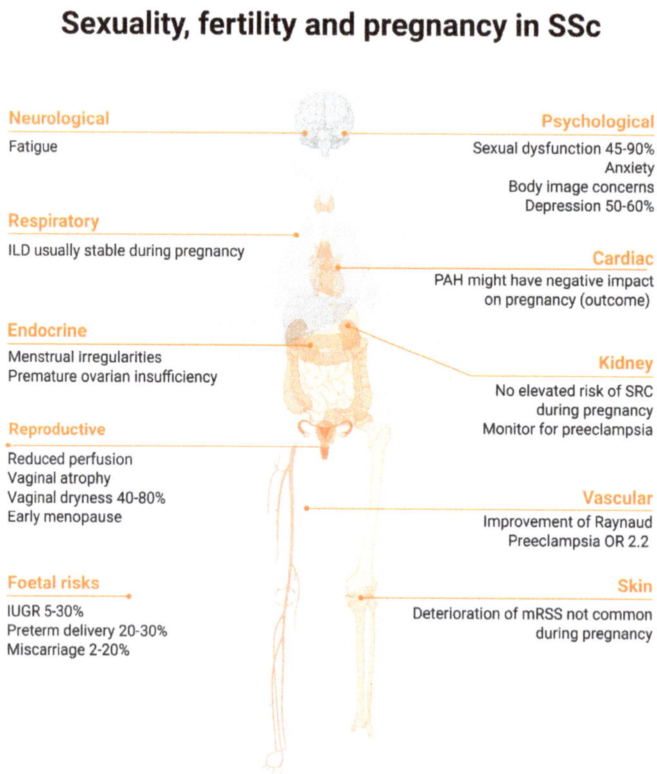

Figure 1. Summary of the effects of systemic sclerosis (SSc) on sexuality, fertility, and pregnancy. (created with BioRender.com).

When a partner becomes a caregiver, this can change the roles in the relationship and put a strain on the sexual relationship. Such changes can cause feelings of dependency or loss of equality, making intimacy even more difficult. Openness to talk about sexual problems is often difficult, which can lead to misunderstandings or a lack of support in partnerships. A lack of communication about needs and fears increases the emotional burden. These emotional factors are closely linked to physical symptoms and should be taken into account when treating sexual dysfunction. Therefore, the help of professional talk/sex/couples therapists is a useful addition [14].

The psychological burden of dealing with SSc can significantly affect the aspects of women's health. Coping with a chronic illness often leads to feelings of isolation, stress, and anxiety, which can exacerbate issues related to sexual health, intimacy, and reproductive decisions. Individuals with SSc may experience changes in their body image due to skin thickening, weight changes, or visible scarring, which can negatively affect their sexual self-esteem and willingness to engage in sexual activity. Counselling, sexual therapy, and support groups may therefore play a crucial role in helping individuals address the psychological impacts of the disease. Providing resources for sexual health and fertility counselling can assist patients in making informed decisions about their reproductive health. Also, the open communication between partners is vital in addressing SDF and maintaining intimacy. Couples may benefit from education and therapy that helps them navigate the challenges posed by systemic sclerosis.

Fertility in SSc patients seems to be reduced compared to healthy controls [22]; therefore, it is of high importance to address family planning early and to define the ideal timepoint for a pregnancy together with our patients.

Pregnancy in the context of SSc necessitates careful management in view of the potential for complications, namely, increased rates of hypertension, preeclampsia, and cases of renal crisis have been reported. It is considered ideal to achieve remission or low levels of disease activity for a period of 3–6 months prior to conception. It is also important to consider the potential risks to the foetus. Women with SSc are at an increased risk of preterm birth and IUGR. Furthermore, miscarriage may also be more prevalent. However, due to difficulties such as underreporting, differences in populations and definitions, as well as inconsistent data collection methods, obtaining meaningful data on pregnancy losses is challenging. Pregnancy risks are frequently associated with vascular complications, such as insufficient placental blood flow. The process of invasion by extravillous trophoblasts into the decidua, accompanied by remodelling of the arteries, is contingent upon the integrity of vascular health. Vascular abnormalities might result in placental insufficiency, which may consequently lead to IUGR, low birth weight, and an elevated risk of stillbirth. Indeed, findings in placental biopsies demonstrated placental vasculopathy [62]. Therefore, interdisciplinary care involving rheumatologists and obstetricians is crucial when counselling SSc patients with wish to become pregnant and during pregnancy. Adjustments in immunosuppressive therapies and close monitoring improve outcomes, and careful monitoring of maternal organ function (renal, cardiopulmonary) is essential. Early diagnosis and treatment of complications, such as hypertension or renal issues, can improve outcomes for both mother and baby. Medication use during pregnancy must be carefully considered, as many immunosuppressive drugs used in SSc are contraindicated during pregnancy [41]. Alternatives must be explored to manage the disease while minimising foetal risks. Azathioprine and low-dose glucocorticoids are considered to be safe for use during pregnancy; in severe cases, B-cell depletion with rituximab might be considered [41,63].

Premature menopause is common in SSc, and as patients with SSc have a higher risk for osteoporosis [57,58], we strongly recommend bone density assessment in all SSc patients on a regular basis. Continued research is needed to explore the full extent of these impacts and to develop better strategies for managing the condition's influence on sexual and reproductive health.

In conclusion, SSc as a systemic disease also has a huge influence on all aspects of women's health, and we as the treating physicians would all do well to be aware of that. Interdisciplinarity, therefore, is a cornerstone of treating patients with SSc, and learning from each other and listening to the patients' complaints will improve all aspects of SSc care.

Funding: This research received no external funding.

Conflicts of Interest: The authors declare no conflict of interest.

References

1. Denton, C.P.; Khanna, D. Systemic sclerosis. *Lancet* **2017**, *390*, 1685–1699. [CrossRef] [PubMed]
2. Good, S.D.; Lee, J.Y.; Johnson, R.E.; Volkmann, E.R. A scoping review of the epidemiology of systemic sclerosis and its organ manifestations: 2018–2024. *Curr. Opin. Rheumatol.* **2025**, *37*, 103–112. [CrossRef] [PubMed]
3. Elhai, M.; Meune, C.; Boubaya, M.; Avouac, J.; Hachulla, E.; Balbir-Gurman, A.; Riemekasten, G.; Airo, P.; Joven, B.; Vettori, S.; et al. Mapping and predicting mortality from systemic sclerosis. *Ann. Rheum. Dis.* **2017**, *76*, 1897–1905. [CrossRef] [PubMed]
4. Gigante, A.; Navarini, L.; Margiotta, D.; Barbano, B.; Afeltra, A.; Rosato, E. Female sexual dysfunction in systemic sclerosis: The role of endothelial growth factor and endostatin. *J. Scleroderma Relat. Disord.* **2019**, *4*, 71–76. [CrossRef]

5. Schmalzing, M.; Nau, L.F.; Gernert, M.; Froehlich, M.; Schwaneck, E.C.; Pecher, A.C.; Saur, S.; Tony, H.P.; Henes, M.; Henes, J. Sexual function in German women with systemic sclerosis compared to women with systemic lupus erythematosus and evaluation of a screening test. *Clin. Exp. Rheumatol.* **2020**, *38* (Suppl. S125), 59–64.
6. Dag, A.; Ak, T.; Kaya, E.; Tulek, Z.; Poyraz, B.C.; Ugurlu, S.; Melikoglu, M.; Fresko, I.; Seyahi, E. Sexual dysfunction among female patients with rheumatic diseases. *Rheumatol. Int.* **2024**, *44*, 2099–2109. [CrossRef]
7. Rosen, R.; Brown, C.; Heiman, J.; Leiblum, S.; Meston, C.; Shabsigh, R.; Ferguson, D.; D'Agostino, R., Jr. The Female Sexual Function Index (FSFI): A multidimensional self-report instrument for the assessment of female sexual function. *J. Sex Marital Ther.* **2000**, *26*, 191–208. [CrossRef]
8. Gossec, L.; Solano, C.; Paternotte, S.; Beauvais, C.; Gaudin, P.; von Krause, G.; Sordet, C.; Perdriger, A. Elaboration and validation of a questionnaire (Qualisex) to assess the impact of rheumatoid arthritis on sexuality with patient involvement. *Clin. Exp. Rheumatol.* **2012**, *30*, 505–513.
9. Beck, A.T.; Ward, C.H.; Mendelson, M.; Mock, J.; Erbaugh, J. An inventory for measuring depression. *Arch. Gen. Psychiatry* **1961**, *4*, 561–571. [CrossRef]
10. Lazzaroni, M.G.; Moschetti, L.; Pedretti, E.; Andreoli, L.; Ramazzotto, F.; Zatti, S.; Galetti, I.; Airo, P.; Tincani, A.; Franceschini, F. The impact of systemic sclerosis on women's health evaluated with an ad hoc-developed patient-reported questionnaire. *J. Scleroderma Relat. Disord.* **2025**, *online ahead of print*. [CrossRef]
11. Ruffolo, A.F.; Serati, M.; Casiraghi, A.; Benini, V.; Scancarello, C.; Di Dedda, M.C.; Garbagnati, C.; Braga, A.; Candiani, M.; Salvatore, S. The Impact of Systemic Sclerosis on Sexual Health: An Italian Survey. *Healthcare* **2023**, *11*, 2346. [CrossRef]
12. Hermankova, B.; Spiritovic, M.; Smucrova, H.; Oreska, S.; Storkanova, H.; Komarc, M.; Pavelka, K.; Senolt, L.; Vencovsky, J.; Becvar, R.; et al. Female Sexual Dysfunction and Pelvic Floor Muscle Function Associated with Systemic Sclerosis: A Cross-Sectional Study. *Int. J. Environ. Res. Public Health* **2022**, *19*, 612. [CrossRef] [PubMed]
13. Ucar, I.; Turgay, B.; Kucuksahin, O.; Ozkan Ucar, E.; Turgay, M. Sexual dysfunction in patients with systemic sclerosis. *Turk. J. Med. Sci.* **2018**, *48*, 1104–1108. [CrossRef] [PubMed]
14. Marcoccia, A.; Guarino, A.; Cocchiaro, T.; Modesti, M.; Cianfrocca, C.; Privitera, R.; Isabelli, S.; Vizzini, M.A.S.; Rago, R.; Renzi, A.; et al. Psychopathological symptoms and their association with the quality of life and the sexual functioning in women affected by systemic scleroderma: A preliminary investigation. *Eur. Rev. Med. Pharmacol. Sci.* **2024**, *28*, 288–297. [CrossRef]
15. Sanchez, K.; Denys, P.; Giuliano, F.; Palazzo, C.; Berezne, A.; Abid, H.; Rannou, F.; Poiraudeau, S.; Mouthon, L. Systemic sclerosis: Sexual dysfunction and lower urinary tract symptoms in 73 patients. *Presse Med.* **2016**, *45*, e79–e89. [CrossRef]
16. Grossmann, B.; Saur, S.; Rall, K.; Pecher, A.C.; Hubner, S.; Henes, J.; Henes, M. Prevalence of autoimmune disease in women with premature ovarian failure. *Eur. J. Contracept. Reprod. Health Care* **2020**, *25*, 72–75. [CrossRef] [PubMed]
17. Zhang, C.; Yu, D.; Mei, Y.; Liu, S.; Shao, H.; Sun, Q.; Lu, Q.; Hu, J.; Gu, H. Single-cell RNA sequencing of peripheral blood reveals immune cell dysfunction in premature ovarian insufficiency. *Front. Endocrinol.* **2023**, *14*, 1129657. [CrossRef]
18. Costenbader, K.H.; Feskanich, D.; Stampfer, M.J.; Karlson, E.W. Reproductive and menopausal factors and risk of systemic lupus erythematosus in women. *Arthritis Rheum.* **2007**, *56*, 1251–1262. [CrossRef]
19. Motta, F.; Di Simone, N.; Selmi, C. The Impact of Menopause on Autoimmune and Rheumatic Diseases. *Clin. Rev. Allergy Immunol.* **2025**, *68*, 32. [CrossRef]
20. Silman, A.J.; Black, C. Increased incidence of spontaneous abortion and infertility in women with scleroderma before disease onset: A controlled study. *Ann. Rheum. Dis.* **1988**, *47*, 441–444. [CrossRef]
21. Steen, V.D.; Conte, C.; Day, N.; Ramsey-Goldman, R.; Medsger, T.A., Jr. Pregnancy in women with systemic sclerosis. *Arthritis Rheumatol.* **1989**, *32*, 151–157. [CrossRef]
22. Pecher, A.C.; Henes, J.C.; Demin, A.; Staufenberg, E.M.; Henes, M. Ovarian reserve alteration in premenopausal women with systemic sclerosis. *Rheumatol. Int.* **2024**, *44*, 3087–3092. [CrossRef]
23. Jutiviboonsuk, A.; Salang, L.; Eamudomkarn, N.; Mahakkanukrauh, A.; Suwannaroj, S.; Foocharoen, C. Prevalence and clinical associations with premature ovarian insufficiency, early menopause, and low ovarian reserve in systemic sclerosis. *Clin. Rheumatol.* **2021**, *40*, 2267–2275. [CrossRef] [PubMed]
24. Kharbanda, R.; Naveen, R.; Misra, D.P.; Gupta, L.; Agarwal, V. Poor maternal and foetal outcomes in women with systemic sclerosis: An interview-based study at a tertiary centre. *Rheumatol. Int.* **2021**, *41*, 1133–1142. [CrossRef] [PubMed]
25. Dai, L.; Xu, D.; Li, X.; Huang, S.; Duan, X.; Zheng, A.; Yang, J.; Zhao, J.; Zeng, L.; Mu, R. Reproductive health in female patients with systemic sclerosis: A cross-sectional study. *Rheumatology* **2024**, *63*, 1911–1916. [CrossRef] [PubMed]
26. Henes, M.; Froeschlin, J.; Taran, F.A.; Brucker, S.; Rall, K.K.; Xenitidis, T.; Igney-Oertel, A.; Lawrenz, B.; Henes, J.C. Ovarian reserve alterations in premenopausal women with chronic inflammatory rheumatic diseases: Impact of rheumatoid arthritis, Behcet's disease and spondyloarthritis on anti-Mullerian hormone levels. *Rheumatology* **2015**, *54*, 1709–1712. [CrossRef]
27. Lawrenz, B.; Henes, J.; Henes, M.; Neunhoeffer, E.; Schmalzing, M.; Fehm, T.; Kitter, I. Impact of systemic lupus erythematosus on ovarian reserve in premenopausal women: Evaluation by using anti-Muellerian hormone. *Lupus* **2011**, *20*, 1193–1197. [CrossRef]

28. Mont'Alverne, A.R.; Pereira, R.M.; Yamakami, L.Y.; Viana, V.S.; Baracat, E.C.; Bonfa, E.; Silva, C.A. Reduced ovarian reserve in patients with Takayasu arteritis. *J. Rheumatol.* **2014**, *41*, 2055–2059. [CrossRef]
29. Blagojevic, J.; AlOdhaibi, K.A.; Aly, A.M.; Bellando-Randone, S.; Lepri, G.; Bruni, C.; Moggi-Pignone, A.; Guiducci, S.; Mecacci, F.; Matucci-Cerinic, M.; et al. Pregnancy in Systemic Sclerosis: Results of a Systematic Review and Metaanalysis. *J. Rheumatol.* **2020**, *47*, 881–887. [CrossRef]
30. Steen, V.D. Pregnancy in women with systemic sclerosis. *Obstet. Gynecol.* **1999**, *94*, 15–20. [CrossRef]
31. Brown, A.N.; Bolster, M.B. Scleroderma renal crisis in pregnancy associated with massive proteinuria. *Clin. Exp. Rheumatol.* **2003**, *21*, 114–116.
32. Gore, J.E.; Brown, A.N. Scleroderma renal crisis sine scleroderma in pregnancy: A case report. *Clin. Exp. Rheumatol.* **2006**, *24*, 87–88. [PubMed]
33. Mok, C.C.; Kwan, T.H.; Chow, L. Scleroderma renal crisis sine scleroderma during pregnancy. *Scand. J. Rheumatol.* **2003**, *32*, 55–57. [CrossRef] [PubMed]
34. Steen, V.D.; Medsger, T.A., Jr. Fertility and pregnancy outcome in women with systemic sclerosis. *Arthritis Rheumatol.* **1999**, *42*, 763–768. [CrossRef] [PubMed]
35. Rubio-Rivas, M.; Pestana-Fernandez, M. Prevalence of the limited vs. extensive scleroderma-related interstitial lung disease at the time of diagnosis of SSc-ILD based on Goh et al. criteria. Systematic review and meta-analysis. *Rev. Clin. Esp.* **2024**, *224*, 189–196. [CrossRef]
36. Clowse, M.E.B.; Rajendran, A.; Eudy, A.; Giattino, S.; Swaminathan, A.; James, A.H. Pregnancy Outcomes in Patients With Interstitial Lung Disease. *Arthritis Care Res.* **2023**, *75*, 1166–1174. [CrossRef]
37. Colbenson, G.A.; Rose, C.H.; Ernste, F.C.; Ryu, J.H. Successful Pregnancy Outcome With Connective Tissue Disease-Associated Interstitial Lung Disease: A Case Series. *J. Clin. Rheumatol.* **2022**, *28*, e305–e307. [CrossRef]
38. Lapinsky, S.E.; Tram, C.; Mehta, S.; Maxwell, C.V. Restrictive lung disease in pregnancy. *Chest* **2014**, *145*, 394–398. [CrossRef]
39. Duarte, A.G.; Thomas, S.; Safdar, Z.; Torres, F.; Pacheco, L.D.; Feldman, J.; deBoisblanc, B. Management of pulmonary arterial hypertension during pregnancy: A retrospective, multicenter experience. *Chest* **2013**, *143*, 1330–1336. [CrossRef]
40. Luo, J.; Shi, H.; Xu, L.; Su, W.; Li, J. Pregnancy outcomes in patients with pulmonary arterial hypertension: A retrospective study. *Medicine* **2020**, *99*, e20285. [CrossRef]
41. Ruegg, L.; Pluma, A.; Hamroun, S.; Cecchi, I.; Perez-Garcia, L.F.; Anderson, P.O.; Andreoli, L.; Wirstrom, S.B.; Boyadhzieva, V.; Chambers, C.; et al. EULAR recommendations for use of antirheumatic drugs in reproduction, pregnancy, and lactation: 2024 update. *Ann. Rheum. Dis.* **2025**, *84*, 910–926. [CrossRef]
42. Bedard, E.; Dimopoulos, K.; Gatzoulis, M.A. Has there been any progress made on pregnancy outcomes among women with pulmonary arterial hypertension? *Eur. Heart J.* **2009**, *30*, 256–265. [CrossRef]
43. Barilaro, G.; Castellanos, A.; Gomez-Ferreira, I.; Lledo, G.M.; Della Rocca, C.; Fernandez-Blanco, L.; Cervera, R.; Banos, N.; Figueras, F.; Espinosa, G. Systemic sclerosis and pregnancy outcomes: A retrospective study from a single center. *Arthritis Res. Ther.* **2022**, *24*, 91. [CrossRef] [PubMed]
44. Crisafulli, F.; Lazzaroni, M.G.; Nalli, C.; Orabona, R.; Franceschini, F.; Tincani, A. Reproductive Health in Scleroderma, Vasculitis, and Sjogren Syndrome. *J. Clin. Rheumatol.* **2024**, *30*, S49–S55. [CrossRef]
45. Kamper-Jorgensen, M.; Gammill, H.S.; Nelson, J.L. Preeclampsia and scleroderma: A prospective nationwide analysis. *Acta Obstet. Gynecol. Scand.* **2018**, *97*, 587–590. [CrossRef] [PubMed]
46. Taraborelli, M.; Ramoni, V.; Brucato, A.; Airo, P.; Bajocchi, G.; Bellisai, F.; Biasi, D.; Blagojevic, J.; Canti, V.; Caporali, R.; et al. Brief report: Successful pregnancies but a higher risk of preterm births in patients with systemic sclerosis: An Italian multicenter study. *Arthritis Rheumatol.* **2012**, *64*, 1970–1977. [CrossRef] [PubMed]
47. Kawano, Y.; Kolstad, K.D.; Li, S.; Simard, J.F.; Chung, L. Trends in adverse pregnancy outcomes among women with systemic sclerosis in the United States. *Semin. Arthritis Rheum.* **2023**, *63*, 152252. [CrossRef]
48. Bankole, A.; Nwaonu, J. A review of neonatal lupus syndrome. *Sci. Prog.* **2024**, *107*, 368504241278476. [CrossRef]
49. Mierau, R.; Moinzadeh, P.; Riemekasten, G.; Melchers, I.; Meurer, M.; Reichenberger, F.; Buslau, M.; Worm, M.; Blank, N.; Hein, R.; et al. Frequency of disease-associated and other nuclear autoantibodies in patients of the German Network for Systemic Scleroderma: Correlation with characteristic clinical features. *Arthritis Res. Ther.* **2011**, *13*, R172. [CrossRef]
50. Chicharo, A.T.; Lopes, A.R.; Barreira, S.; Martins, P.; Cruz-Machado, A.R.; Pinto, L.; Capela, S. Pregnancy outcomes in systemic sclerosis: Experience of a rheumatology-obstetric multidisciplinary clinic. *ARP Rheumatol.* **2025**, *4*, 66–68. [CrossRef]
51. Sieiro Santos, C.; Ordas Martinez, J.; Moriano Morales, C.; Alvarez Castro, C.; Diez Alvarez, E. Pregnancy outcomes in connective tissue diseases: A 30-year study of 465 cases from a single-center Spanish registry with insights on hydroxychloroquine use. *ARP Rheumatol.* **2025**, *4*, 29–36. [CrossRef]
52. Alrifai, N.; Puttur, A.; Ghanem, F.; Dhital, Y.; Jabri, A.; Al-Abdouh, A.; Alhuneafat, L. Maternal and fetal outcomes in those with autoimmune connective tissue disease. *Clin. Rheumatol.* **2025**, *44*, 391–401. [CrossRef] [PubMed]

53. Singh, M.; Wambua, S.; Lee, S.I.; Okoth, K.; Wang, Z.; Fayaz, F.F.A.; Eastwood, K.A.; Nelson-Piercy, C.; Reynolds, J.A.; Nirantharakumar, K.; et al. Autoimmune diseases and adverse pregnancy outcomes: An umbrella review. *BMC Med.* **2024**, *22*, 94. [CrossRef] [PubMed]
54. Perkovic, D.; Martinovic Kaliterna, D.; Jurisic, Z.; Lalovac, M.; Radic, M. Androgens in post-menopausal patients with systemic sclerosis. *Rheumatology* **2015**, *54*, 744–746. [CrossRef]
55. Ciaffi, J.; van Leeuwen, N.M.; Schoones, J.W.; Huizinga, T.W.J.; de Vries-Bouwstra, J.K. Sex hormones and sex hormone-targeting therapies in systemic sclerosis: A systematic literature review. *Semin. Arthritis Rheum.* **2020**, *50*, 140–148. [CrossRef]
56. Patasova, K.; Dehara, M.; Mantel, A.; Bixo, M.; Arkema, E.; Holmqvist, M. Menopausal hormone therapy and the risk of systemic lupus erythematosus and systemic sclerosis: A population-based nested case-control study. *Rheumatology* **2025**, *64*, 3563–3570. [CrossRef]
57. Tu, X.; Li, C.; Zhuang, M.; Liu, L.; Xu, C.; Wang, J. High prevalence and risk factors for osteoporosis in 1839 patients with systemic sclerosis: A systematic review and meta-analysis. *Clin. Rheumatol.* **2023**, *42*, 1087–1099. [CrossRef] [PubMed]
58. Lillpers, K.; McGuigan, F.; Andreasson, K.; Hesselstrand, R.; Kapetanovic, M.C.; Akesson, K.E. Increased prevalence of osteopenia and osteoporosis in systemic sclerosis patients, including in men and young women-a case-control study. *Rheumatology* **2025**, *64*, 2783–2791. [CrossRef]
59. Chuealee, W.; Foocharoen, C.; Mahakkanukrauh, A.; Suwannaroj, S.; Pongchaiyakul, C.; Nanagara, R. Prevalence and predictive factors of osteoporosis in Thai systemic sclerosis. *Sci. Rep.* **2021**, *11*, 9424. [CrossRef]
60. Ferreira, C.H.; Dwyer, P.L.; Davidson, M.; De Souza, A.; Ugarte, J.A.; Frawley, H.C. Does pelvic floor muscle training improve female sexual function? A systematic review. *Int. Urogynecology J.* **2015**, *26*, 1735–1750. [CrossRef]
61. Hermankova, B.; Spiritovic, M.; Oreska, S.; Storkanova, H.; Mann, H.; Pavelka, K.; Senolt, L.; Vencovsky, J.; Becvar, R.; Tomcik, M. Effect of an 8-Week Tailored Physiotherapy Program on Sexual Health in Women with Scleroderma and Myositis: A Controlled Pilot Study. *Rheumatol. Ther.* **2023**, *10*, 1089–1105. [CrossRef]
62. Ibba-Manneschi, L.; Manetti, M.; Milia, A.F.; Miniati, I.; Benelli, G.; Guiducci, S.; Mecacci, F.; Mello, G.; Di Lollo, S.; Matucci-Cerinic, M. Severe fibrotic changes and altered expression of angiogenic factors in maternal scleroderma: Placental findings. *Ann. Rheum. Dis.* **2010**, *69*, 458–461. [CrossRef] [PubMed]
63. Pluma, A.; Hamroun, S.; Ruegg, L.; Cecchi, I.; Kramer, M.; Perez-Garcia, L.F.; Rivero, T.; Finckh, A.; Meissner, Y.; Forger, F. Antirheumatic drugs in reproduction, pregnancy, and lactation: A systematic literature review informing the 2024 update of the EULAR recommendations. *Ann. Rheum. Dis.* **2025**, *online ahead of print*. [CrossRef]

sclerosis

Review

The Evolving Landscape of Systemic Sclerosis Pathogenesis: From Foundational Mechanisms to Organ-Specific Modifiers

Toshiya Takahashi and Yoshihide Asano *

Department of Dermatology, Tohoku University Graduate School of Medicine, 1-1 Seiryo-Machi, Aoba-Ku, Sendai 980-8574, Japan; toshiya.takahashi.c8@tohoku.ac.jp
* Correspondence: yasano@derma.med.tohoku.ac.jp; Tel.: +81-22-717-7271; Fax: +81-22-717-7361

Abstract: Systemic sclerosis (SSc) is a multifaceted autoimmune disease in which the complex interplay of genetic predisposition and environmental factors triggers aberrant immune responses, ultimately leading to vasculopathy and fibrosis. This review offers a comprehensive overview of current perspectives on SSc pathogenesis, integrating classical concepts with recent breakthroughs enabled by advanced analytical techniques. We delve into the foundational trans-organ pathophysiology of SSc, encompassing epigenetic dysregulation, chronic inflammation, vascular injury, vasculopathy, and fibrosis. Furthermore, we explore the organ-specific modifiers that contribute to the heterogeneity of SSc manifestations across different organ systems, including the skin, gastrointestinal tract, lungs, and heart. Recent studies employing single-cell transcriptomics, spatial proteomics, and epigenomic profiling are highlighted, demonstrating how these technologies are revolutionizing our understanding of SSc cellular and molecular pathology. This evolving landscape of SSc pathogenesis research is critical for identifying novel therapeutic targets and advancing personalized medicine approaches for SSc patients.

Keywords: systemic sclerosis; pathogenesis; fibrosis; vasculopathy; immune dysfunction; skin; single-cell analysis; transcriptomics; proteomics; epigenetics

1. Introduction

Systemic sclerosis (SSc) is a multisystem connective tissue disorder of unknown origin, defined by three core pathological features: dysregulated immune activity, vascular injury followed by defective neovascularization and vessel remodeling, and the resulting fibrosis of the skin and various internal organs [1]. The etiology of SSc is still unknown, and there is currently no single hypothesis that uniquely explains the variety of pathophysiologic manifestations of the disease. However, our insight into its pathogenesis is rapidly growing, driven by clinical investigations of patient-derived samples, basic science research with animal models, and progress in targeted molecular treatments. Recent breakthroughs in sophisticated analytical methods, particularly single-cell analysis, have revolutionized the field. These advancements are vital for confirming disease mechanisms in patient tissues and for facilitating the discovery of new therapeutic approaches. This manuscript provides a summary of current perspectives on SSc pathogenesis, with a focus on the latest advancements.

 https://doi.org/10.3390/sclerosis3020020

2. Systemic Sclerosis Pathogenesis: Foundational Trans-Organ Pathophysiology

2.1. "Genetics" in SSc

Etiological research suggests that SSc results from a combination of genetic and environmental influences. While family history is the leading risk factor [2], concordance for SSc among twins is low, with comparable rates in both monozygotic (4.2%) and dizygotic (5.6%) pairs. One critical finding, however, is that the concordance for possessing autoantibodies is markedly higher in the unaffected monozygotic twin of an SSc patient (95%), compared to a dizygotic twin (60%, $p < 0.05$) [3]. This observation suggests that genetic factors are associated with autoimmunity, thereby increasing SSc susceptibility, but are insufficient for the development of clinically definite SSc. Consistent with this notion, the majority of SSc susceptibility genes are Human Leukocyte Antigen (HLA) haplotypes and non-HLA genes implicated in immunity and inflammation, which are also implicated in other connective tissue diseases such as rheumatoid arthritis and systemic lupus erythematosus (SLE) [4,5]. Beyond influencing susceptibility, genetic factors also determine the severity of SSc. This is demonstrated by multiple case-control and genome-wide association studies showing that variations like single-nucleotide polymorphisms (SNPs) in certain genes correlate with the disease course [6–9]. For instance, a specific SNP linked to lower levels of interferon regulatory factor 5 (IRF5) is more prevalent among SSc patients with less severe clinical manifestations [10].

2.2. "Epigenetics" in SSc

Epigenetics refers to the mechanisms by which cells regulate and transmit gene expression without alterations to the DNA base sequence. It also encompasses the field of study dedicated to these mechanisms. The pathogenesis of SSc is investigated from three perspectives: immune dysregulation, vasculopathy, and fibrosis. However, the ultimate goal of these investigations is to elucidate the mechanisms through which fibroblasts maintain a persistently activated state across various organs. While fibroblast activation is generally considered a response to the cumulative stimuli from the extracellular microenvironment in vivo, fibroblasts isolated from the skin and lungs of SSc patients retain their activated phenotype even after in vitro serial passage. This observation suggests the existence of a mechanism for maintaining a "pathological memory" intrinsic to these cells. Epigenetics is considered to be one such mechanism. DNA methylation, histone acetylation and methylation, microRNAs (miRNAs), and long non-coding RNAs (lncRNAs) have been identified as epigenetic modifications implicated in sustaining the activated state of fibroblasts derived from SSc patients.

Focusing on genetic factors, genome-wide association studies, as noted earlier, have identified that most susceptibility genes for SSc are located within the HLA region and in non-HLA immune-related genes. This suggests that genetically determined immune abnormalities play a central role in the development of SSc [5]. Indeed, antinuclear antibodies are detected in over 90% of SSc patients, and numerous other autoantibodies with pathogenic functions have been identified [11,12]. In the lesional skin of patients with early-stage SSc, perivascular lymphocytic infiltration is observed. This inflammation is thought to induce structural abnormalities in blood vessels characteristic of SSc, such as the loss of capillaries and thickening of small artery walls. Furthermore, it activates fibroblasts, leading to fibrosis. Although the precise mechanisms remain to be fully elucidated, it is proposed that SSc-specific phenotypic changes arise in various cells through epigenetic regulation influenced by environmental factors and are potentially shaped by genetic predisposition. These changes result in the breakdown of immune tolerance, excessive inflammatory responses, impaired vascular remodeling, and persistent and aberrant activation of vascular endothelial cells and fibroblasts. Consequently, these processes contribute to the complex pathogenesis of this disease [13]. Moreover, epigenetic modifications are deeply implicated in the mechanisms by which various cells maintain their pathological phenotypes within the highly fibrotic environment. In summary, epigenetics is considered to be involved in cellular phenotypic changes from two perspectives: the responses to external environmental factors that trigger SSc onset and the mechanisms maintaining pathological homeostasis against the internal microenvironment.

In SSc, the transcription factor FLI1 was the first gene identified as being under epigenetic control of its expression. Wang et al. [14] reported that, in both cultured SSc dermal fibroblasts and lesional SSc skin, CpG methylation is markedly increased in the *FLI1* promoter region. Furthermore, in cultured SSc dermal fibroblasts, significant decreases in histone H3 and H4 acetylation have been observed. Immunohistochemical analysis of skin tissue revealed that FLII expression in fibroblasts and vascular endothelial cells is mildly reduced in non-lesional SSc skin compared to healthy skin. A more pronounced reduction was observed in lesional SSc skin [15]. In the skin of $Fli1^{+/-}$ mice, fibroblasts are constitutively activated and exhibit increased type I collagen production; however, dermal thickening is not histologically apparent. Furthermore, mild structural abnormalities are present in skin microvessels, and phenotypic alterations resembling those in SSc skin vascular endothelial cells are evident at the molecular level [16]. Conversely, when bleomycin-induced SSc model mice are generated using $Fli1^{+/-}$ mice, an exacerbation of SSc-like phenotypes is observed across all aspects: inflammation, vasculopathy, and fibrosis [17]. These findings indicate that reduced FLI1 expression can induce activation of immune cells, vascular endothelial cells, and fibroblasts, molecularly resembling SSc, but this anomaly alone is insufficient to trigger SSc onset.

KLF5 is a crucial transcription factor regulating diverse fibrotic responses, acting as a pro-fibrotic factor in cardiac fibroblasts and a fibrosis-suppressing factor in renal tubular cells [18,19]. DNA microarray analysis has revealed that the expression of this transcription factor is downregulated in lesional SSc skin [20]. A study using cultured SSc dermal fibroblasts has revealed a marked downregulation of KLF5 expression at both the mRNA and protein levels. It was demonstrated that the application of an epigenetic inhibitor could recover KLF5 expression to levels comparable to those in healthy cells. Moreover, increased CpG methylation in the KLF5 promoter region was also detected [16]. These findings elucidate that KLF5 expression is robustly suppressed by epigenetic mechanisms in SSc dermal fibroblasts.

Building upon these findings, $Klf5^{+/-}$; $Fli1^{+/-}$ mice were generated to serve as a model for skin fibrosis. Notably, these mice not only faithfully recapitulated skin and lung fibrosis pathologies of SSc but also mirrored SSc vasculopathy, inflammation, and autoimmunity. Importantly, inflammation and autoimmunity emerged at 4 weeks of age, vasculopathy at 4–8 weeks, and skin fibrosis at 8–12 weeks. The temporal sequence of these major pathologies mirrored that observed in SSc [16]. Thus, $Klf5^{+/-}$; $Fli1^{+/-}$ mice can be considered a novel SSc model that spontaneously develops the three major SSc pathologies in a manner temporally similar to human SSc. This research highlights a significant finding: by focusing on factors governing pathological memory in SSc patient-derived cells, we can potentially identify key players in the pathogenesis of this disease.

Analyses of DNA methylation, histone modifications, miRNAs, and lncRNAs have been conducted in various cell types derived from SSc patients, including fibroblasts, vascular endothelial cells, $CD4^+$ T cells, B cells, and plasmacytoid dendritic cells (pDCs). Consequently, a substantial number of epigenetic aberrations have been reported. Detailed descriptions of individual findings are omitted in this paper, as they are summarized in several review articles; readers are referred to these for further details [21–27].

2.3. Genetic Polymorphisms of FLI1 and SSc Susceptibility

Yamashita et al. [4] conducted a case-control study in a Japanese population, directly genotyping this *FLI1* (GA)*n* microsatellite. Their findings revealed a significant association between extended repeat alleles of the *FLI1* (GA)*n* microsatellite and increased susceptibility to SSc. Specifically, alleles with 22 or more GA repeats (L alleles) were more frequent in SSc patients compared to healthy controls. Furthermore, these L alleles were associated with reduced *FLI1* mRNA levels in healthy individuals, suggesting a functional consequence of this genetic polymorphism on gene expression. This genetic association with *FLI1* further strengthens the evidence implicating *FLI1* as a key player in SSc pathogenesis, acting not only through epigenetic modifications but also through inherent genetic predispositions that influence its expression and potentially its function. These findings suggest that *FLI1* genetic variants, particularly microsatellite polymorphisms, may contribute to the "missing heritability" in SSc.

2.4. Inflammation and Immunological Dysfunction in SSc

As previously described, the interaction between endothelial cells and circulating immune cells, mediated by cell adhesion molecules and chemokines, facilitates the activation of inflammatory cells and their infiltration into SSc-affected organs. Typically, infiltration by T cells, macrophages, and mast cells predominates in SSc-involved skin, whereas B-cell infiltration is comparatively limited [28–31]. In contrast, numerous lymphoid aggregates, characterized by a substantial accumulation of B cells and relatively fewer T cells and macrophages, are commonly observed in the lung tissue of patients with SSc-associated interstitial lung disease (ILD) [32]. Notably, genes associated with activated B cells are upregulated in SSc-involved skin [20], and the B-cell count in the skin correlates with the progression of skin fibrosis [31]. Consequently, while the composition of infiltrating cell types may vary across different affected organs, increased infiltration of B cells, T cells, and innate immune cells is a shared feature in the organs involved in SSc.

Alterations in T cell subsets are a well-documented feature of SSc. The balance of Th1/Th2 and Th17/Treg immune responses is skewed toward Th2 and Th17 dominance [33–36], and regulatory T cell (Treg) function is impaired during the active phase of SSc [37]. In the early stage of diffuse cutaneous SSc (dcSSc), serum levels of interleukin-6 (IL-6) and IL-10 are significantly elevated, whereas they decrease to normal levels in the late stage of dcSSc, which is characterized by the regression of skin sclerosis [38]. The cytokine profile in dcSSc displays dynamic changes over time. Initially, IL-4 levels are normal, and they decline as the skin sclerosis resolves. In contrast, serum IL-12 is low in early dcSSc but rises with disease duration, eventually exceeding normal levels in the late stage [33]. The Th17 pathway is also clearly involved; in early dcSSc skin lesions, the expression of IL-17A, IL-21, and IL-22 is increased, though IL-17F is not [36,39]. Systemically, the frequency of circulating Th17 cells and their IL-17 production are elevated, with Th17 counts corresponding to disease activity [34]. Within the skin, the Treg population is also altered, showing an increased proportion of Th2-like Tregs [30].

Currently, the direct role of SSc-related antinuclear antibodies (ANAs), including antibodies against topoisomerase I (topo I), centromere, and RNA polymerase III (RNAP III) antigens, is not fully understood, although a potential role for anti-topoisomerase I antibodies has been suggested (described below). Nevertheless, the strong correlation of these ANAs with clinical manifestations implies that altered B-cell phenotypes may be associated with the core abnormality driving disease progression.

On the other hand, the potential pathogenic role of so-called functional vascular antibodies, particularly those targeting the angiotensin II type 1 receptor (AT1R) and the endothelin-1 type A receptor (ETAR), has been a subject of discussion. However, compelling evidence for their direct contribution to pathophysiology is still lacking, and the clinical utility of testing for these antibodies remains unclear [40,41]. The ultimate proof that an antibody is causative is when passive transfer in an animal model (possibly with a specific genetic background) results in disease features.

Aberrant activation of B cells could occur through genetic and epigenetic mechanisms shared across cell types and/or through complex interactions with other immune and non-immune cells. In SSc, B cells are in a state of continuous activation, demonstrated by increased surface expression of the co-receptor CD19 [42] and the activation markers CD80 and CD86 on memory B cells [43]. This is significant because, in addition to producing antibodies, B cells contribute to pathogenesis through cytokine secretion, antigen presentation, and regulation of macrophages and lymphoid tissue [44]. The critical role of B cells is supported by the efficacy of rituximab, an anti-CD20 antibody that improves skin fibrosis and ILD by depleting B cells, as shown in multiple case series and open-label studies [45–48]. Furthermore, several case reports and case series have documented the amelioration of calcinosis, digital ulcers (DUs), and arterial stiffness following rituximab therapy [49–51]. CD19-targeted Chimeric Antigen Receptor (CAR) T-cell therapy is an emerging investigational treatment for severe and refractory SSc. Initial case studies and small series have demonstrated promising clinical responses, including improvements in skin fibrosis, ILD, and cardiac function, often accompanied by reduced autoantibody levels and disease activity. Supporting data show decreased TGF-β levels in dermal biopsies, improved skin elasticity on elastography, and amelioration of lung and heart fibrosis on imaging and through markers like KL-6. These benefits sometimes allow cessation of other immunosuppressive treatments, with generally manageable safety profiles reported [52–55]. Thus, B cells contribute to the activation of vascular and fibrotic processes, in addition to immune system activation in SSc, reinforcing the concept that immune cells are upstream mediators in the SSc-specific disease cascade.

Beyond adaptive immune cells, innate immune cells are also abundantly present in SSc-involved organs. In SSc lesional skin, mast cells secrete excessive levels of transforming growth factor-β (TGF-β) [56]. Moreover, M2 macrophages appear to be critical regulators of tissue fibrosis, as the M2 macrophage-associated gene program, which is upregulated in the skin of early SSc patients, is suppressed in conjunction with the resolution of skin fibrosis following treatment with tocilizumab (an anti-IL-6 receptor antibody) [57].

In SSc-affected skin, a specific sequence of events is thought to drive excess IFN-α production by plasmacytoid dendritic cells (pDCs). First, pDCs are recruited to the area around dermal small vessels by elevated levels of the chemoattractant chemerin [58,59]. Concurrently, endothelial cell death provides a source of self-DNA, which interacts with increased local concentrations of LL-37 [60]. This process forms stimulatory self-DNA/LL-37 complexes that are hypothesized to activate pDCs via TLR7 and 9, resulting in high local production of IFN-α.

Furthermore, disease-associated autoantibodies, particularly anti-topoisomerase I antibodies, may contribute to this process. Anti-topoisomerase I antibodies react with nuclear antigens from endothelial cells, and immune complexes formed with nucleic acids, especially RNA, induce IFN-α production from pDCs [61]. The idea that IFN-α contributes to SSc development is supported by clinical and experimental data. A trial using recombinant IFN-α for SSc reported higher withdrawal rates than placebo, with many discontinuing patients showing worsened ILD [62]. Moreover, administering IFN-α for other disorders, like multiple sclerosis or chronic hepatitis C, can trigger SSc or similar symptoms [63–68]. This may be explained by a self-amplifying cycle in which continuous IFN-α exposure causes endothelial senescence [69], providing self-DNA that stimulates pDCs to produce more IFN-α, thus driving vascular injury and immune activation. Recently, the discovery of ectopic TLR8 expression on SSc pDCs, a key RNA sensor linked to experimental fibrosis, has added another layer to this mechanism [70]. In addition to their role in IFN-α production, recent findings indicate that pDCs can also contribute to fibrosis through endoplasmic reticulum (ER) stress-mediated mechanisms, as demonstrated by Ferreira et al. [71] who revealed that ER stress induction in pDCs promotes fibroblast activation via direct cell–cell contact, suggesting a novel pathway contributing to fibrosis development in SSc. Collectively, the continuous release of autoantigens from damaged and senescent endothelial cells serves as a fundamental driver of SSc pathology, acting through the induction of chronic inflammation.

2.5. Vascular Injury in SSc

As previously discussed, the pathogenesis of SSc begins with immune dysregulation, while histopathologically detectable structural abnormalities first manifest as vascular damage [72–74]. Indeed, vasculopathy is a critical element in the early clinical picture of SSc, manifesting in patient-reported symptoms such as Raynaud's phenomenon and digital edema [75]. Crucially, the presence of disease-specific autoantibodies, hallmarks of SSc's autoimmune nature, can be detected even before these initial clinical manifestations emerge, highlighting the early involvement of autoimmunity in vascular injury [75–77]. Following this initial vascular insult, the vasculature in SSc undergoes significant structural abnormalities [78]. These changes arise from a combination of dysfunctional vascular remodeling processes and the development of various vascular functional impairments [78].

In the early stages of SSc, capillary fragility leads to capillary dilation, which in turn results in the extravasation of erythrocytes [75]. The observation of dilated and hemorrhaging nailfold capillaries is diagnostically significant, serving as an important early indicator of the disease [76]. As SSc progresses, a progressive loss of capillaries occurs, with capillary numbers gradually diminishing and eventually being replaced by fibrotic tissue [76]. In parallel with this capillary rarefaction and fibrotic replacement, vascular endothelial cells and pericytes, which are crucial components of blood vessels, undergo differentiation into myofibroblasts through processes known as endothelial-to-mesenchymal transition (EndoMT) and pericyte-to-mesenchymal transition (PMT), respectively [78,79]. These transformed cells acquire resistance to apoptosis, or programmed cell death, and exhibit cellular senescence phenotypes. This altered cellular behavior significantly contributes to the establishment and perpetuation of the extensive fibrosis characteristic of SSc [78]. The ensuing loss of capillaries leads to tissue hypoxia, a state of oxygen deficiency, which in turn acts as a potent stimulus for further myofibroblast activation and promotes the fibrotic process across a range of organs, including the skin, lungs, heart, and intestines [78]. In contrast, within arterioles and small to medium-sized arteries, the vascular endothelial cells, when injured, also undergo differentiation into myofibroblasts [78]. Furthermore, the proliferative capacity of vascular smooth muscle cells, another key cell type in blood vessels, and their ability to produce extracellular matrix (ECM) components, are enhanced, culminating in fibrotic stenosis, or narrowing of the blood vessels [78]. The characteristic arterial lesions of SSc arise from an abnormal gathering of myofibroblasts within the vessel wall. This accumulation creates fibroproliferative changes that subsequently impair vascular perfusion [78].

The vascular functional derangements in SSc are multifaceted and encompass a range of abnormalities. These include diminished vascular endothelial function, which refers to the impaired ability of the endothelium to regulate vascular tone and permeability; a reduced capacity for thrombus inhibition, increasing the risk of blood clot formation; impaired physiological anticoagulation mechanisms, further exacerbating the pro-thrombotic state; aberrant expression of cell adhesion molecules and chemokines, which contribute to chronic inflammation and immune cell recruitment to the vessel wall; and an augmented generation of reactive oxygen species (ROS), leading to oxidative stress and cellular damage [17,80,81]. These functional aberrations play a crucial role in activating fibroblasts, the primary effector cells in fibrosis, mainly by promoting tissue hypoxia and chronic inflammation [17,80–83]. Vasospasm affecting arterioles and arteries, clinically manifested as Raynaud's phenomenon, further exacerbates fibroblast activation through ischemia–reperfusion injury, a process involving tissue damage caused by alternating periods of insufficient blood supply and reperfusion [84]. Fibroblasts themselves undergo phenotypic modulation, acquiring a profibrotic phenotype, and exhibit dysregulated responses to inflammatory signals. Notably, they demonstrate excessive ECM synthesis, contributing to the tissue fibrosis [78]. The cellular origins of myofibroblasts in SSc are diverse, encompassing not only resident tissue fibroblasts but also vascular wall-resident endothelial cells and pericytes, epithelial cells, adipocytes, and bone marrow-derived fibrocytes [78]. Myofibroblasts originating from this heterogeneous array of cellular sources collectively orchestrate the pathogenesis of the extensive fibrosis observed in SSc [78]. The preceding discussion elucidates the fundamental pathophysiology of SSc, highlighting a shared mechanistic basis that operates across various organs affected by fibrosis, and thus can be conceptualized as a foundational trans-organ pathophysiology [72,73].

2.6. Fibrosis in SSc

The key effector cells driving SSc fibrosis are α-smooth muscle actin (α-SMA)-positive myofibroblasts, which secrete excessive ECM in affected tissues. These cells derive from a heterogeneous population of precursors, including local fibroblasts, circulating fibrocytes [85], and cells undergoing epithelial–mesenchymal [86], and endothelial–mesenchymal transition (EndoMT) [87,88], and adipocyte–myofibroblast transdifferentiation [89]. This state of fibroblast activation is the final outcome of the SSc pathogenic process, and the cells maintain their activated phenotype through a combination of intrinsic and extrinsic mechanisms.

A primary growth factor driving dermal fibroblast activation in SSc is TGF-β, which induces the production of ECM components like fibrillar collagens (types I, III, and V). Its expression is high in early, active disease and diminishes in established fibrosis. The localization of its isoforms suggests a role in the disease's inflammatory phase; specifically, TGF-β1 and TGF-β2 are prominently expressed around dermal vessels in connection with perivascular mononuclear infiltrates, while all three isoforms are detectable throughout the ECM [90–92]. Consequently, in the early stages of SSc, TGF-β appears to promote inflammation by recruiting leukocytes through the modulation of cell adhesion molecules and the establishment of chemokine gradients, by activating leukocytes, and by inducing various proinflammatory cytokines and mediators. Conversely, in the sclerotic phase, SSc dermal fibroblasts exhibit constitutive activation with a profibrotic phenotype, resembling that of normal fibroblasts treated with TGF-β1, even when TGF-β expression is diminished or undetectable in the skin [93]. This suggests that SSc fibroblasts possess a self-activation system, one at least partially mediated via autocrine TGF-β signaling. The increased expression of latent TGF-β receptors, including integrin αVβ3, integrin αVβ5, and thrombospondin-1, contributes to this process in SSc fibroblasts [94–98]. These receptors recruit and activate latent TGF-β on the cell surface, efficiently increasing the concentration of active TGF-β in the cellular microenvironment. Further expanding on the mechanisms of TGF-β-driven fibrosis, Meng et al. [99] identified ADAM19 as a significantly upregulated metalloproteinase in SSc skin fibrosis, demonstrating its role in promoting TGF-β-induced ECM deposition and fibroblast activation through the shedding of pro-fibrotic neuregulin-1 (NRG1), thereby contributing to the development of skin fibrosis in SSc. Thus, dermal fibroblasts are constitutively activated, at least partially, through autocrine TGF-β signaling, in SSc lesional skin.

SSc dermal fibroblasts respond differently to T-cell stimuli, relative to healthy fibroblasts. Normally, collagen production is downregulated by Th1 cells via IFN-γ [100], and by Th2 cells via membrane-associated tumor necrosis factor-α (TNF-α) [101], which counter the profibrotic effect of IL-4. In SSc, however, fibroblasts are resistant to this suppression, especially that from the Th2 cells [100,101]. One proposed reason is the high secretion of progranulin, a TNF receptor antagonist that negates the anti-fibrotic effect of TNF-α [102]. This specific lack of response to Th2-mediated suppression is thought to be a critical driver of fibroblast activation during the early, Th2-polarized phase of dcSSc. Adding to the complexity of fibroblast activation, Bergmann et al. [103] discovered a mutual amplification loop between GLI2/Hedgehog and JUN/AP-1 signaling pathways within SSc fibroblasts, where these pathways synergistically enhance each other's activity, resulting in sustained fibroblast activation and collagen production, highlighting a potential target for combined therapeutic interventions.

The interaction is bidirectional, as SSc dermal fibroblasts also shape the differentiation of inflammatory cells. For example, they direct the transdifferentiation of Tregs into Th2-like cells via IL-33 in the skin [30,104]. By overproducing galectin-9, they also inhibit IFN-γ expression in skin-infiltrating CD4+ T cells, which fosters fibrosis within the Th2/Th17-dominant microenvironment [105]. These findings suggest SSc fibroblasts affect skin immunity more extensively than previously thought.

Collectively, SSc fibroblasts perpetuate their activation through autocrine signaling and feedforward loops with other cells, culminating in the irreversible fibrotic remodeling of multiple organs.

3. Verification of Pathogenesis Hypotheses: Insights from Recent Analytical Innovations

Pathogenesis hypotheses of SSc, as previously outlined, have been largely formulated based on conventional clinical and basic research methodologies, utilizing clinical samples from SSc patients (primarily lesional skin and lung biopsy tissues, and peripheral blood) and animal models. However, recent years have witnessed a transformative shift with the advent of cutting-edge analytical techniques, including single-cell RNA sequencing (scRNA-seq), spatial transcriptomics, imaging mass cytometry, and single-nucleus assay for transposase-accessible chromatin with sequencing (snATAC-seq), particularly in the context of lesional skin analysis. These advanced technologies have provided unprecedented opportunities for the successive validation and refinement of the aforementioned pathogenesis hypotheses. Representative studies employing these innovative approaches are introduced below.

3.1. *Scleroderma-Associated Fibroblast (ScAF) Identification via scRNA-Seq Analysis*

In a landmark study in 2022, Gur et al. [106] leveraged scRNA-seq to analyze skin tissues from a large cohort comprising 97 patients with SSc and 56 healthy individuals, subsequently publishing transformative findings. Their comprehensive analysis led to the refined classification of skin fibroblasts into 10 distinct cellular subpopulations. Notably, myofibroblasts, which have historically been considered central effector cells in the pathogenesis of SSc, were found to represent only a minor fraction, constituting approximately 1% of the total cellular population. Conversely, the most abundant fibroblast subpopulation was identified as LGR5 (Leucine-rich repeat-containing G-protein coupled Receptor 5)-positive fibroblasts, which account for approximately 30% of the cells in healthy individuals. Gene expression pattern analysis indicated that this LGR5+ fibroblast population plays a critical homeostatic role in maintaining normal skin architecture. However, a significant reduction in the abundance of this cell population was observed in SSc patients. Furthermore, these Scleroderma-Associated Fibroblasts (ScAFs) exhibited a constellation of molecular characteristics consistent with previously described SSc skin fibroblasts, including the following: 1, pathologically excessive ECM production coupled with suppressed degradation; 2, aberrant activation of Type I interferon signaling, TGF-β pathway, and IL-1 pathway; 3, dysregulation of Wnt signaling and IGF1 signaling, and abnormal expression of CCN1 family proteins; 4, pathologically activated angiogenesis, increased vascular fragility, and enhanced coagulation and platelet aggregation; 5, diminished antioxidation and adipogenesis capacity; and 6, overexpression of CDKN2A (p16) and CDKN1A (p21), indicative of enhanced cellular senescence. Notably, the study also demonstrated a significant inverse correlation between the cellular density of this ScAF population and skin score. These compelling findings suggest that ScAFs, identified as the principal fibroblast subpopulation orchestrating the fibrotic pathology of SSc, may represent promising novel therapeutic targets. Conversely, the investigation also revealed a concomitant increase in vascular endothelial cells and pericytes alongside the progression of skin sclerosis. In particular, RGS5 (Regulator of G-protein Signaling 5)-positive vascular pericytes demonstrated a positive correlation with skin score. These observations may be interpreted as providing support for conventional pathogenesis hypotheses that posit vascular endothelial cells and pericytes as primary cellular origins of pathogenic fibroblasts in SSc.

3.2. Spatial Transcriptomics Analysis

Ma et al. [107] performed an in-depth analysis of SSc pathogenesis using single-cell and spatial transcriptomics. They analyzed scRNA-seq data from skin biopsies of twenty-two SSc patients and eighteen healthy controls, alongside spatial RNA-seq data from four SSc patients, to map disease-associated cells and their interactions within SSc lesions. The study reported four key observations. First, fibroblasts, vascular endothelial cells, and pericytes were diffusely present in fibrotic areas of SSc skin. Second, fibroblasts were classified into seven distinct populations; SFRP2$^+$ fibroblasts activated and differentiated into COL8A1$^+$ fibroblasts (with myofibroblast features) during fibrosis progression. Third, vascular endothelial cells demonstrated heterogeneity, with categorization into seven distinct subpopulations, including arteriolar endothelial cells (EC2) and activated endothelial cells (EC5). EndoMT maturity served as a differentiating factor among these subpopulations, with EC2 identified as the dominant subpopulation within SSc lesions. Fourth, ligand–receptor network analysis indicated that fibroblast–vascular endothelial cell interactions were most pronounced, with EC2 and COL8A1$^+$ myofibroblast-like fibroblasts being the key communicators. These results reinforce existing pathogenesis models implicating vascular wall cells as myofibroblast origins in SSc.

3.3. Integrated Analysis: scRNA-Seq and snATAC-Seq, Focusing on Vascular Endothelial Cells

In their 2024 study, Huang et al. [108] performed a comprehensive analysis using scRNA-seq and snATAC-seq data to investigate SSc vasculopathy. Analyzing skin biopsies from twenty-seven SSc patients and ten healthy controls via scRNA-seq, and snATAC-seq data from eight SSc patients and six controls, they explored the role of transcription factors in SSc-associated vascular pathology. The scRNA-seq analysis of lesional SSc skin revealed two key observations: first, increased apoptosis and decreased cell numbers in arteriolar endothelial cells; and second, an elevation in tip and stalk cell populations, indicative of constitutively enhanced angiogenesis in dermal microvascular endothelial cells. These findings align with established pathogenesis hypotheses of SSc, particularly regarding destructive vasculopathy and angiogenic abnormalities. Furthermore, snATAC-seq analysis indicated increased chromatin accessibility at the ETS motif in SSc vascular endothelial cells, supporting the involvement of ETS transcription factors, especially FLI1, in SSc vasculopathy, consistent with prior research. These integrated analyses using scRNA-seq and snATAC-seq reinforce the conventional understanding of SSc pathogenesis by highlighting the roles of vascular endothelial cell apoptosis, dysregulated angiogenesis, and ETS transcription factors in the development of SSc vasculopathy (Figure 1).

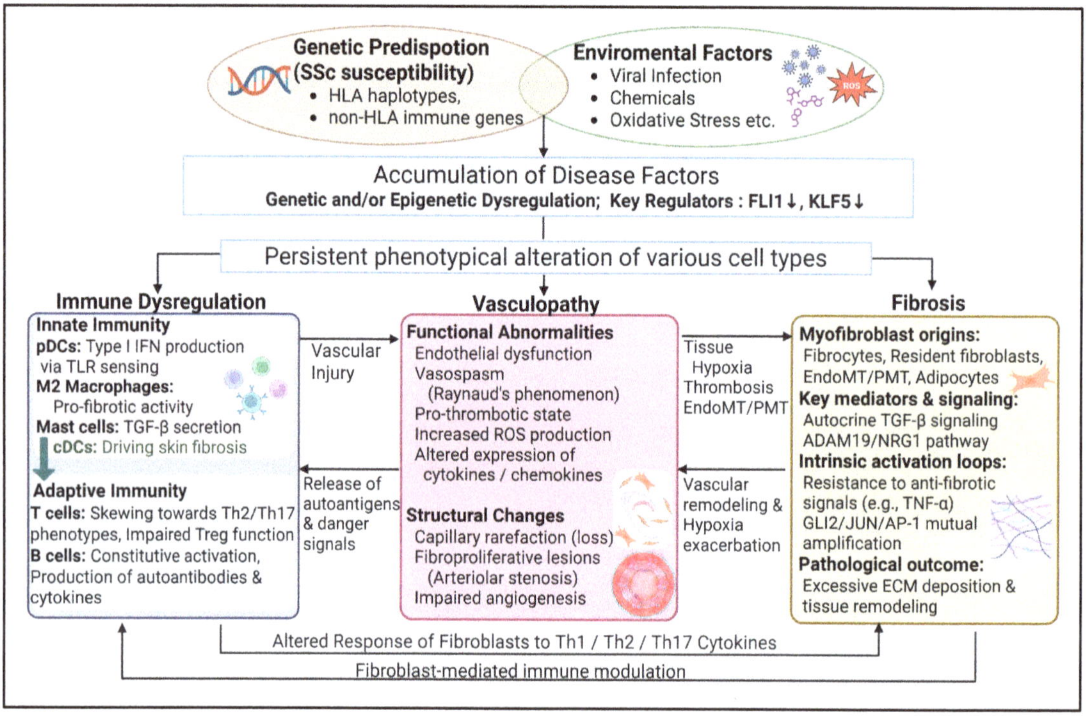

Figure 1. An integrated view of the pathogenesis of systemic sclerosis (SSc). The disease is initiated by genetic predisposition and environmental factors that, via epigenetic dysregulation (e.g., reduced FLI1/KLF5), drive three interconnected pathologies. These are immune dysregulation, involving key innate and adaptive effector cells; vasculopathy, comprising functional and structural abnormalities like endothelial dysfunction and capillary loss; and fibrosis, characterized by activated myofibroblasts and excessive ECM deposition. These pillars are linked by vicious cycles, as depicted by the arrows. Immune-mediated vascular injury is amplified by the subsequent release of autoantigens. Vasculopathy promotes fibrosis through tissue hypoxia and EndoMT/PMT. Activated fibroblasts modulate the immune response, while simultaneously showing an altered response to immune signals, creating a self-perpetuating disease state.

3.4. *Vascular Niche Analysis by Spatial Proteomics Using Imaging Mass Cytometry*

Rius Rigau et al. [109] employed imaging mass cytometry to conduct a vascular niche analysis in skin samples from 19 SSc patients and 14 healthy individuals. Their spatial proteomics-based approach identified seven subpopulations of vascular endothelial cells based on their unique protein expression profiles. In SSc patients, the researchers reported an increased population of $CD34^+$;αSMA^+;$CD31^+$ cells alongside a reduction in vascular endothelial progenitor cells. The perivascular microenvironment of $CD34^+$;αSMA^+;$CD31^+$ cells was characterized by a significant presence of immune cells, predominantly $CD4^+$ T cells and myeloid cells, as well as myofibroblasts. Moreover, $CD34^+$;αSMA^+;$CD31^+$ cells exhibited markers of EndoMT, such as SNAI1, SNAI2, TWIST, and ZEB1. The density of CD34^{+};αSMA^{+};CD31^{+} cells was found to correlate with the clinical progression of skin sclerosis. These observations reinforce the established pathogenesis model wherein vascular endothelial cells contribute to the myofibroblast population through EndoMT in SSc-related fibrosis.

3.5. Novel Pathogenesis Mechanism of SSc Skin Fibrosis Suggested by Epigenetic Analysis Using ATAC-Seq

Liu et al. [110] conducted an epigenetic analysis to explore novel pathogenesis mechanisms in SSc skin fibrosis, employing ATAC-seq. Using flow cytometry, they isolated eight skin-resident cell types—fibroblasts, vascular endothelial cells, epidermal cells, CD4^{+} T cells, CD8^{+} T cells, dendritic cells, Langerhans cells, and macrophages—from the healthy, lesional, and non-lesional SSc skin of seven SSc patients and six healthy controls, totaling 19 samples. Leveraging the known enrichment of disease-susceptibility SNPs in non-coding regulatory DNA, they hypothesized that cell-type-specific chromatin accessibility analysis at SSc-associated SNP loci could pinpoint pathogenic cell types. Their analysis revealed significantly increased chromatin accessibility in SSc-associated SNP regions specifically within dendritic cells (DCs), compared to other skin cell types. Re-analysis of time-series RNA-seq data from SSc lesions further supported this, showing a strong positive correlation between the DC gene signature and skin fibrosis score. Specifically, conventional DCs (cDCs) were identified as a key cellular population. Immunohistochemical validation using ZBTB46, a cDC marker, confirmed significant infiltration of ZBTB46^{+} cells into SSc lesions. These epigenetic findings suggest a previously unappreciated role for cDCs in SSc skin fibrosis, offering a novel perspective on SSc pathogenesis beyond conventional hypotheses. The importance of dendritic cells in the pathogenesis of SSc is also demonstrated in the following articles [111,112]

3.6. Novel Therapeutic Targets Identified by Gene Expression Meta-Analysis of Lung Tissue

Yang et al. [113] published a gene expression meta-analysis of lung tissue, examining 38 patients with SSc-ILD and 18 healthy controls. Their analysis, utilizing three public datasets (GSE48149, GSE81292, GSE76808), identified the activation of epithelial–mesenchymal transition, cellular senescence, coagulation, and DNA repair pathways as characteristic changes in SSc-ILD lung tissue. Consistent with an aging phenotype, telomere length in type II alveolar epithelial cells from SSc-ILD lungs was found to be reduced, indicating enhanced cellular senescence. The current therapeutic development for SSc-ILD primarily targets myofibroblasts and inflammation/autoimmunity. However, this study suggests that cellular senescence and coagulation pathways could offer novel therapeutic avenues for SSc-ILD.

Plasminogen Activator Inhibitor-1 (PAI-1) is a serpin that inhibits tissue-type Plasminogen Activator (tPA) and urokinase-type Plasminogen Activator (uPA), and regulates the plasmin activation and the fibrinolytic system [114]. Emerging research underscores the significance of PAI-1 in regulating cellular senescence, with findings demonstrating that PAI-1 not only serves as a senescence marker but also actively mediates senescence pathways, impacting lifespan and age-related pathologies [115–117]. The tPA, uPA, and PAI-1 are thought to play an important role in the maintenance of endothelial homeostasis, and are associated with the endothelial dysfunction of SSc [118,119]. Therefore, PAI-1 inhibition may be therapeutic for SSc-ILD.

4. Organ-Specific Pathophysiology Modifiers: Refining the Landscape of SSc Organ Involvement

To fully elucidate the organ-specific manifestations of SSc, it is essential to consider organ-specific pathophysiology modifiers, in addition to the broadly acting trans-organ basic pathophysiology. The following sections detail the principal organ-specific modifiers across major organ systems affected by SSc [13].

4.1. Cutaneous Pathology

Epidermal cells and adipocytes function as key pathophysiology modifiers in the skin in SSc (Figure 2).

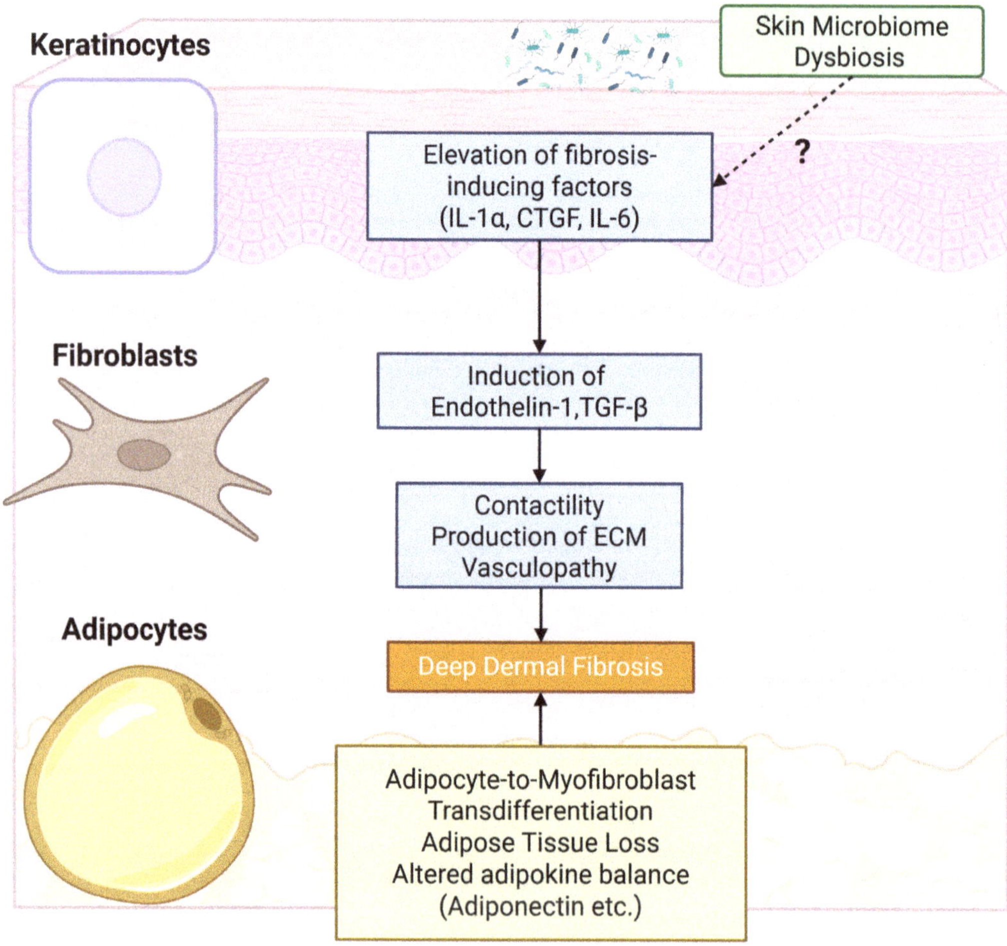

Figure 2. Keratinocytes and adipocytes as key modifiers of skin pathophysiology in systemic sclerosis (SSc). This concept map illustrates the multifaceted roles of keratinocytes and adipocytes in the pathogenesis of SSc skin involvement. Dysfunctional keratinocytes upregulate various disease-associated molecules, contributing to dermal fibroblast activation and fibrosis. Epithelial cell-specific Fli1 deficiency leads to keratinocyte activation, inducing dermal fibrosis, and thymus dysfunction. While the interaction with skin microbiota remains unclear in SSc, it may modulate keratinocyte function and immunity. Adipocytes contribute to dermal fibrosis through adipocyte-to-myofibroblast transition and altered adipokine production, collectively driving SSc skin pathology.

4.1.1. Keratinocytes

The epidermis in SSc is an active participant in the disease process, as evidenced by research identifying the upregulation of numerous molecules in affected skin. These include growth factors (e.g., TGF-β, VEGF, and CTGF), cytokines (e.g., IL-1α, IL-6, and TNF-α), and chemokines (e.g., CCL2, CCL5), in addition to other proteins like endothelin-1, IL-21 receptor, specific keratins, psoriasin, and galectin-7 [120–129]. As several of these molecules—notably IL-1α, CTGF, and IL-6—have strong pro-fibrotic properties, it is probable that SSc keratinocytes play a role in activating dermal fibroblasts.

Experiments using a recently developed mouse model of SSc have suggested a role for various epithelial cells in the disease's development, including keratinocytes, esophageal stratified squamous epithelia, and medullary thymic epithelial cells [130]. Deficiency of the transcription factor Fli1, a potential SSc susceptibility factor [14], induces SSc-like properties in various cell types, including fibroblasts, endothelial cells, keratinocytes, T cells, B cells, cDC, and macrophages [17,130–134]. Notably, epithelial cell-specific *Fli1* knockout mice (*Fli1*$^{flox/flox}$; *K14-Cre*$^{+/-}$ mice), which exhibit SSc-like phenotypic features in epithelial cells, spontaneously develop dermal and esophageal fibrosis due to epithelial cell activation in the skin and esophagus. Furthermore, these mice develop ILD, mediated at least in part by T cells autoreactive to lung antigens, resulting from impaired negative selection and Treg development in the thymus. One component of this impaired central tolerance is attributed to the downregulation of autoimmune regulator (Aire), which modulates the processing and presentation of self-antigens in medullary thymic epithelial cells [135,136]. Importantly, epithelial cell-specific *Fli1* knockout mice lacking an acquired immune system (*Rag1*$^{-/-}$; *Fli1*$^{flox/flox}$; *K14-Cre*$^{+/-}$ mice) spontaneously develop dermal and esophageal fibrosis, along with mast cell infiltration in the skin, but do not develop ILD [137]. This suggests that epithelial cell activation alone can induce tissue fibrosis through the activation of innate immunity. This novel murine model indicates that abnormally activated epithelial cells underlie selective organ fibrosis and autoimmunity in SSc.

Another potential aspect of the keratinocyte-dependent regulation of dermal fibrosis is the interplay between the immune system and the skin microbiota. This area of research has recently garnered significant attention regarding inflammatory skin diseases, such as atopic dermatitis [138] and SLE [139]. This dialogue begins when keratinocytes detect pathogen-associated molecular patterns by the use of microbes using pattern-recognition receptors. This recognition prompts the keratinocytes to release antimicrobial peptides (AMPs), which can kill or inactivate microorganisms and activate other cells like dermal fibroblasts and endothelial cells [140]. The expression of these AMPs can be either constant or temporary, with the latter being regulated by the skin's microbial community. The specific impact of the skin microbiota on keratinocyte function and immunity in SSc is not yet established, but the finding of microbiome dysbiosis in affected skin suggests it may be a contributing factor [141].

4.1.2. Adipocytes

Recently, subcutaneous adipose tissue has been increasingly implicated in the development of skin fibrosis in SSc. This is histologically significant, as the skin is characterized by a large, adjacent layer of fat. The concept that adipose tissue could be a source of fibrotic cells is consistent with the knowledge that myofibroblasts can be derived from non-fibroblast precursors in a pro-fibrotic environment [142]. According to lineage-tracing studies [143], subcutaneous adipocytes are highly plastic cells capable of transdifferentiating into myofibroblasts [144]. Indeed, a significant proportion of activated myofibroblasts in SSc-involved skin appear to derive from adipocytes located adjacent to the deep dermis [89,145].

Adipocytes also influence the disease by producing a range of signaling molecules called adipokines [146]. When adipocyte loss or dysfunction alters the balance of these adipokines, it may contribute to the characteristic inflammation, vasculopathy, and fibrosis of SSc [147–157]. The role of adiponectin, a well-studied example, illustrates this connection; its serum and tissue levels are inversely related to skin score in patients [147,156,158]. Moreover, mice lacking adiponectin show reduced dermal fibrosis after bleomycin challenge [159], and AdipoRon, a drug that inhibits adiponectin signaling, lessens SSc-like features in mouse models [160]. Taken together, these findings indicate that subcutaneous adipose tissue is a significant driver of skin fibrosis in SSc.

4.2. Gastrointestinal Pathology

Affecting approximately 90% of patients, gastrointestinal (GI) issues are a leading cause of morbidity in SSc, stemming from impaired motility and deficient enzyme secretion throughout the digestive system [161–163]. The esophagus is the most commonly affected site, resulting in a high prevalence (70–90%) of upper GI symptoms like GERD and dysphagia. Following the esophagus, the anorectal region, small bowel, stomach, and colon are also frequently involved. This leads to a variety of lower GI symptoms (seen in 20–70% of patients), which can include small intestinal bacterial overgrowth, malabsorption, diarrhea, pseudo-obstruction, and fecal incontinence [164].

Consistent with observations in the skin and other internal organs, the common SSc-specific pathological cascade broadly impacts the GI system, ultimately leading to extensive atrophy and fibrosis of the gastrointestinal smooth muscle [165]. Additionally, SSc exhibits a GI organ-specific pathology relevant to the complex and highly organized enteric nervous system. Vascular structural changes, such as capillary rarefaction and arteriolar stenosis, induce tissue hypoxia throughout the GI tract, resulting in autonomic axonal degeneration [166]. Thus, SSc-associated GI involvement is attributed to the hypomotility and dysmotility stemming from extensive atrophy and fibrosis of the enteric smooth muscle, as well as disturbances in the enteric nervous system. Indeed, SSc-associated esophageal dysfunction comprises three pathological components: (i) reduced lower esophageal sphincter pressure; (ii) ineffective esophageal body peristalsis, particularly in the lower esophagus; and (iii) discoordination of peristaltic and lower esophageal sphincter function [161,165,167–169]. Ultimately, the long-term course of SSc-associated GI involvement often culminates in atrophic and fibrotic changes within the gastrointestinal smooth muscle. The precise temporal dynamics and predisposing factors associated with this progression are complex, with recent evidence suggesting that while esophageal dysfunction can occur early, the overall worsening of GI symptoms over extended periods may be influenced more by characteristics like patient sex and specific autoantibody profiles, such as ACA, rather than strictly by cutaneous subtypes [170].

The neuropathy in SSc-related GI dysfunction may be partly driven by pathogenic autoantibodies. For instance, some patients have antibodies against myenteric neurons [171], including those specific for the muscarinic acetylcholine receptor M3 [172,173]. These are considered pathogenic because they disrupt peristalsis in animal experiments [171,172], and in SSc patients, their levels are associated with more severe GI disease [174], suggesting a pathogenic role for these antibodies in humans. Consistent with this, the motility of the pharynx and proximal esophagus, which is regulated by the somatic nervous system, remains normal in SSc [174,175]. Overall, current evidence supports the concept that a combination of autoimmunity, vasculopathy, and fibrosis underlies GI involvement in SSc.

Drawing a parallel with the skin, the esophagus's stratified squamous epithelia may directly drive fibrosis in SSc. This idea is supported by the *Fli1*$^{flox/flox}$; *K14-Cre*$^{+/-}$ mice, where the esophagus displays SSc-like molecular features, including increased IL-8 and prominent IL-1β expression. This epithelial dysfunction could also explain symptoms, as epithelium-derived cytokines are thought to cause refractory GERD-related and functional heartburn [176]. This is particularly relevant, because SSc patients' symptoms often do not correlate with objective physiological findings [161,177]. Thus, an abnormal epithelial phenotype is a plausible, though not yet proven, contributor to both fibrosis and heartburn in SSc.

The gut microbiota is also a key component of GI-specific pathology in SSc. It is known to modulate the immune system and is implicated in autoimmune diseases through immune dysfunction [178–180]. In SSc, studies show that the intestinal microbial composition is different from that in healthy individuals, with a decrease in commensal bacteria (e.g., *Faecalibacterium, Clostridium*) and an increase in pathobionts (e.g., *Fusobacterium*) [181,182]. It is not yet clear whether these changes are a cause or a consequence of SSc or its treatments. However, a report that fecal microbiota transplantation reduced lower GI symptoms suggests a direct role [183]. More research is needed to clarify the mechanisms by which the gut microbiota interacts with inflammatory and fibrotic pathways in SSc.

In conclusion, the abnormally activated stratified squamous epithelia and enteric nervous system dysfunction constitute organ-specific pathological processes within the GI tract in SSc (Figure 3).

4.3. Pulmonary Pathology

Pulmonary involvement, encompassing ILD and pulmonary hypertension (PH), represents the primary cause of SSc-related mortality [184,185]. ILD in SSc arises from the common SSc-specific pathological cascade and can be further influenced by microaspiration of gastric contents due to GERD. Pulmonary arterial hypertension (PAH) in SSc is attributed to pulmonary arteriolar stenosis resulting from occlusive vascular fibrosis.

The World Health Organization (WHO) classification categorizes PH into five groups: Group 1, PAH characterized by pre-capillary pulmonary vasculopathy involving small pulmonary arterioles; Group 2, PH due to left heart disease; Group 3, PH due to lung diseases and/or hypoxia (including ILD); Group 4, PH due to pulmonary artery obstructions (e.g., chronic thromboembolic pulmonary hypertension, CTEPH); and Group 5, PH with unclear multifactorial mechanisms [186]. SSc-associated pulmonary hypertension (SSc-PH) most commonly falls into Group 1 (PAH), Group 2, or Group 3 [187,188]. Additionally, SSc patients with associated antiphospholipid antibody syndrome may be at risk for developing Group 4 PH. It has been observed that PAH (Group 1) is the most frequent form of PH when associated with connective tissue diseases like SSc [189]. These distinct pathologies, particularly PAH and ILD, can indeed coexist to varying extents in SSc patients. The presence of concomitant ILD in PAH-SSc patients has been shown to worsen hemodynamics and pulmonary function tests, making the clinical classification and management more challenging [189]. Such coexistence of PAH and ILD is a significant concern, as these are the two leading causes of mortality in SSc [189].

Historically, SSc-PAH was considered more prevalent in patients with limited cutaneous SSc (lcSSc) and those with ACA [190,191]. However, the understanding of these associations continues to evolve with larger and more contemporary cohort studies. For instance, a meta-analysis by Rubio-Rivas et al. [192] reported an overall PAH prevalence in SSc of 6.4%, with a prevalence of 7.7% in lcSSc and 6.3% in dcSSc, supporting a higher prevalence in lcSSc. Survival for patients with Group 1 SSc-PAH has shown improvement in the most recent decade, potentially due to earlier detection through screening programs and more effective therapeutic strategies, including upfront combination therapy [188,193].

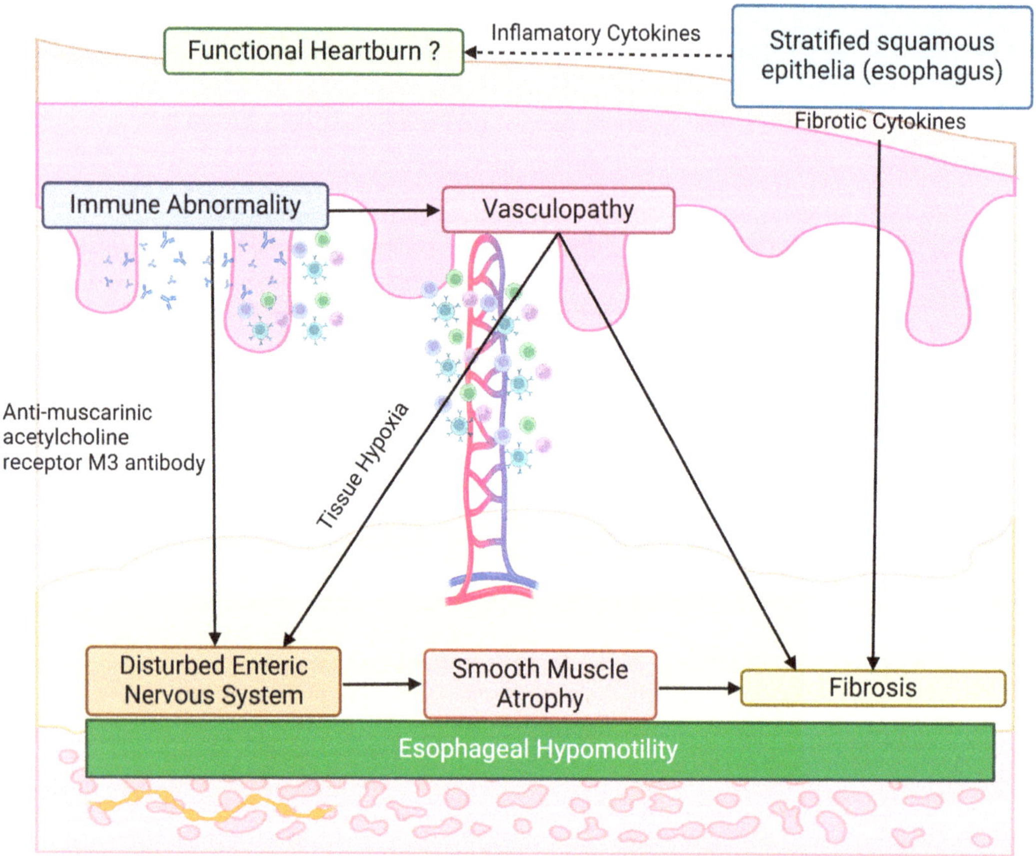

Figure 3. Pathophysiological mechanisms of esophageal involvement in systemic sclerosis (SSc). This schematic illustrates the multi-factorial pathogenesis of gastrointestinal (GI) manifestations in SSc. The cascade is initiated by immune abnormality, including the presence of anti-muscarinic acetylcholine receptor M3 antibodies, and vasculopathy. Both of these pathological processes contribute to disturbed enteric nervous system function, ultimately resulting in esophageal hypomotility. A disturbed enteric nervous system induces smooth muscle atrophy, further contributing to esophageal hypomotility and leading to fibrosis of the esophagus. Esophageal stratified squamous epithelia can produce inflammatory and fibrotic cytokines, further promoting fibrosis. Functional heartburn may also occur, potentially linked to inflammatory cytokines produced by the esophageal stratified squamous epithelia. These interconnected pathways highlight the complex interplay of immune, vascular, epithelial, and neural factors in SSc-related GERD.

In a more focused sense, SSc-PAH is histologically characterized by a proliferative and obliterative vasculopathy predominantly affecting the pulmonary arterioles. This is considered a consequence of the shared SSc-specific pathological cascade involving endothelial dysfunction, inflammation, and fibrotic remodeling [190]. The vascular lesions in SSc-PAH often feature perivascular lymphocytic infiltrates and significant intimal fibrosis. Notably, classical plexiform lesions, which are characteristic of idiopathic PAH, are less commonly observed in SSc-PAH [190].

Furthermore, the clinical picture of SSc-PAH can be frequently complicated by, or mimicked by, conditions such as pulmonary veno-occlusive disease (PVOD) or PAH with overt features of venous/capillaries involvement. PVOD is also classified under WHO

Group 1 PH but represents a distinct pathological entity primarily affecting pulmonary venules and capillaries. PVOD arising in a background of connective tissue disease such as SSc (PVOD-like changes) is a rare but critical condition, often underdiagnosed in SSc due to its symptomatic similarity to PAH. A key distinguishing concern with regard to PVOD-like changes is its particularly poor prognosis and the significant risk of precipitating acute pulmonary edema with the use of PAH-specific vasodilator therapies. Therefore, careful diagnostic evaluation is paramount. High-resolution computed tomography (HRCT) plays a vital role when PVOD-like changes is suspected, with characteristic findings including centrilobular ground-glass opacities, interlobular septal thickening, and mediastinal lymph node enlargement [187,194].

Therefore, understanding and managing SSc-PH necessitates a comprehensive approach that considers all components of the pulmonary circulation. Given that SSc is a disease characterized by multi-organ involvement, a thorough evaluation of all elements related to pulmonary circulation is essential when addressing PH in these patients (Figure 4).

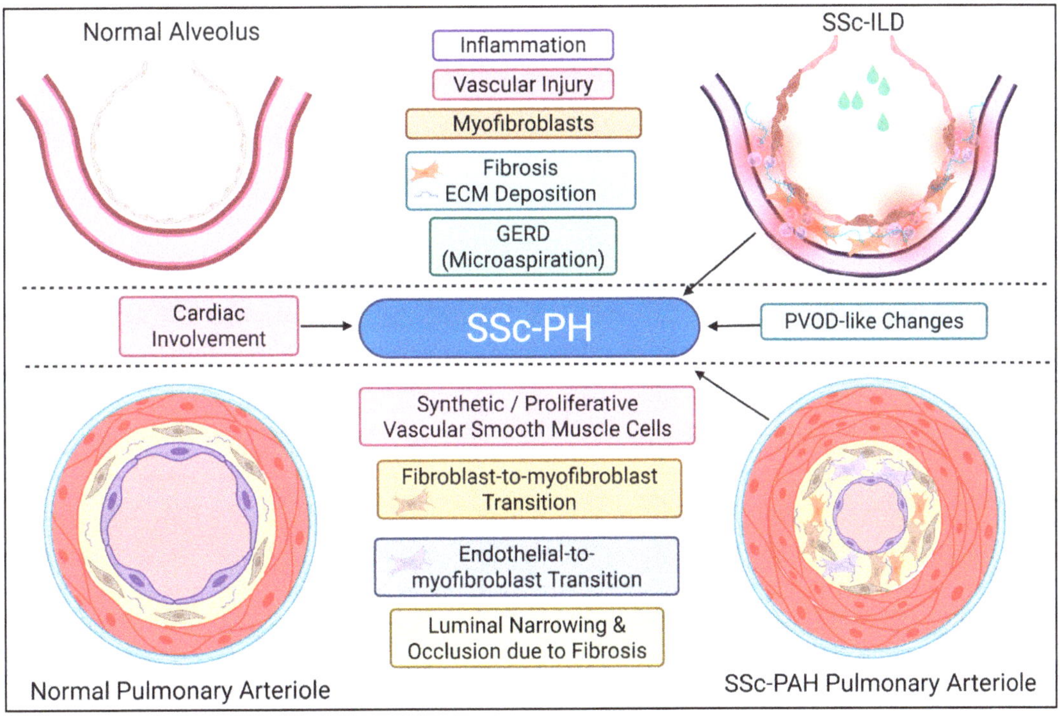

Figure 4. Schematic diagram of the complex pulmonary pathology in SSc, encompassing both ILD and PH. [Upper panel: Interstitial Lung Disease (ILD)] SSc-ILD pathogenesis is driven by the common SSc-specific pathological cascade, leading to distinct histological stages of nonspecific interstitial pneumonia (NSIP), and in some cases, usual interstitial pneumonia (UIP). Gastroesophageal reflux disease (GERD) acts as an organ-specific modifier, potentially exacerbating ILD progression through microaspiration and contributing to centrilobular fibrosis (CLF). [Lower panel: Pulmonary Hypertension (PH)] SSc-PH encompasses pulmonary arterial hypertension (PAH) due to pulmonary arteriolar fibrosis (Group 1 WHO classification), as well as PH related to cardiac involvement (Group 2) or ILD (Group 3). SSc-PAH is characterized by pulmonary arteriole occlusion and may coexist with pulmonary veno-occlusive disease (PVOD)-like changes.

ILD is detectable in 50–60% of SSc patients via HRCT [195,196]. Risk factors for the development of SSc-ILD encompass dcSSc [197], African American ethnicity [198], shorter disease duration [199], older age at disease onset [197], and the presence of anti-topoisomerase I antibody and/or absence of ACA [197]. ILD typically manifests early in the course of dcSSc, particularly within the first 3 years of disease onset [197,199,200], while in lcSSc patients, ILD can arise at any point during the disease course [201]. The clinical trajectory of SSc-ILD is heterogeneous; some patients maintain stable forced vital capacity (FVC), whereas others experience a progressive decline in pulmonary function [202]. ILD progression is generally most pronounced within the initial 4 years following SSc onset, subsequently slowing or ceasing entirely, even without therapeutic intervention [203]. Severe ILD, defined by an FVC decline below 50%, is reported to affect approximately 15% of the total SSc population [203,204]. The predominant histological pattern in SSc-ILD is nonspecific interstitial pneumonia (NSIP), observed in roughly two-thirds of patients [205]. Usual interstitial pneumonia (UIP) is present in a smaller proportion of SSc-ILD cases [205–207] and may correlate with less favorable prognoses [208].

Histologically, nonspecific interstitial pneumonia (NSIP) in SSc-ILD is categorized into four stages [209]:

- * Stage 1 (Initial): Characterized by microvessel overdevelopment with structural abnormalities, and alveolar septal thickening with numerous α-SMA-positive myofibroblasts. The overdeveloped microvessels contain blood cells within their lumina, indicating maintained functional circulation.
- * Stage 2 (Progressive ECM Deposition): Marked by substantial and progressive ECM deposition, irregular and indistinct alveolar septal borders, further structural disorganization of microvessels, and obliteration of larger blood vessels. Disarray or partial loss of the alveolar epithelium is also evident.
- * Stage 3 (Extensive Fibrosis): Progression of fibrosis extensively damages vital lung structures, including alveoli and vasculature.
- * Stage 4 (Final): The lung transforms into a contracted fibrous organ devoid of alveoli and vasculature.

The early microvascular alterations and subsequent progressive fibrotic changes reinforce the concept that SSc-ILD is driven by the common SSc-specific pathological cascade, similar to other organ involvements.

Above pathological findings suggest the presence of foundational trans-organ pathophysiology in the lung tissue.

Microaspiration of gastric contents due to GERD is a potential factor driving the progression of SSc-ILD. Clinical data, histological analyses, and animal studies support this hypothesis. Several clinical studies have shown a positive correlation between increased lung fibrosis severity and more frequent reflux episodes, as well as greater proximal extension of refluxate [210]. In a rat GERD model, pulmonary parenchymal fibrosis was induced by introducing gastric content into the lungs [211]. Analysis of lung biopsy specimens identified a distinct histological pattern of lung disease, centrilobular fibrosis (CLF), particularly prevalent in SSc patients with severe GERD [212]. CLF is characterized by a predominantly bronchocentric distribution of lesions and the presence of intraluminal basophilic material and foreign bodies within the bronchi, sometimes accompanied by multinucleated giant cell reactions. In a prior study examining open lung biopsies from 22 SSc-ILD patients [213], isolated CLF was observed in 21% of cases, and a CLF pattern was present in 84% of patients with a predominant NSIP pattern, suggesting that GERD may exacerbate underlying NSIP in SSc-ILD. Although clinical trial data have not yet demonstrated pulmonary function improvement in SSc-ILD following aggressive GERD management, aggressive GERD treatment may still benefit the majority of SSc patients. Overall, GERD acts as an organ-specific disease modifier in SSc-ILD (Figure 4).

4.4. Cardiovascular Pathology

Histological examination of autopsy tissues from SSc patients without prior clinical cardiac symptoms reveals evidence of myocardial disease in all cases [214]. Thus, cardiac involvement is nearly ubiquitous in SSc patients, although often clinically silent [215,216]. Once clinically manifest, however, cardiac involvement carries a poor prognosis [215,217–219]. Primary cardiac involvement in SSc encompasses a wide spectrum of clinical manifestations, including arrhythmias, conduction system defects, myocarditis, pericarditis, systolic and diastolic ventricular dysfunction, and heart failure [220,221]. Primary myocardial involvement is estimated to account for approximately 30% of deaths in SSc patients [185,219,222].

In a study employing cardiovascular magnetic resonance (CMR) parametric mapping in SSc patients, Purevsuren et al. [223] demonstrated that native T1 mapping effectively detects early myocardial changes and correlates with left-ventricular diastolic dysfunction, with more pronounced myocardial involvement observed in dcSSc compared to lcSSc. This finding of early diffuse myocardial edema-like lesions on contrast-enhanced MRI mirrors the edematous induration seen in early skin lesions of SSc, suggesting a parallel pathological process, affecting both skin and internal organs, in the initial stages of the disease.

Although the precise molecular mechanisms of SSc-related cardiomyopathy remain incompletely understood [220,224–226], the prevailing consensus attributes a central role to microvascular disease. The proposed mechanism is that structural microvascular defects, including capillary rarefaction and arteriolar stenosis, result in tissue hypoxia. This oxygen deprivation is believed to subsequently trigger inflammation and excessive ECM synthesis by cardiac fibroblasts [215]. This model is supported by histological findings from SSc autopsy specimens, which show increased inflammation, vascular damage, and ECM deposition compared to controls [214]. The microvascular origin is further indicated by the patchy, non-coronary distribution of fibrosis throughout the ventricles [224,227].

In addition to structural damage, abnormal vasoreactivity of small cardiac vessels, known as "myocardial Raynaud's phenomenon," contributes to cardiac involvement in SSc. This concept is supported by multiple lines of evidence. For instance, cold exposure can induce this phenomenon in approximately 30% of SSc patients with a history of Raynaud's, and the effect is preventable with calcium channel blockers (CCBs) [228]. The therapeutic benefit of vasodilators like nifedipine, nicardipine, and captopril, which acutely improve myocardial perfusion and function [229–232], also points to a vasospastic component. Finally, the absence of prior CCB therapy is an independent factor associated with left-ventricular dysfunction.

Thus, from a management perspective, the cardiac involvement in SSc must be viewed as being a result of two distinct categories of vascular change. One category is structural, encompassing capillary rarefaction and arteriolar stenosis, while the other is functional, specifically the myocardial Raynaud's phenomenon.

4.5. Scleroderma Renal Crisis

One frequent form of renal involvement in SSc patients is a subclinical renal vasculopathy, characterized by vascular damage and normal renal function [233]. Scleroderma renal crisis (SRC) complicates the course of 5–10% of SSc patients [234–237], presenting most commonly within the first few years of disease onset, particularly in those with dcSSc [234,236]. Key risk factors include rapidly progressive skin thickening, the presence of anti-RNA polymerase III antibodies [234,236,238–240], and recent high-dose corticosteroid therapy (>15 mg/day) [234–237,241,242]. While strongly associated with anti-RNA polymerase III antibodies, SRC can rarely occur in patients with lcSSc, including those positive for ACA [239,241,243,244].

Clinically, SRC typically manifests suddenly, with an abrupt onset of accelerated hypertension (often > 150/85 mmHg or a significant rise from baseline) and acute kidney injury (AKI), frequently accompanied by headache, visual changes, or signs of hypertensive encephalopathy or cardiopulmonary failure [234,236,245]. Approximately 10–11% of cases manifest as normotensive SRC, which may be associated with corticosteroid use and has been linked to a poorer prognosis, possibly due to delayed diagnosis or a potentially more severe underlying pathology [234,236,241,245]. Laboratory findings may include microangiopathic hemolytic anemia (MAHA) and thrombocytopenia, features overlapping with hemolytic uremic syndrome (HUS)/thrombotic microangiopathy (TMA) [234,236,241,245].

The core pathogenesis involves endothelial injury in renal arterioles, leading to intimal accumulation of myxoid material, subsequent intimal proliferation resulting in luminal narrowing ("onion-skin" lesions), thrombosis, and fibrinoid necrosis [234,236,241,245]. Renal biopsy findings, such as the extent of vascular thrombosis, severe glomerular ischemic collapse, and peritubular capillary C4d deposits, may predict failure to recover renal function [245]. This vascular damage triggers activation of the renin–angiotensin–aldosterone system (RAAS), causing hyperreninemia and creating a vicious cycle of worsening hypertension and renal ischemia [234,236,241]. Renal vasospasm ("renal Raynaud's") is also thought to contribute significantly to the reduced renal perfusion [234,236]. Historically, it has been reported that SSc patients already on angiotensin-converting enzyme (ACE) inhibitor therapy at the time of SRC onset may experience worse outcomes [236,246,247]. More recently, studies have indicated that prior exposure to ACE inhibitors might not only be associated with poorer SRC prognosis, but could also represent an independent risk factor for the development of SRC itself, particularly in hypertensive SSc patients [248]. These findings have led to the recommendation against the prophylactic use of ACE inhibitors to prevent SRC in patients, without a clear indication for these drugs, such as established hypertension [236,247]. This evolving understanding of the complex relationship between ACE inhibitor use and SRC may offer new insights into the underlying pathogenetic mechanisms of this severe SSc complication.

SRC, along with DUs and SSc-PAH, is considered a manifestation of the systemic, non-organ-specific vasculopathy underlying SSc, primarily driven by arteriolar stenosis affecting different vascular territories [13].

5. Conclusions

The current understanding of SSc pathogenesis, bolstered by advanced analytical methods, has been the focus of this review. The skin's frequent affliction and ease of sampling have made it a cornerstone for pathogenetic investigations. Future research, extending these sophisticated analytical tools to internal organs like the lungs, holds considerable promise for refining our comprehension of the fundamental, widespread pathophysiology and the specific factors that modulate organ involvement in SSc. This improved insight is vital for tailoring more effective treatments, and thereby enhancing disease management and patient prognosis and opening new therapeutic avenues. It is acknowledged that SSc treatment strategies are varied, adapt to specific pathological manifestations, and are the subject of numerous clinical investigations; however, these are not detailed here, and specialized reviews can offer further information [249–252].

Central to deciphering SSc's complex cross-organ impact is the identification of its core pathogenic driver. Although immune dysfunction is characteristic of its autoimmune nature and "sclerosis" underscores fibrosis, we propose vasculopathy as the pivotal intermediary linking aberrant immunity to fibrotic outcomes. This view is informed by clinical patterns in which vascular alterations are often the first indicators of SSc, as seen with Raynaud's phenomenon, and potentially represent the final opportunity for impactful therapeutic modulation, contrasting with early immune dysregulation, which may be subclinical, and established fibrosis, which is typically irreversible.

Author Contributions: Conceptualization, T.T. and Y.A.; Writing—Original Draft Preparation, T.T.; Writing—Review and Editing, T.T. and Y.A.; Supervision, Y.A. All authors have read and agreed to the published version of the manuscript.

Funding: This research received no external funding.

Institutional Review Board Statement: Not applicable.

Informed Consent Statement: Not applicable.

Data Availability Statement: Not applicable.

Acknowledgments: Figures have been Created in https://BioRender.com.

Conflicts of Interest: The authors declare no conflicts of interest.

References

1. Denton, C.P.; Khanna, D. Systemic Sclerosis. *Lancet* **2017**, *390*, 1685–1699. [CrossRef]
2. Arnett, F.C.; Cho, M.; Chatterjee, S.; Aguilar, M.B.; Reveille, J.D.; Mayes, M.D. Familial Occurrence Frequencies and Relative Risks for Systemic Sclerosis (Scleroderma) in Three United States Cohorts. *Arthritis Rheum.* **2001**, *44*, 1359–1362. [CrossRef] [PubMed]
3. Feghali-Bostwick, C.; Medsger, T.A., Jr.; Wright, T.M. Analysis of Systemic Sclerosis in Twins Reveals Low Concordance for Disease and High Concordance for the Presence of Antinuclear Antibodies. *Arthritis Rheum.* **2003**, *48*, 1956–1963. [CrossRef]
4. Yamashita, K.; Kawasaki, A.; Matsushita, T.; Furukawa, H.; Kondo, Y.; Okiyama, N.; Nagaoka, S.; Shimada, K.; Sugii, S.; Katayama, M.; et al. Association of Functional (GA)n Microsatellite Polymorphism in the FLI1 Gene with Susceptibility to Human Systemic Sclerosis. *Rheumatology* **2020**, *59*, 3553–3562. [CrossRef]
5. Agarwal, S.K. The Genetics of Systemic Sclerosis. *Discov. Med.* **2010**, *10*, 134–143. [PubMed]
6. Dieudé, P.; Guedj, M.; Wipff, J.; Avouac, J.; Fajardy, I.; Diot, E.; Granel, B.; Sibilia, J.; Cabane, J.; Mouthon, L.; et al. Association between the IRF5 Rs2004640 Functional Polymorphism and Systemic Sclerosis: A New Perspective for Pulmonary Fibrosis. *Arthritis Rheum.* **2009**, *60*, 225–233. [CrossRef]
7. Ito, I.; Kawaguchi, Y.; Kawasaki, A.; Hasegawa, M.; Ohashi, J.; Hikami, K.; Kawamoto, M.; Fujimoto, M.; Takehara, K.; Sato, S.; et al. Association of a Functional Polymorphism in the IRF5 Region with Systemic Sclerosis in a Japanese Population. *Arthritis Rheum.* **2009**, *60*, 1845–1850. [CrossRef]
8. Radstake, T.R.D.J.; Gorlova, O.; Rueda, B.; Martin, J.-E.; Alizadeh, B.Z.; Palomino-Morales, R.; Coenen, M.J.; Vonk, M.C.; Voskuyl, A.E.; Schuerwegh, A.J.; et al. Genome-Wide Association Study of Systemic Sclerosis Identifies CD247 as a New Susceptibility Locus. *Nat. Genet.* **2010**, *42*, 426–429. [CrossRef] [PubMed]
9. Tang, L.; Chen, B.; Ma, B.; Nie, S. Association between IRF5 Polymorphisms and Autoimmune Diseases: A Meta-Analysis. *Genet. Mol. Res.* **2014**, *13*, 4473–4485. [CrossRef]
10. Sharif, R.; Mayes, M.D.; Tan, F.K.; Gorlova, O.Y.; Hummers, L.K.; Shah, A.A.; Furst, D.E.; Khanna, D.; Martin, J.; Bossini-Castillo, L.; et al. IRF5 Polymorphism Predicts Prognosis in Patients with Systemic Sclerosis. *Ann. Rheum. Dis.* **2012**, *71*, 1197–1202. [CrossRef]
11. Benfaremo, D.; Svegliati Baroni, S.; Manfredi, L.; Moroncini, G.; Gabrielli, A. Putative Functional Pathogenic Autoantibodies in Systemic Sclerosis. *Eur. J. Rheumatol.* **2020**, *7*, S181–S186. [CrossRef] [PubMed]
12. Senécal, J.-L.; Hoa, S.; Yang, R.; Koenig, M. Pathogenic Roles of Autoantibodies in Systemic Sclerosis: Current Understandings in Pathogenesis. *J. Scleroderma Relat. Disord.* **2020**, *5*, 103–129. [CrossRef] [PubMed]
13. Asano, Y. The Pathogenesis of Systemic Sclerosis: An Understanding Based on a Common Pathologic Cascade across Multiple Organs and Additional Organ-Specific Pathologies. *J. Clin. Med.* **2020**, *9*, 2687. [CrossRef] [PubMed]
14. Wang, Y.; Fan, P.-S.; Kahaleh, B. Association between Enhanced Type I Collagen Expression and Epigenetic Repression of the FLI1 Gene in Scleroderma Fibroblasts. *Arthritis Rheum.* **2006**, *54*, 2271–2279. [CrossRef]

15. Kubo, M.; Czuwara-Ladykowska, J.; Moussa, O.; Markiewicz, M.; Smith, E.; Silver, R.M.; Jablonska, S.; Blaszczyk, M.; Watson, D.K.; Trojanowska, M. Persistent Down-Regulation of Fli1, a Suppressor of Collagen Transcription, in Fibrotic Scleroderma Skin. *Am. J. Pathol.* **2003**, *163*, 571–581. [CrossRef]
16. Noda, S.; Asano, Y.; Nishimura, S.; Taniguchi, T.; Fujiu, K.; Manabe, I.; Nakamura, K.; Yamashita, T.; Saigusa, R.; Akamata, K.; et al. Simultaneous Downregulation of KLF5 and Fli1 Is a Key Feature Underlying Systemic Sclerosis. *Nat. Commun.* **2014**, *5*, 5797. [CrossRef]
17. Taniguchi, T.; Asano, Y.; Akamata, K.; Noda, S.; Takahashi, T.; Ichimura, Y.; Toyama, T.; Trojanowska, M.; Sato, S. Fibrosis, Vascular Activation, and Immune Abnormalities Resembling Systemic Sclerosis in Bleomycin-Treated Fli-1-Haploinsufficient Mice: SSc Phenotype Induction by Bleomycin in Fli-1+/−Mice. *Arthritis Rheumatol.* **2015**, *67*, 517–526. [CrossRef]
18. Takeda, N.; Manabe, I.; Uchino, Y.; Eguchi, K.; Matsumoto, S.; Nishimura, S.; Shindo, T.; Sano, M.; Otsu, K.; Snider, P.; et al. Cardiac Fibroblasts Are Essential for the Adaptive Response of the Murine Heart to Pressure Overload. *J Clin Investig.* **2010**, *120*, 254–265. [CrossRef]
19. Fujiu, K.; Manabe, I.; Nagai, R. Renal Collecting Duct Epithelial Cells Regulate Inflammation in Tubulointerstitial Damage in Mice. *J. Clin. Investig.* **2011**, *121*, 3425–3441. [CrossRef]
20. Whitfield, M.L.; Finlay, D.R.; Murray, J.I.; Troyanskaya, O.G.; Chi, J.-T.; Pergamenschikov, A.; McCalmont, T.H.; Brown, P.O.; Botstein, D.; Connolly, M.K. Systemic and Cell Type-Specific Gene Expression Patterns in Scleroderma Skin. *Proc. Natl. Acad. Sci. USA* **2003**, *100*, 12319–12324. [CrossRef]
21. Yu, J.; Tang, R.; Ding, K. Epigenetic Modifications in the Pathogenesis of Systemic Sclerosis. *Int. J. Gen. Med.* **2022**, *15*, 3155–3166. [CrossRef]
22. Riemekasten, G.; Distler, J.H.W. A Broad Look into the Future of Systemic Sclerosis. *Ther. Adv. Musculoskelet. Dis.* **2022**, *14*, 1759720X221109404. [CrossRef]
23. Angiolilli, C.; Marut, W.; van der Kroef, M.; Chouri, E.; Reedquist, K.A.; Radstake, T.R.D.J. New Insights into the Genetics and Epigenetics of Systemic Sclerosis. *Nat. Rev. Rheumatol.* **2018**, *14*, 657–673. [CrossRef] [PubMed]
24. Altorok, N.; Kahaleh, B. Epigenetics and Systemic Sclerosis. *Semin. Immunopathol.* **2015**, *37*, 453–462. [CrossRef]
25. Gao, L.; Lu, Q. The Critical Importance of Epigenetics in Autoimmune-Related Skin Diseases. *Front. Med.* **2023**, *17*, 43–57. [CrossRef] [PubMed]
26. Truchetet, M.E.; Brembilla, N.C.; Chizzolini, C. Current Concepts on the Pathogenesis of Systemic Sclerosis. *Clin. Rev. Allergy Immunol.* **2023**, *64*, 262–283. [CrossRef]
27. Zhang, Y.; Maskan Bermudez, N.; Sa, B.; Maderal, A.D.; Jimenez, J.J. Epigenetic Mechanisms Driving the Pathogenesis of Systemic Lupus Erythematosus, Systemic Sclerosis and Dermatomyositis. *Exp. Dermatol.* **2024**, *33*, e14986. [CrossRef] [PubMed]
28. Higashi-Kuwata, N.; Jinnin, M.; Makino, T.; Fukushima, S.; Inoue, Y.; Muchemwa, F.C.; Yonemura, Y.; Komohara, Y.; Takeya, M.; Mitsuya, H.; et al. Characterization of Monocyte/Macrophage Subsets in the Skin and Peripheral Blood Derived from Patients with Systemic Sclerosis. *Arthritis Res. Ther.* **2010**, *12*, R128. [CrossRef] [PubMed]
29. Yukawa, S.; Yamaoka, K.; Sawamukai, N.; Shimajiri, S.; Kubo, S.; Miyagawa, I.; Sonomoto, K.; Saito, K.; Tanaka, Y. Dermal Mast Cell Density in Fingers Reflects Severity of Skin Sclerosis in Systemic Sclerosis. *Mod. Rheumatol.* **2013**, *23*, 1151–1157. [CrossRef]
30. MacDonald, K.G.; Dawson, N.A.J.; Huang, Q.; Dunne, J.V.; Levings, M.K.; Broady, R. Regulatory T Cells Produce Profibrotic Cytokines in the Skin of Patients with Systemic Sclerosis. *J. Allergy Clin. Immunol.* **2015**, *135*, 946–955.e9. [CrossRef]
31. Bosello, S.; Angelucci, C.; Lama, G.; Alivernini, S.; Proietti, G.; Tolusso, B.; Sica, G.; Gremese, E.; Ferraccioli, G. Characterization of Inflammatory Cell Infiltrate of Scleroderma Skin: B Cells and Skin Score Progression. *Arthritis Res. Ther.* **2018**, *20*, 75. [CrossRef] [PubMed]
32. Lafyatis, R.; O'Hara, C.; Feghali-Bostwick, C.A.; Matteson, E. B Cell Infiltration in Systemic Sclerosis-Associated Interstitial Lung Disease. *Arthritis Rheum.* **2007**, *56*, 3167–3168. [CrossRef] [PubMed]
33. Matsushita, T.; Hasegawa, M.; Hamaguchi, Y.; Takehara, K.; Sato, S. Longitudinal Analysis of Serum Cytokine Concentrations in Systemic Sclerosis: Association of Interleukin 12 Elevation with Spontaneous Regression of Skin Sclerosis. *J. Rheumatol.* **2006**, *33*, 275–284.
34. Yang, X.; Yang, J.; Xing, X.; Wan, L.; Li, M. Increased Frequency of Th17 Cells in Systemic Sclerosis Is Related to Disease Activity and Collagen Overproduction. *Arthritis Res. Ther.* **2014**, *16*, R4. [CrossRef]
35. Murata, M.; Fujimoto, M.; Matsushita, T.; Hamaguchi, Y.; Hasegawa, M.; Takehara, K.; Komura, K.; Sato, S. Clinical Association of Serum Interleukin-17 Levels in Systemic Sclerosis: Is Systemic Sclerosis a Th17 Disease? *J. Dermatol. Sci.* **2008**, *50*, 240–242. [CrossRef] [PubMed]
36. Zhou, Y.; Hou, W.; Xu, K.; Han, D.; Jiang, C.; Mou, K.; Li, Y.; Meng, L.; Lu, S. The Elevated Expression of Th17-Related Cytokines and Receptors Is Associated with Skin Lesion Severity in Early Systemic Sclerosis. *Hum. Immunol.* **2015**, *76*, 22–29. [CrossRef]
37. Frantz, C.; Auffray, C.; Avouac, J.; Allanore, Y. Regulatory T Cells in Systemic Sclerosis. *Front. Immunol.* **2018**, *9*, 2356. [CrossRef]
38. Sato, S.; Hasegawa, M.; Takehara, K. Serum Levels of Interleukin-6 and Interleukin-10 Correlate with Total Skin Thickness Score in Patients with Systemic Sclerosis. *J. Dermatol. Sci.* **2001**, *27*, 140–146. [CrossRef]

39. Nakashima, T.; Jinnin, M.; Yamane, K.; Honda, N.; Kajihara, I.; Makino, T.; Masuguchi, S.; Fukushima, S.; Okamoto, Y.; Hasegawa, M.; et al. Impaired IL-17 Signaling Pathway Contributes to the Increased Collagen Expression in Scleroderma Fibroblasts. *J. Immunol.* **2012**, *188*, 3573–3583. [CrossRef]
40. Bankamp, L.; Preuß, B.; Pecher, A.-C.; Beucke, N.; Henes, J.; Klein, R. Functionally Active Antibodies to the Angiotensin II Type 1-Receptor Measured by a Luminometric Bioassay Do Not Correlate with Clinical Manifestations in Systemic Sclerosis: A Comparison with Antibodies to Vascular Receptors and Topoisomerase I Detected by ELISA. *Front. Immunol.* **2021**, *12*, 786039.
41. van Oostveen, W.M.; Hoekstra, E.M.; Levarht, E.W.N.; Kotliar, I.B.; Sakmar, T.P.; Toes, R.E.M.; de Vries-Bouwstra, J.K.; Heitman, L.H.; Fehres, C.M. Absence of Functional Autoantibodies Targeting Angiotensin II Receptor Type 1 and Endothelin-1 Type A Receptor in Circulation and Purified IgG from Patients with Systemic Sclerosis. *Arthritis Rheumatol.* **2024**. [CrossRef] [PubMed]
42. Sato, S.; Hasegawa, M.; Fujimoto, M.; Tedder, T.F.; Takehara, K. Quantitative Genetic Variation in CD19 Expression Correlates with Autoimmunity. *J. Immunol.* **2000**, *165*, 6635–6643. [CrossRef]
43. Sato, S.; Fujimoto, M.; Hasegawa, M.; Takehara, K. Altered Blood B Lymphocyte Homeostasis in Systemic Sclerosis: Expanded Naive B Cells and Diminished but Activated Memory B Cells. *Arthritis Rheum.* **2004**, *50*, 1918–1927. [CrossRef]
44. Yoshizaki, A. B Lymphocytes in Systemic Sclerosis: Abnormalities and Therapeutic Targets. *J. Dermatol.* **2016**, *43*, 39–45. [CrossRef]
45. Jordan, S.; Distler, J.H.W.; Maurer, B.; Huscher, D.; van Laar, J.M.; Allanore, Y.; Distler, O.; EUSTAR Rituximab study group. Effects and Safety of Rituximab in Systemic Sclerosis: An Analysis from the European Scleroderma Trial and Research (EUSTAR) Group. *Ann. Rheum. Dis.* **2015**, *74*, 1188–1194. [CrossRef] [PubMed]
46. Daoussis, D.; Melissaropoulos, K.; Sakellaropoulos, G.; Antonopoulos, I.; Markatseli, T.E.; Simopoulou, T.; Georgiou, P.; Andonopoulos, A.P.; Drosos, A.A.; Sakkas, L.; et al. A Multicenter, Open-Label, Comparative Study of B-Cell Depletion Therapy with Rituximab for Systemic Sclerosis-Associated Interstitial Lung Disease. *Semin. Arthritis Rheum.* **2017**, *46*, 625–631. [CrossRef]
47. Bosello, S.L.; De Luca, G.; Rucco, M.; Berardi, G.; Falcione, M.; Danza, F.M.; Pirronti, T.; Ferraccioli, G. Long-Term Efficacy of B Cell Depletion Therapy on Lung and Skin Involvement in Diffuse Systemic Sclerosis. *Semin. Arthritis Rheum.* **2015**, *44*, 428–436. [CrossRef] [PubMed]
48. Ebata, S.; Yoshizaki, A.; Fukasawa, T.; Miura, S.; Takahashi, T.; Sumida, H.; Asano, Y.; Sato, S. Rituximab Therapy Is More Effective than Cyclophosphamide Therapy for Japanese Patients with Anti-Topoisomerase I-Positive Systemic Sclerosis-Associated Interstitial Lung Disease. *J. Dermatol.* **2019**, *46*, 1006–1013. [CrossRef]
49. Daoussis, D.; Antonopoulos, I.; Liossis, S.-N.C.; Yiannopoulos, G.; Andonopoulos, A.P. Treatment of Systemic Sclerosis-Associated Calcinosis: A Case Report of Rituximab-Induced Regression of CREST-Related Calcinosis and Review of the Literature. *Semin. Arthritis Rheum.* **2012**, *41*, 822–829. [CrossRef]
50. Khor, C.-G.; Chen, X.L.-F.; Lin, T.-S.; Lu, C.-H.; Hsieh, S.-C. Rituximab for Refractory Digital Infarcts and Ulcers in Systemic Sclerosis. *Clin. Rheumatol.* **2014**, *33*, 1019–1020. [CrossRef]
51. Maslyanskiy, A.; Lapin, S.; Kolesova, E.; Peñín, I.; Cheshuina, M.D.; Feist, E.; Konradi, A. Effects of Rituximab Therapy on Elastic Properties of Vascular Wall in Patients with Progressive Systemic Sclerosis. *Clin. Exp. Rheumatol.* **2014**, *32*, S-228. [PubMed]
52. Bergmann, C.; Müller, F.; Distler, J.H.W.; Györfi, A.-H.; Völkl, S.; Aigner, M.; Kretschmann, S.; Reimann, H.; Harrer, T.; Bayerl, N.; et al. Treatment of a Patient with Severe Systemic Sclerosis (SSc) Using CD19-Targeted CAR T Cells. *Ann. Rheum. Dis.* **2023**, *82*, 1117–1120. [CrossRef] [PubMed]
53. Müller, F.; Taubmann, J.; Bucci, L.; Wilhelm, A.; Bergmann, C.; Völkl, S.; Aigner, M.; Rothe, T.; Minopoulou, I.; Tur, C.; et al. CD19 CAR T-Cell Therapy in Autoimmune Disease—A Case Series with Follow-Up. *N. Engl. J. Med.* **2024**, *390*, 687–700. [CrossRef] [PubMed]
54. Wang, X.; Wu, X.; Tan, B.; Zhu, L.; Zhang, Y.; Lin, L.; Xiao, Y.; Sun, A.; Wan, X.; Liu, S.; et al. Allogeneic CD19-Targeted CAR-T Therapy in Patients with Severe Myositis and Systemic Sclerosis. *Cell* **2024**, *187*, 4890–4904.e9. [CrossRef]
55. Merkt, W.; Freitag, M.; Claus, M.; Kolb, P.; Falcone, V.; Röhrich, M.; Rodon, L.; Deicher, F.; Andreeva, I.; Tretter, T.; et al. Third-Generation CD19.CAR-T Cell-Containing Combination Therapy in Scl70+ Systemic Sclerosis. *Ann. Rheum. Dis.* **2024**, *83*, 543–546. [CrossRef]
56. Hügle, T.; Hogan, V.; White, K.E.; van Laar, J.M. Mast Cells Are a Source of Transforming Growth Factor β in Systemic Sclerosis. *Arthritis Rheum.* **2011**, *63*, 795–799. [CrossRef]
57. Khanna, D.; Denton, C.P.; Jahreis, A.; van Laar, J.M.; Frech, T.M.; Anderson, M.E.; Baron, M.; Chung, L.; Fierlbeck, G.; Lakshminarayanan, S.; et al. Safety and Efficacy of Subcutaneous Tocilizumab in Adults with Systemic Sclerosis (FaSScinate): A Phase 2, Randomised, Controlled Trial. *Lancet* **2016**, *387*, 2630–2640. [CrossRef]
58. Akamata, K.; Asano, Y.; Taniguchi, T.; Yamashita, T.; Saigusa, R.; Nakamura, K.; Noda, S.; Aozasa, N.; Toyama, T.; Takahashi, T.; et al. Increased Expression of Chemerin in Endothelial Cells Due to Fli1 Deficiency May Contribute to the Development of Digital Ulcers in Systemic Sclerosis. *Rheumatology* **2015**, *54*, 1308–1316. [CrossRef]
59. Duan, H.; Fleming, J.; Pritchard, D.K.; Amon, L.M.; Xue, J.; Arnett, H.A.; Chen, G.; Breen, P.; Buckner, J.H.; Molitor, J.A.; et al. Combined Analysis of Monocyte and Lymphocyte Messenger RNA Expression with Serum Protein Profiles in Patients with Scleroderma. *Arthritis Rheum.* **2008**, *58*, 1465–1474. [CrossRef]

60. Takahashi, T.; Asano, Y.; Nakamura, K.; Yamashita, T.; Saigusa, R.; Ichimura, Y.; Toyama, T.; Taniguchi, T.; Yoshizaki, A.; Tamaki, Z.; et al. A Potential Contribution of Antimicrobial Peptide LL-37 to Tissue Fibrosis and Vasculopathy in Systemic Sclerosis. *Br. J. Dermatol.* **2016**, *175*, 1195–1203. [CrossRef]
61. Kim, D.; Peck, A.; Santer, D.; Patole, P.; Schwartz, S.M.; Molitor, J.A.; Arnett, F.C.; Elkon, K.B. Induction of Interferon-Alpha by Scleroderma Sera Containing Autoantibodies to Topoisomerase I: Association of Higher Interferon-Alpha Activity with Lung Fibrosis. *Arthritis Rheum.* **2008**, *58*, 2163–2173. [CrossRef]
62. Black, C.M.; Silman, A.J.; Herrick, A.I.; Denton, C.P.; Wilson, H.; Newman, J.; Pompon, L.; Shi-Wen, X. Interferon-Alpha Does Not Improve Outcome at One Year in Patients with Diffuse Cutaneous Scleroderma: Results of a Randomized, Double-Blind, Placebo-Controlled Trial. *Arthritis Rheum.* **1999**, *42*, 299–305. [CrossRef] [PubMed]
63. Hügle, T.; Gratzl, S.; Daikeler, T.; Frey, D.; Tyndall, A.; Walker, U.A. Sclerosing Skin Disorders in Association with Multiple Sclerosis. Coincidence, Underlying Autoimmune Pathology or Interferon Induced? *Ann. Rheum. Dis.* **2009**, *68*, 47–50. [CrossRef] [PubMed]
64. Pelidou, S.-H.; Tsifetaki, N.; Giannopoulos, S.; Deretzi, G.; Voulgari, P.; Kyritsis, A. Multiple Sclerosis Associated with Systemic Sclerosis. *Rheumatol. Int.* **2007**, *27*, 771–773. [CrossRef]
65. Spadaro, A.; Sensi, F.; Barrella, M.; Francia, A. Systemic Sclerosis and Multiple Sclerosis. *J. Neurol.* **1999**, *246*, 497–499. [CrossRef]
66. Tahara, H.; Kojima, A.; Hirokawa, T.; Oyama, T.; Naganuma, A.; Maruta, S.; Okada, K.; Ban, S.; Yoshida, K.; Takagi, H.; et al. Systemic Sclerosis after Interferon Alphacon-1 Therapy for Hepatitis C. *Intern. Med.* **2007**, *46*, 473–476. [CrossRef] [PubMed]
67. Esteban, I.; Vilardell, M.R.; Solans, J.A. Bosch. *Clin. Exp. Rheumatol.* **2004**, *22*, 625–628.
68. Beretta, L.; Caronni, M.; Vanoli, M.; Scorza, R. Systemic Sclerosis after Interferon-Alfa Therapy for Myeloproliferative Disorders. *Br. J. Dermatol.* **2002**, *147*, 385–386. [CrossRef]
69. Pammer, J.; Reinisch, C.; Birner, P.; Pogoda, K.; Sturzl, M.; Tschachler, E. Interferon-Alpha Prevents Apoptosis of Endothelial Cells after Short-Term Exposure but Induces Replicative Senescence after Continuous Stimulation. *Lab. Investig.* **2006**, *86*, 997–1007. [CrossRef]
70. Ah Kioon, M.D.; Tripodo, C.; Fernandez, D.; Kirou, K.A.; Spiera, R.F.; Crow, M.K.; Gordon, J.K.; Barrat, F.J. Plasmacytoid Dendritic Cells Promote Systemic Sclerosis with a Key Role for TLR8. *Sci. Transl. Med.* **2018**, *10*, eaam8458. [CrossRef]
71. Ferreira, B.H.; Silva, I.S.; Mendes, A.; Leite-Pinheiro, F.; Paton, A.W.; Paton, J.C.; Duarte, I.F.; Pierre, P.; Almeida, C.R. Promoting ER Stress in a Plasmacytoid Dendritic Cell Line Drives Fibroblast Activation. *Cell Commun. Signal.* **2025**, *23*, 66. [CrossRef]
72. Abraham, D.J.; Krieg, T.; Distler, J.; Distler, O. Overview of Pathogenesis of Systemic Sclerosis. *Rheumatology* **2009**, *48* (Suppl. S3), iii3–iii7. [CrossRef]
73. Asano, Y. Future Treatments in Systemic Sclerosis. *J. Dermatol.* **2010**, *37*, 54–70. [CrossRef]
74. Asano, Y.; Sato, S. Vasculopathy in Scleroderma. *Semin. Immunopathol.* **2015**, *37*, 489–500. [CrossRef]
75. Prescott, R.J.; Freemont, A.J.; Jones, C.J.; Hoyland, J.; Fielding, P. Sequential Dermal Microvascular and Perivascular Changes in the Development of Scleroderma. *J. Pathol.* **1992**, *166*, 255–263. [CrossRef] [PubMed]
76. Sgonc, R.; Gruschwitz, M.S.; Dietrich, H.; Recheis, H.; Gershwin, M.E.; Wick, G. Endothelial Cell Apoptosis Is a Primary Pathogenetic Event Underlying Skin Lesions in Avian and Human Scleroderma. *J. Clin. Investig.* **1996**, *98*, 785–792. [CrossRef] [PubMed]
77. Burbelo, P.D.; Gordon, S.M.; Waldman, M.; Edison, J.D.; Little, D.J.; Stitt, R.S.; Bailey, W.T.; Hughes, J.B.; Olson, S.W. Autoantibodies Are Present before the Clinical Diagnosis of Systemic Sclerosis. *PLoS ONE* **2019**, *14*, e0214202. [CrossRef] [PubMed]
78. Ihn, H. Scleroderma, Fibroblasts, Signaling, and Excessive Extracellular Matrix. *Curr. Rheumatol. Rep.* **2005**, *7*, 156–162. [CrossRef] [PubMed]
79. Romano, E.; Rosa, I.; Fioretto, B.S.; Matucci-Cerinic, M.; Manetti, M. New Insights into Profibrotic Myofibroblast Formation in Systemic Sclerosis: When the Vascular Wall Becomes the Enemy. *Life* **2021**, *11*, 610. [CrossRef]
80. Takahashi, T.; Asano, Y.; Amiya, E.; Hatano, M.; Tamaki, Z.; Takata, M.; Ozeki, A.; Watanabe, A.; Kawarasaki, S.; Taniguchi, T.; et al. Clinical Correlation of Brachial Artery Flow-Mediated Dilation in Patients with Systemic Sclerosis. *Mod. Rheumatol.* **2014**, *24*, 106–111. [CrossRef]
81. Cerinic, M.M.; Valentini, G.; Sorano, G.G.; D'Angelo, S.; Cuomo, G.; Fenu, L.; Generini, S.; Cinotti, S.; Morfini, M.; Pignone, A.; et al. Blood Coagulation, Fibrinolysis, and Markers of Endothelial Dysfunction in Systemic Sclerosis. *Semin. Arthritis Rheum.* **2003**, *32*, 285–295. [CrossRef] [PubMed]
82. Ihn, H. Autocrine TGF-Beta Signaling in the Pathogenesis of Systemic Sclerosis. *J. Dermatol. Sci.* **2008**, *49*, 103–113. [CrossRef] [PubMed]
83. Bhattacharyya, S.; Kelley, K.; Melichian, D.S.; Tamaki, Z.; Fang, F.; Su, Y.; Feng, G.; Pope, R.M.; Budinger, G.R.S.; Mutlu, G.M.; et al. Toll-like Receptor 4 Signaling Augments Transforming Growth Factor-β Responses: A Novel Mechanism for Maintaining and Amplifying Fibrosis in Scleroderma. *Am. J. Pathol.* **2013**, *182*, 192–205. [CrossRef]
84. Kahaleh, M. Raynaud's Phenomenon and Vascular Disease in Scleroderma. *Curr. Opin. Rheumatol.* **1994**, *6*, 621–627. [CrossRef]

85. Tourkina, E.; Bonner, M.; Oates, J.; Hofbauer, A.; Richard, M.; Znoyko, S.; Visconti, R.P.; Zhang, J.; Hatfield, C.M.; Silver, R.M.; et al. Altered Monocyte and Fibrocyte Phenotype and Function in Scleroderma Interstitial Lung Disease: Reversal by Caveolin-1 Scaffolding Domain Peptide. *Fibrogenesis Tissue Repair* **2011**, *4*, 15. [CrossRef]
86. Nikitorowicz-Buniak, J.; Denton, C.P.; Abraham, D.; Stratton, R. Partially Evoked Epithelial-Mesenchymal Transition (EMT) Is Associated with Increased TGFβ Signaling within Lesional Scleroderma Skin. *PLoS ONE* **2015**, *10*, e0134092. [CrossRef]
87. Mendoza, F.A.; Piera-Velazquez, S.; Farber, J.L.; Feghali-Bostwick, C.; Jiménez, S.A. Endothelial Cells Expressing Endothelial and Mesenchymal Cell Gene Products in Lung Tissue from Patients with Systemic Sclerosis-Associated Interstitial Lung Disease. *Arthritis Rheumatol.* **2016**, *68*, 210–217. [CrossRef]
88. Manetti, M.; Romano, E.; Rosa, I.; Guiducci, S.; Bellando-Randone, S.; De Paulis, A.; Ibba-Manneschi, L.; Matucci-Cerinic, M. Endothelial-to-Mesenchymal Transition Contributes to Endothelial Dysfunction and Dermal Fibrosis in Systemic Sclerosis. *Ann. Rheum. Dis.* **2017**, *76*, 924–934. [CrossRef] [PubMed]
89. Marangoni, R.G.; Korman, B.D.; Wei, J.; Wood, T.A.; Graham, L.V.; Whitfield, M.L.; Scherer, P.E.; Tourtellotte, W.G.; Varga, J. Myofibroblasts in Murine Cutaneous Fibrosis Originate from Adiponectin-Positive Intradermal Progenitors: Adipocyte-Myofibroblast Transition in Skin Fibrosis. *Arthritis Rheumatol.* **2015**, *67*, 1062–1073. [CrossRef]
90. Gruschwitz, M.; Müller, P.U.; Sepp, N.; Hofer, E.; Fontana, A.; Wick, G. Transcription and Expression of Transforming Growth Factor Type Beta in the Skin of Progressive Systemic Sclerosis: A Mediator of Fibrosis? *J. Investig. Dermatol.* **1990**, *94*, 197–203. [CrossRef]
91. Querfeld, C.; Eckes, B.; Huerkamp, C.; Krieg, T.; Sollberg, S. Expression of TGF-Beta 1, -Beta 2 and -Beta 3 in Localized and Systemic Scleroderma. *J. Dermatol. Sci.* **1999**, *21*, 13–22. [CrossRef] [PubMed]
92. Kulozik, M.; Hogg, A.; Lankat-Buttgereit, B.; Krieg, T. Co-Localization of Transforming Growth Factor Beta 2 with Alpha 1(I) Procollagen MRNA in Tissue Sections of Patients with Systemic Sclerosis. *J. Clin. Investig.* **1990**, *86*, 917–922. [CrossRef]
93. Asano, Y.; Ihn, H.; Yamane, K.; Kubo, M.; Tamaki, K. Impaired Smad7-Smurf-Mediated Negative Regulation of TGF-Beta Signaling in Scleroderma Fibroblasts. *J. Clin. Investig.* **2004**, *113*, 253–264. [CrossRef]
94. Asano, Y.; Ihn, H.; Yamane, K.; Jinnin, M.; Mimura, Y.; Tamaki, K. Increased Expression of Integrin Alpha(v)Beta3 Contributes to the Establishment of Autocrine TGF-Beta Signaling in Scleroderma Fibroblasts. *J. Immunol.* **2005**, *175*, 7708–7718. [CrossRef]
95. Asano, Y.; Ihn, H.; Yamane, K.; Kubo, M.; Tamaki, K. Increased Expression Levels of Integrin Alphavbeta5 on Scleroderma Fibroblasts. *Am. J. Pathol.* **2004**, *164*, 1275–1292. [CrossRef] [PubMed]
96. Asano, Y.; Ihn, H.; Yamane, K.; Jinnin, M.; Mimura, Y.; Tamaki, K. Involvement of Alphavbeta5 Integrin-Mediated Activation of Latent Transforming Growth Factor Beta1 in Autocrine Transforming Growth Factor Beta Signaling in Systemic Sclerosis Fibroblasts. *Arthritis Rheum.* **2005**, *52*, 2897–2905. [CrossRef] [PubMed]
97. Asano, Y.; Ihn, H.; Yamane, K.; Jinnin, M.; Tamaki, K. Increased Expression of Integrin Alphavbeta5 Induces the Myofibroblastic Differentiation of Dermal Fibroblasts. *Am. J. Pathol.* **2006**, *168*, 499–510. [CrossRef]
98. Mimura, Y.; Ihn, H.; Jinnin, M.; Asano, Y.; Yamane, K.; Tamaki, K. Constitutive Thrombospondin-1 Overexpression Contributes to Autocrine Transforming Growth Factor-Beta Signaling in Cultured Scleroderma Fibroblasts. *Am. J. Pathol.* **2005**, *166*, 1451–1463. [CrossRef]
99. Meng, Q.; Bao, D.; Liu, S.; Huang, J.; Guo, M.; Dai, B.; Ding, L.; Xie, S.; Meng, M.; Lv, C.; et al. ADAM Metallopeptidase Domain 19 Promotes Skin Fibrosis in Systemic Sclerosis via Neuregulin-1. *Mol. Med.* **2024**, *30*, 269. [CrossRef]
100. Chizzolini, C.; Rezzonico, R.; Ribbens, C.; Burger, D.; Wollheim, F.A.; Dayer, J.M. Inhibition of Type I Collagen Production by Dermal Fibroblasts upon Contact with Activated T Cells: Different Sensitivity to Inhibition between Systemic Sclerosis and Control Fibroblasts. *Arthritis Rheum.* **1998**, *41*, 2039–2047. [CrossRef]
101. Chizzolini, C.; Parel, Y.; De Luca, C.; Tyndall, A.; Akesson, A.; Scheja, A.; Dayer, J.-M. Systemic Sclerosis Th2 Cells Inhibit Collagen Production by Dermal Fibroblasts via Membrane-Associated Tumor Necrosis Factor Alpha: Th2 Cells Inhibit Collagen Synthesis by Dermal Fibroblasts. *Arthritis Rheum.* **2003**, *48*, 2593–2604. [CrossRef] [PubMed]
102. Ichimura, Y.; Asano, Y.; Akamata, K.; Noda, S.; Taniguchi, T.; Takahashi, T.; Toyama, T.; Tada, Y.; Sugaya, M.; Sato, S.; et al. Progranulin Overproduction Due to Fli-1 Deficiency Contributes to the Resistance of Dermal Fibroblasts to Tumor Necrosis Factor in Systemic Sclerosis: THE ROLE OF PROGRANULIN IN SSc. *Arthritis Rheumatol.* **2015**, *67*, 3245–3255. [CrossRef] [PubMed]
103. Bergmann, C.; Chenguiti Fakhouri, S.; Trinh-Minh, T.; Filla, T.; Rius Rigau, A.; Ekici, A.B.; Merlevede, B.; Hallenberger, L.; Zhu, H.; Dees, C.; et al. Mutual Amplification of GLI2/Hedgehog and Transcription Factor JUN/AP-1 Signaling in Fibroblasts in Systemic Sclerosis: Potential Implications for Combined Therapies. *Arthritis Rheumatol.* **2025**, *77*, 92–98. [CrossRef] [PubMed]
104. Saigusa, R.; Asano, Y.; Taniguchi, T.; Hirabayashi, M.; Nakamura, K.; Miura, S.; Yamashita, T.; Takahashi, T.; Ichimura, Y.; Toyama, T.; et al. Fli1-Haploinsufficient Dermal Fibroblasts Promote Skin-Localized Transdifferentiation of Th2-like Regulatory T Cells. *Arthritis Res. Ther.* **2018**, *20*, 23. [CrossRef]
105. Saigusa, R.; Asano, Y.; Nakamura, K.; Hirabayashi, M.; Miura, S.; Yamashita, T.; Taniguchi, T.; Ichimura, Y.; Takahashi, T.; Yoshizaki, A.; et al. Systemic Sclerosis Dermal Fibroblasts Suppress Th1 Cytokine Production via Galectin-9 Overproduction Due to Fli1 Deficiency. *J. Investig. Dermatol.* **2017**, *137*, 1850–1859. [CrossRef]

106. Gur, C.; Wang, S.-Y.; Sheban, F.; Zada, M.; Li, B.; Kharouf, F.; Peleg, H.; Aamar, S.; Yalin, A.; Kirschenbaum, D.; et al. LGR5 Expressing Skin Fibroblasts Define a Major Cellular Hub Perturbed in Scleroderma. *Cell* **2022**, *185*, 1373–1388.e20. [CrossRef]
107. Ma, F.; Tsou, P.-S.; Gharaee-Kermani, M.; Plazyo, O.; Xing, X.; Kirma, J.; Wasikowski, R.; Hile, G.A.; Harms, P.W.; Jiang, Y.; et al. Systems-Based Identification of the Hippo Pathway for Promoting Fibrotic Mesenchymal Differentiation in Systemic Sclerosis. *Nat. Commun.* **2024**, *15*, 210. [CrossRef]
108. Huang, M.; Tabib, T.; Khanna, D.; Assassi, S.; Domsic, R.; Lafyatis, R. Single-Cell Transcriptomes and Chromatin Accessibility of Endothelial Cells Unravel Transcription Factors Associated with Dysregulated Angiogenesis in Systemic Sclerosis. *Ann. Rheum. Dis.* **2024**, *83*, 1335–1344. [CrossRef]
109. Rius Rigau, A.; Li, Y.-N.; Matei, A.-E.; Györfi, A.-H.; Bruch, P.-M.; Koziel, S.; Devakumar, V.; Gabrielli, A.; Kreuter, A.; Wang, J.; et al. Characterization of Vascular Niche in Systemic Sclerosis by Spatial Proteomics. *Circ. Res.* **2024**, *134*, 875–891. [CrossRef]
110. Liu, Q.; Zaba, L.C.; Satpathy, A.T.; Longmire, M.; Zhang, W.; Li, K.; Granja, J.; Guo, C.; Lin, J.; Li, R.; et al. Chromatin Accessibility Landscapes of Skin Cells in Systemic Sclerosis Nominate Dendritic Cells in Disease Pathogenesis. *Nat. Commun.* **2020**, *11*, 5843. [CrossRef]
111. Miura, S.; Asano, Y.; Saigusa, R.; Yamashita, T.; Taniguchi, T.; Takahashi, T.; Ichimura, Y.; Toyama, T.; Yoshizaki, A.; Sato, S.; et al. Regulation of Skin Fibrosis by RALDH1-Producing Dermal Dendritic Cells via Retinoic Acid-Mediated Regulatory T Cell Induction: A Role in Scleroderma. *J. Dermatol. Sci.* **2020**, *97*, 125–134. [CrossRef] [PubMed]
112. Miura, S.; Watanabe, Y.; Saigusa, R.; Yamashita, T.; Nakamura, K.; Hirabayashi, M.; Miyagawa, T.; Yoshizaki, A.; Trojanowska, M.; Sato, S.; et al. Fli1 Deficiency Suppresses RALDH1 Activity of Dermal Dendritic Cells and Related Induction of Regulatory T Cells: A Possible Role in Scleroderma. *Arthritis Res. Ther.* **2021**, *23*, 137. [CrossRef]
113. Yang, M.M.; Lee, S.; Neely, J.; Hinchcliff, M.; Wolters, P.J.; Sirota, M. Gene Expression Meta-Analysis Reveals Aging and Cellular Senescence Signatures in Scleroderma-Associated Interstitial Lung Disease. *Front. Immunol.* **2024**, *15*, 1326922. [CrossRef] [PubMed]
114. Vaughan, D.E.; Rai, R.; Khan, S.S.; Eren, M.; Ghosh, A.K. Plasminogen Activator Inhibitor-1 Is a Marker and a Mediator of Senescence. *Arterioscler. Thromb. Vasc. Biol.* **2017**, *37*, 1446–1452. [CrossRef]
115. Rana, T.; Jiang, C.; Liu, G.; Miyata, T.; Antony, V.; Thannickal, V.J.; Liu, R.-M. PAI-1 Regulation of TGF-B1-Induced Alveolar Type II Cell Senescence, SASP Secretion, and SASP-Mediated Activation of Alveolar Macrophages. *Am. J. Respir. Cell Mol. Biol.* **2020**, *62*, 319–330. [CrossRef]
116. Eren, M.; Boe, A.E.; Murphy, S.B.; Place, A.T.; Nagpal, V.; Morales-Nebreda, L.; Urich, D.; Quaggin, S.E.; Budinger, G.R.S.; Mutlu, G.M.; et al. PAI-1-Regulated Extracellular Proteolysis Governs Senescence and Survival in Klotho Mice. *Proc. Natl. Acad. Sci. USA* **2014**, *111*, 7090–7095. [CrossRef] [PubMed]
117. Khan, S.S.; Shah, S.J.; Klyachko, E.; Baldridge, A.S.; Eren, M.; Place, A.T.; Aviv, A.; Puterman, E.; Lloyd-Jones, D.M.; Heiman, M.; et al. A Null Mutation in SERPINE1 Protects against Biological Aging in Humans. *Sci. Adv.* **2017**, *3*, eaao1617. [CrossRef]
118. Kanno, Y. The Role of Fibrinolytic Regulators in Vascular Dysfunction of Systemic Sclerosis. *Int. J. Mol. Sci.* **2019**, *20*, 619. [CrossRef] [PubMed]
119. Kanno, Y. The UPA/UPAR System Orchestrates the Inflammatory Response, Vascular Homeostasis, and Immune System in Fibrosis Progression. *Int. J. Mol. Sci.* **2023**, *24*, 1796. [CrossRef]
120. Vancheeswaran, R.; Azam, A.; Black, C.; Dashwood, M.R. Localization of Endothelin-1 and Its Binding Sites in Scleroderma Skin. *J. Rheumatol.* **1994**, *21*, 1268–1276.
121. Rudnicka, L.; Varga, J.; Christiano, A.M.; Iozzo, R.V.; Jimenez, S.A.; Uitto, J. Elevated Expression of Type VII Collagen in the Skin of Patients with Systemic Sclerosis. Regulation by Transforming Growth Factor-Beta. *J. Clin. Investig.* **1994**, *93*, 1709–1715. [CrossRef] [PubMed]
122. Distler, O.; Pap, T.; Kowal-Bielecka, O.; Meyringer, R.; Guiducci, S.; Landthaler, M.; Schölmerich, J.; Michel, B.A.; Gay, R.E.; Matucci-Cerinic, M.; et al. Overexpression of Monocyte Chemoattractant Protein 1 in Systemic Sclerosis: Role of Platelet-Derived Growth Factor and Effects on Monocyte Chemotaxis and Collagen Synthesis. *Arthritis Rheum.* **2001**, *44*, 2665–2678. [CrossRef]
123. Davies, C.A.; Jeziorska, M.; Freemont, A.J.; Herrick, A.L. The Differential Expression of VEGF, VEGFR-2, and GLUT-1 Proteins in Disease Subtypes of Systemic Sclerosis. *Hum. Pathol.* **2006**, *37*, 190–197. [CrossRef]
124. Distler, J.H.W.; Jüngel, A.; Kowal-Bielecka, O.; Michel, B.A.; Gay, R.E.; Sprott, H.; Matucci-Cerinic, M.; Chilla, M.; Reich, K.; Kalden, J.R.; et al. Expression of Interleukin-21 Receptor in Epidermis from Patients with Systemic Sclerosis: Altered Expression Pattern of Keratinocytes in SSc. *Arthritis Rheum.* **2005**, *52*, 856–864. [CrossRef] [PubMed]
125. Aden, N.; Nuttall, A.; Shiwen, X.; de Winter, P.; Leask, A.; Black, C.M.; Denton, C.P.; Abraham, D.J.; Stratton, R.J. Epithelial Cells Promote Fibroblast Activation via IL-1alpha in Systemic Sclerosis. *J. Investig. Dermatol.* **2010**, *130*, 2191–2200. [CrossRef] [PubMed]
126. Nikitorowicz-Buniak, J.; Shiwen, X.; Denton, C.P.; Abraham, D.; Stratton, R. Abnormally Differentiating Keratinocytes in the Epidermis of Systemic Sclerosis Patients Show Enhanced Secretion of CCN2 and S100A9. *J. Investig. Dermatol.* **2014**, *134*, 2693–2702. [CrossRef]

127. McCoy, S.S.; Reed, T.J.; Berthier, C.C.; Tsou, P.-S.; Liu, J.; Gudjonsson, J.E.; Khanna, D.; Kahlenberg, J.M. Scleroderma Keratinocytes Promote Fibroblast Activation Independent of Transforming Growth Factor Beta. *Rheumatology* **2017**, *56*, 1970–1981. [CrossRef]
128. Takahashi, T.; Asano, Y.; Yamashita, T.; Nakamura, K.; Saigusa, R.; Miura, S.; Ichimura, Y.; Toyama, T.; Hirabayashi, M.; Taniguchi, T.; et al. A Potential Contribution of Psoriasin to Vascular and Epithelial Abnormalities and Inflammation in Systemic Sclerosis. *J. Eur. Acad. Dermatol. Venereol.* **2018**, *32*, 291–297. [CrossRef]
129. Saigusa, R.; Yamashita, T.; Miura, S.; Hirabayashi, M.; Nakamura, K.; Miyagawa, T.; Fukui, Y.; Yoshizaki, A.; Sato, S.; Asano, Y. A Potential Contribution of Decreased Galectin-7 Expression in Stratified Epithelia to the Development of Cutaneous and Oesophageal Manifestations in Systemic Sclerosis. *Exp. Dermatol.* **2019**, *28*, 536–542. [CrossRef]
130. Takahashi, T.; Asano, Y.; Sugawara, K.; Yamashita, T.; Nakamura, K.; Saigusa, R.; Ichimura, Y.; Toyama, T.; Taniguchi, T.; Akamata, K.; et al. Epithelial Fli1 Deficiency Drives Systemic Autoimmunity and Fibrosis: Possible Roles in Scleroderma. *J. Exp. Med.* **2017**, *214*, 1129–1151. [CrossRef]
131. Asano, Y.; Stawski, L.; Hant, F.; Highland, K.; Silver, R.; Szalai, G.; Watson, D.K.; Trojanowska, M. Endothelial Fli1 Deficiency Impairs Vascular Homeostasis: A Role in Scleroderma Vasculopathy. *Am. J. Pathol.* **2010**, *176*, 1983–1998. [CrossRef] [PubMed]
132. Asano, Y.; Markiewicz, M.; Kubo, M.; Szalai, G.; Watson, D.K.; Trojanowska, M. Transcription Factor Fli1 Regulates Collagen Fibrillogenesis in Mouse Skin. *Mol. Cell. Biol.* **2009**, *29*, 425–434. [CrossRef] [PubMed]
133. Bujor, A.M.; El Adili, F.; Parvez, A.; Marden, G.; Trojanowska, M. Fli1 Downregulation in Scleroderma Myeloid Cells Has Profibrotic and Proinflammatory Effects. *Front. Immunol.* **2020**, *11*, 800. [CrossRef]
134. Taniguchi, T.; Miyagawa, T.; Toyama, S.; Yamashita, T.; Nakamura, K.; Saigusa, R.; Ichimura, Y.; Takahashi, T.; Toyama, T.; Yoshizaki, A.; et al. CXCL13 Produced by Macrophages Due to Fli1 Deficiency May Contribute to the Development of Tissue Fibrosis, Vasculopathy and Immune Activation in Systemic Sclerosis. *Exp. Dermatol.* **2018**, *27*, 1030–1037. [CrossRef]
135. Anderson, M.S.; Venanzi, E.S.; Klein, L.; Chen, Z.; Berzins, S.P.; Turley, S.J.; von Boehmer, H.; Bronson, R.; Dierich, A.; Benoist, C.; et al. Projection of an Immunological Self Shadow within the Thymus by the Aire Protein. *Science* **2002**, *298*, 1395–1401. [CrossRef]
136. Mathis, D.; Benoist, C. Aire. *Annu. Rev. Immunol.* **2009**, *27*, 287–312. [CrossRef]
137. Saigusa, R.; Asano, Y.; Yamashita, T.; Takahashi, T.; Nakamura, K.; Miura, S.; Ichimura, Y.; Toyama, T.; Taniguchi, T.; Sumida, H.; et al. Systemic Sclerosis Complicated with Localized Scleroderma-like Lesions Induced by Köbner Phenomenon. *J. Dermatol. Sci.* **2018**, *89*, 282–289. [CrossRef] [PubMed]
138. Byrd, A.L.; Belkaid, Y.; Segre, J.A. The Human Skin Microbiome. *Nat. Rev. Microbiol.* **2018**, *16*, 143–155. [CrossRef]
139. Terui, H.; Yamasaki, K.; Wada-Irimada, M.; Onodera-Amagai, M.; Hatchome, N.; Mizuashi, M.; Yamashita, R.; Kawabe, T.; Ishii, N.; Abe, T.; et al. Staphylococcus Aureus Skin Colonization Promotes SLE-like Autoimmune Inflammation via Neutrophil Activation and the IL-23/IL-17 Axis. *Sci. Immunol.* **2022**, *7*, eabm9811. [CrossRef]
140. Grice, E.A.; Segre, J.A. The Skin Microbiome. *Nat. Rev. Microbiol.* **2011**, *9*, 244–253. [CrossRef]
141. Johnson, M.E.; Franks, J.M.; Cai, G.; Mehta, B.K.; Wood, T.A.; Archambault, K.; Pioli, P.A.; Simms, R.W.; Orzechowski, N.; Arron, S.; et al. Microbiome Dysbiosis Is Associated with Disease Duration and Increased Inflammatory Gene Expression in Systemic Sclerosis Skin. *Arthritis Res. Ther.* **2019**, *21*, 49. [CrossRef] [PubMed]
142. Bhattacharyya, S.; Wei, J.; Varga, J. Understanding Fibrosis in Systemic Sclerosis: Shifting Paradigms, Emerging Opportunities. *Nat. Rev. Rheumatol.* **2011**, *8*, 42–54. [CrossRef]
143. Lynch, M.D.; Watt, F.M. Fibroblast Heterogeneity: Implications for Human Disease. *J. Clin. Investig.* **2018**, *128*, 26–35. [CrossRef]
144. Zhang, Z.; Shao, M.; Hepler, C.; Zi, Z.; Zhao, S.; An, Y.A.; Zhu, Y.; Ghaben, A.L.; Wang, M.-Y.; Li, N.; et al. Dermal Adipose Tissue Has High Plasticity and Undergoes Reversible Dedifferentiation in Mice. *J. Clin. Investig.* **2019**, *129*, 5327–5342. [CrossRef]
145. Varga, J.; Marangoni, R.G. Systemic Sclerosis in 2016: Dermal White Adipose Tissue Implicated in SSc Pathogenesis: Systemic Sclerosis in 2016. *Nat. Rev. Rheumatol.* **2017**, *13*, 71–72. [CrossRef] [PubMed]
146. Matsuzawa, Y.; Shimomura, I.; Kihara, S.; Funahashi, T. Importance of Adipocytokines in Obesity-Related Diseases. *Horm. Res.* **2003**, *60* (Suppl. S3), 56–59. [CrossRef] [PubMed]
147. Masui, Y.; Asano, Y.; Shibata, S.; Noda, S.; Aozasa, N.; Akamata, K.; Yamada, D.; Tamaki, Z.; Tada, Y.; Sugaya, M.; et al. Serum Adiponectin Levels Inversely Correlate with the Activity of Progressive Skin Sclerosis in Patients with Diffuse Cutaneous Systemic Sclerosis: Significance of Serum Adiponectin Levels in SSc. *J. Eur. Acad. Dermatol. Venereol.* **2012**, *26*, 354–360. [CrossRef]
148. Masui, Y.; Asano, Y.; Takahashi, T.; Shibata, S.; Akamata, K.; Aozasa, N.; Noda, S.; Taniguchi, T.; Ichimura, Y.; Toyama, T.; et al. Clinical Significance of Monitoring Serum Adiponectin Levels during Intravenous Pulse Cyclophosphamide Therapy in Interstitial Lung Disease Associated with Systemic Sclerosis. *Mod. Rheumatol.* **2013**, *23*, 323–329. [CrossRef]
149. Masui, Y.; Asano, Y.; Shibata, S.; Noda, S.; Akamata, K.; Aozasa, N.; Taniguchi, T.; Takahashi, T.; Ichimura, Y.; Toyama, T.; et al. A Possible Contribution of Visfatin to the Resolution of Skin Sclerosis in Patients with Diffuse Cutaneous Systemic Sclerosis via a Direct Anti-Fibrotic Effect on Dermal Fibroblasts and Th1 Polarization of the Immune Response. *Rheumatology* **2013**, *52*, 1239–1244. [CrossRef]

150. Aozasa, N.; Asano, Y.; Akamata, K.; Noda, S.; Masui, Y.; Yamada, D.; Tamaki, Z.; Tada, Y.; Sugaya, M.; Kadono, T.; et al. Serum Apelin Levels: Clinical Association with Vascular Involvements in Patients with Systemic Sclerosis: Significance of Serum Apelin Levels in SSc. *J. Eur. Acad. Dermatol. Venereol.* **2013**, *27*, 37–42. [CrossRef]
151. Masui, Y.; Asano, Y.; Akamata, K.; Aozasa, N.; Noda, S.; Taniguchi, T.; Takahashi, T.; Ichimura, Y.; Toyama, T.; Sumida, H.; et al. Serum Resistin Levels: A Possible Correlation with Pulmonary Vascular Involvement in Patients with Systemic Sclerosis. *Rheumatol. Int.* **2014**, *34*, 1165–1170. [CrossRef] [PubMed]
152. Toyama, T.; Asano, Y.; Takahashi, T.; Aozasa, N.; Akamata, K.; Noda, S.; Taniguchi, T.; Ichimura, Y.; Sumida, H.; Tamaki, Z.; et al. Clinical Significance of Serum Retinol Binding Protein-4 Levels in Patients with Systemic Sclerosis: Significance of Serum RBP4 Levels in SSc. *J. Eur. Acad. Dermatol. Venereol.* **2013**, *27*, 337–344. [CrossRef] [PubMed]
153. Takahashi, T.; Asano, Y.; Noda, S.; Aozasa, N.; Akamata, K.; Taniguchi, T.; Ichimura, Y.; Toyama, T.; Sumida, H.; Kuwano, Y.; et al. A Possible Contribution of Lipocalin-2 to the Development of Dermal Fibrosis, Pulmonary Vascular Involvement and Renal Dysfunction in Systemic Sclerosis. *Br. J. Dermatol.* **2015**, *173*, 681–689. [CrossRef] [PubMed]
154. Miura, S.; Asano, Y.; Saigusa, R.; Yamashita, T.; Taniguchi, T.; Takahashi, T.; Ichimura, Y.; Toyama, T.; Tamaki, Z.; Tada, Y.; et al. Serum Omentin Levels: A Possible Contribution to Vascular Involvement in Patients with Systemic Sclerosis. *J. Dermatol.* **2015**, *42*, 461–466. [CrossRef]
155. Miura, S.; Asano, Y.; Saigusa, R.; Yamashita, T.; Taniguchi, T.; Takahashi, T.; Ichimura, Y.; Toyama, T.; Tamaki, Z.; Tada, Y.; et al. Serum Vaspin Levels: A Possible Correlation with Digital Ulcers in Patients with Systemic Sclerosis. *J. Dermatol.* **2015**, *42*, 528–531. [CrossRef]
156. Lakota, K.; Wei, J.; Carns, M.; Hinchcliff, M.; Lee, J.; Whitfield, M.L.; Sodin-Semrl, S.; Varga, J. Levels of Adiponectin, a Marker for PPAR-Gamma Activity, Correlate with Skin Fibrosis in Systemic Sclerosis: Potential Utility as Biomarker? *Arthritis Res. Ther.* **2012**, *14*, R102. [CrossRef]
157. Tomčík, M.; Arima, K.; Hulejová, H.; Kuklová, M.; Filková, M.; Braun, M.; Beláček, J.; Novák, M.; Bečvář, R.; Vencovský, J.; et al. Adiponectin Relation to Skin Changes and Dyslipidemia in Systemic Sclerosis. *Cytokine* **2012**, *58*, 165–168. [CrossRef]
158. Arakawa, H.; Jinnin, M.; Muchemwa, F.C.; Makino, T.; Kajihara, I.; Makino, K.; Honda, N.; Sakai, K.; Fukushima, S.; Ihn, H. Adiponectin Expression Is Decreased in the Involved Skin and Sera of Diffuse Cutaneous Scleroderma Patients: Letter to the Editor. *Exp. Dermatol.* **2011**, *20*, 764–766. [CrossRef]
159. Marangoni, R.G.; Masui, Y.; Fang, F.; Korman, B.; Lord, G.; Lee, J.; Lakota, K.; Wei, J.; Scherer, P.E.; Otvos, L.; et al. Adiponectin Is an Endogenous Anti-Fibrotic Mediator and Therapeutic Target. *Sci. Rep.* **2017**, *7*, 4397. [CrossRef]
160. Yamashita, T.; Lakota, K.; Taniguchi, T.; Yoshizaki, A.; Sato, S.; Hong, W.; Zhou, X.; Sodin-Semrl, S.; Fang, F.; Asano, Y.; et al. An Orally-Active Adiponectin Receptor Agonist Mitigates Cutaneous Fibrosis, Inflammation and Microvascular Pathology in a Murine Model of Systemic Sclerosis. *Sci. Rep.* **2018**, *8*, 11843. [CrossRef]
161. Sjogren, R. Gastrointestinal Features of Scleroderma. *Curr. Opin. Rheumatol.* **1996**, *8*, 569–575. [CrossRef] [PubMed]
162. Poirier, T.; Rankin, G. Gastrointestinal Manifestations of Progressive Systemic Scleroderma Based on a Review of 364 Cases. *Am. J. Gastroenterol.* **1972**, *58*, 30–44. [PubMed]
163. Young, M.A.; Rose, S.; Reynolds, J.C. Gastrointestinal Manifestations of Scleroderma. *Rheum. Dis. Clin. N. Am.* **1996**, *22*, 797–823. [CrossRef]
164. Emmanuel, A. Current Management of the Gastrointestinal Complications of Systemic Sclerosis. *Nat. Rev. Gastroenterol. Hepatol.* **2016**, *13*, 461–472. [CrossRef] [PubMed]
165. Lock, G.; Holstege, A.; Lang, B.; Schölmerich, J. Gastrointestinal Manifestations of Progressive Systemic Sclerosis. *Am. J. Gastroenterol.* **1997**, *92*, 763–771.
166. Malandrini, A.; Selvi, E.; Villanova, M.; Berti, G.; Sabadini, L.; Salvadori, C.; Gambelli, S.; De Stefano, R.; Vernillo, R.; Marcolongo, R.; et al. Autonomic Nervous System and Smooth Muscle Cell Involvement in Systemic Sclerosis: Ultrastructural Study of 3 Cases. *J. Rheumatol.* **2000**, *27*, 1203–1206.
167. Lepri, G.; Guiducci, S.; Bellando-Randone, S.; Giani, I.; Bruni, C.; Blagojevic, J.; Carnesecchi, G.; Radicati, A.; Pucciani, F.; Marco, M.-C. Evidence for Oesophageal and Anorectal Involvement in Very Early Systemic Sclerosis (VEDOSS): Report from a Single VEDOSS/EUSTAR Centre. *Ann. Rheum. Dis.* **2015**, *74*, 124–128. [CrossRef]
168. Weston, S.; Thumshirn, M.; Wiste, J.; Camilleri, M. Clinical and Upper Gastrointestinal Motility Features in Systemic Sclerosis and Related Disorders. *Am. J. Gastroenterol.* **1998**, *93*, 1085–1089. [CrossRef]
169. Roman, S.; Hot, A.; Fabien, N.; Cordier, J.-F.; Miossec, P.; Ninet, J.; Mion, F.; Réseau Sclérodermie des Hospices Civils de Lyon. Esophageal Dysmotility Associated with Systemic Sclerosis: A High-Resolution Manometry Study: Systemic Sclerosis and Esophageal HRM. *Dis. Esophagus* **2011**, *24*, 299–304. [CrossRef]
170. van Leeuwen, N.M.; Boonstra, M.; Fretheim, H.; Brunborg, C.; Midtvedt, Ø.; Garen, T.; Molberg, Ø.; Huizinga, T.W.J.; de Vries-Bouwstra, J.K.; Hoffman-Vold, A.-M. Gastrointestinal Symptom Severity and Progression in Systemic Sclerosis. *Rheumatology* **2022**, *61*, 4024–4034. [CrossRef]

171. Eaker, E.Y.; Kuldau, J.G.; Verne, G.N.; Ross, S.O.; Sallustio, J.E. Myenteric Neuronal Antibodies in Scleroderma: Passive Transfer Evokes Alterations in Intestinal Myoelectric Activity in a Rat Model. *J. Lab. Clin. Med.* **1999**, *133*, 551–556. [CrossRef] [PubMed]
172. Kawaguchi, Y.; Nakamura, Y.; Matsumoto, I.; Nishimagi, E.; Satoh, T.; Kuwana, M.; Sumida, T.; Hara, M. Muscarinic-3 Acetylcholine Receptor Autoantibody in Patients with Systemic Sclerosis: Contribution to Severe Gastrointestinal Tract Dysmotility. *Ann. Rheum. Dis.* **2009**, *68*, 710–714. [CrossRef]
173. Singh, J.; Mehendiratta, V.; Del Galdo, F.; Jimenez, S.A.; Cohen, S.; DiMarino, A.J.; Rattan, S. Immunoglobulins from Scleroderma Patients Inhibit the Muscarinic Receptor Activation in Internal Anal Sphincter Smooth Muscle Cells. *Am. J. Physiol. Gastrointest. Liver Physiol.* **2009**, *297*, G1206–G1213. [CrossRef]
174. Kafaja, S.; Valera, I.; Divekar, A.A.; Saggar, R.; Abtin, F.; Furst, D.E.; Khanna, D.; Singh, R.R. PDCs in Lung and Skin Fibrosis in a Bleomycin-Induced Model and Patients with Systemic Sclerosis. *JCI Insight* **2018**, *3*, e98380. [CrossRef] [PubMed]
175. Dantas, R.O.; Aprile, L.R.O. Esophageal Striated Muscle Contractions in Patients with Gastroesophageal Reflux Symptoms. *Dig. Dis. Sci.* **2002**, *47*, 2586–2590. [CrossRef] [PubMed]
176. Miwa, H.; Kondo, T.; Oshima, T. Gastroesophageal Reflux Disease-Related and Functional Heartburn: Pathophysiology and Treatment. *Curr. Opin. Gastroenterol.* **2016**, *32*, 344–352. [CrossRef]
177. Dessein, P.H.; Joffe, B.I.; Metz, R.M.; Millar, D.L.; Lawson, M.; Stanwix, A.E. Autonomic Dysfunction in Systemic Sclerosis: Sympathetic Overactivity and Instability. *Am. J. Med.* **1992**, *93*, 143–150. [CrossRef]
178. Zhong, D.; Wu, C.; Zeng, X.; Wang, Q. The Role of Gut Microbiota in the Pathogenesis of Rheumatic Diseases. *Clin. Rheumatol.* **2018**, *37*, 25–34. [CrossRef]
179. De Luca, F.; Shoenfeld, Y. The Microbiome in Autoimmune Diseases. *Clin. Exp. Immunol.* **2019**, *195*, 74–85. [CrossRef]
180. Rosser, E.C.; Mauri, C. A Clinical Update on the Significance of the Gut Microbiota in Systemic Autoimmunity. *J. Autoimmun.* **2016**, *74*, 85–93. [CrossRef]
181. Bellocchi, C.; Volkmann, E.R. Update on the Gastrointestinal Microbiome in Systemic Sclerosis. *Curr. Rheumatol. Rep.* **2018**, *20*, 49. [CrossRef] [PubMed]
182. Volkmann, E.R. Intestinal Microbiome in Scleroderma: Recent Progress. *Curr. Opin. Rheumatol.* **2017**, *29*, 553–560. [CrossRef] [PubMed]
183. Fretheim, H.; Chung, B.K.; Didriksen, H.; Bækkevold, E.S.; Midtvedt, Ø.; Brunborg, C.; Holm, K.; Valeur, J.; Tennøe, A.H.; Garen, T.; et al. Fecal Microbiota Transplantation in Systemic Sclerosis: A Double-Blind, Placebo-Controlled Randomized Pilot Trial. *PLoS ONE* **2020**, *15*, e0232739. [CrossRef]
184. Steen, V.D.; Medsger, T.A. Changes in Causes of Death in Systemic Sclerosis, 1972-2002. *Ann. Rheum. Dis.* **2007**, *66*, 940–944. [CrossRef]
185. Elhai, M.; Meune, C.; Boubaya, M.; Avouac, J.; Hachulla, E.; Balbir-Gurman, A.; Riemekasten, G.; Airò, P.; Joven, B.; Vettori, S.; et al. Mapping and Predicting Mortality from Systemic Sclerosis. *Ann. Rheum. Dis.* **2017**, *76*, 1897–1905. [CrossRef]
186. Simonneau, G.; Montani, D.; Celermajer, D.S.; Denton, C.P.; Gatzoulis, M.A.; Krowka, M.; Williams, P.G.; Souza, R. Haemodynamic Definitions and Updated Clinical Classification of Pulmonary Hypertension. *Eur. Respir. J.* **2019**, *53*, 1801913. [CrossRef]
187. Duarte, A.C.; Cordeiro, A.; Loureiro, M.J.; Ferreira, F. Pulmonary Veno-Occlusive Disease: A Probably Underdiagnosed Cause of Pulmonary Hypertension in Systemic Sclerosis. *Clin. Rheumatol.* **2020**, *39*, 1687–1691. [CrossRef]
188. Hassan, H.J.; Naranjo, M.; Ayoub, N.; Housten, T.; Hsu, S.; Balasubramanian, A.; Simpson, C.E.; Damico, R.L.; Mathai, S.C.; Kolb, T.M.; et al. Improved Survival for Patients with Systemic Sclerosis-Associated Pulmonary Arterial Hypertension: The Johns Hopkins Registry. *Am. J. Respir. Crit. Care Med.* **2023**, *207*, 312–322. [CrossRef] [PubMed]
189. Guillén-Del-Castillo, A.; Meseguer, M.L.; Fonollosa-Plá, V.; Giménez, B.S.; Colunga-Argüelles, D.; Revilla-López, E.; Rubio-Rivas, M.; Ropero, M.J.C.; Argibay, A.; Barberà, J.; et al. Impact of Interstitial Lung Disease on the Survival of Systemic Sclerosis with Pulmonary Arterial Hypertension. *Sci. Rep.* **2022**, *12*, 5289. [CrossRef]
190. Zamanian, R.T.; Badesch, D.; Chung, L.; Domsic, R.T.; Medsger, T.; Pinckney, A.; Keyes-Elstein, L.; D'Aveta, C.; Spychala, M.; White, R.J.; et al. Safety and Efficacy of B-Cell Depletion with Rituximab for the Treatment of Systemic Sclerosis-Associated Pulmonary Arterial Hypertension: A Multicenter, Double-Blind, Randomized, Placebo-Controlled Trial. *Am. J. Respir. Crit. Care Med.* **2021**, *204*, 209–221. [CrossRef]
191. Liem, S.I.E.; Boonstra, M.; le Cessie, S.; Riccardi, A.; Airo, P.; Distler, O.; Matucci-Cerinic, M.; Caimmi, C.; Siegert, E.; Allanore, Y.; et al. Sex-Specific Risk of Anti-Topoisomerase Antibodies on Mortality and Disease Severity in Systemic Sclerosis: 10-Year Analysis of the Leiden CCISS and EUSTAR Cohorts. *Lancet Rheumatol.* **2022**, *4*, e699–e709. [CrossRef] [PubMed]
192. Rubio-Rivas, M.; Homs, N.A.; Cuartero, D.; Corbella, X. The Prevalence and Incidence Rate of Pulmonary Arterial Hypertension in Systemic Sclerosis: Systematic Review and Meta-Analysis. *Autoimmun. Rev.* **2021**, *20*, 102713. [CrossRef]
193. Brown, Z.; Proudman, S.; Morrisroe, K.; Stevens, W.; Hansen, D.; Nikpour, M. Screening for the Early Detection of Pulmonary Arterial Hypertension in Patients with Systemic Sclerosis: A Systematic Review and Meta-Analysis of Long-Term Outcomes. *Semin. Arthritis Rheum.* **2021**, *51*, 495–512. [CrossRef]

194. Daraban, A.M.; Enache, R.; Predescu, L.; Platon, P.; Constantinescu, T.; Mihai, C.; Coman, I.M.; Ginghina, C.; Jurcuţ, R. Pulmonary Veno-Occlusive Disease: A Rare Cause of Pulmonary Hypertension in Systemic Sclerosis. Case Presentation and Review of the Literature. *Rom. J. Intern. Med.* **2015**, *53*, 175–183. [CrossRef] [PubMed]
195. Steele, R.; Hudson, M.; Lo, E.; Baron, M.; Canadian Scleroderma Research Group. Clinical Decision Rule to Predict the Presence of Interstitial Lung Disease in Systemic Sclerosis. *Arthritis Care Res.* **2012**, *64*, 519–524. [CrossRef] [PubMed]
196. White, B. Interstitial Lung Disease in Scleroderma. *Rheum. Dis. Clin. N. Am.* **2003**, *29*, 371–390. [CrossRef]
197. Nihtyanova, S.I.; Schreiber, B.E.; Ong, V.H.; Rosenberg, D.; Moinzadeh, P.; Coghlan, J.G.; Wells, A.U.; Denton, C.P. Prediction of Pulmonary Complications and Long-Term Survival in Systemic Sclerosis: Pulmonary Complications and Survival in SSc. *Arthritis Rheumatol.* **2014**, *66*, 1625–1635. [CrossRef]
198. Steen, V.; Domsic, R.T.; Lucas, M.; Fertig, N.; Medsger, T.A., Jr. A Clinical and Serologic Comparison of African American and Caucasian Patients with Systemic Sclerosis. *Arthritis Rheum.* **2012**, *64*, 2986–2994. [CrossRef]
199. Jaeger, V.K.; Wirz, E.G.; Allanore, Y.; Rossbach, P.; Riemekasten, G.; Hachulla, E.; Distler, O.; Airò, P.; Carreira, P.E.; Balbir Gurman, A.; et al. Incidences and Risk Factors of Organ Manifestations in the Early Course of Systemic Sclerosis: A Longitudinal EUSTAR Study. *PLoS ONE* **2016**, *11*, e0163894. [CrossRef]
200. Ostojić, P.; Damjanov, N. Different Clinical Features in Patients with Limited and Diffuse Cutaneous Systemic Sclerosis. *Clin. Rheumatol.* **2006**, *25*, 453–457. [CrossRef]
201. Asano, Y.; Ihn, H.; Yamane, K.; Kubo, M.; Tamaki, K. The Prevalence and Clinical Significance of Anti-U1 RNA Antibodies in Patients with Systemic Sclerosis. *J. Investig. Dermatol.* **2003**, *120*, 204–210. [CrossRef]
202. Man, A.; Davidyock, T.; Ferguson, L.T.; Ieong, M.; Zhang, Y.; Simms, R.W. Changes in Forced Vital Capacity over Time in Systemic Sclerosis: Application of Group-Based Trajectory Modelling. *Rheumatology* **2015**, *54*, 1464–1471. [CrossRef] [PubMed]
203. Steen, V.D.; Conte, C.; Owens, G.R.; Medsger, T.A., Jr. Severe Restrictive Lung Disease in Systemic Sclerosis. *Arthritis Rheum.* **1994**, *37*, 1283–1289. [CrossRef] [PubMed]
204. Morgan, C.; Knight, C.; Lunt, M.; Black, C.M.; Silman, A.J. Predictors of End Stage Lung Disease in a Cohort of Patients with Scleroderma. *Ann. Rheum. Dis.* **2003**, *62*, 146–150. [CrossRef]
205. Bouros, D.; Wells, A.U.; Nicholson, A.G.; Colby, T.V.; Polychronopoulos, V.; Pantelidis, P.; Haslam, P.L.; Vassilakis, D.A.; Black, C.M.; du Bois, R.M. Histopathologic Subsets of Fibrosing Alveolitis in Patients with Systemic Sclerosis and Their Relationship to Outcome. *Am. J. Respir. Crit. Care Med.* **2002**, *165*, 1581–1586. [CrossRef]
206. Kim, D.S.; Yoo, B.; Lee, J.S.; Kim, E.K.; Lim, C.M.; Lee, S.D.; Koh, Y.; Kim, W.S.; Kim, W.D.; Colby, T.V.; et al. The Major Histopathologic Pattern of Pulmonary Fibrosis in Scleroderma Is Nonspecific Interstitial Pneumonia. *Sarcoidosis Vasc. Diffuse Lung Dis.* **2002**, *19*, 121–127.
207. Fischer, A.; Swigris, J.J.; Groshong, S.D.; Cool, C.D.; Sahin, H.; Lynch, D.A.; Curran-Everett, D.; Gillis, J.Z.; Meehan, R.T.; Brown, K.K. Clinically Significant Interstitial Lung Disease in Limited Scleroderma: Histopathology, Clinical Features, and Survival. *Chest* **2008**, *134*, 601–605. [CrossRef]
208. Winstone, T.A.; Assayag, D.; Wilcox, P.G.; Dunne, J.V.; Hague, C.J.; Leipsic, J.; Collard, H.R.; Ryerson, C.J. Predictors of Mortality and Progression in Scleroderma-Associated Interstitial Lung Disease: A Systematic Review. *Chest* **2014**, *146*, 422–436. [CrossRef] [PubMed]
209. Beon, M.; Harley, R.A.; Wessels, A.; Silver, R.M.; Ludwicka-Bradley, A. Myofibroblast Induction and Microvascular Alteration in Scleroderma Lung Fibrosis. *Clin. Exp. Rheumatol.* **2004**, *22*, 733–742.
210. Savarino, E.; Bazzica, M.; Zentilin, P.; Pohl, D.; Parodi, A.; Cittadini, G.; Negrini, S.; Indiveri, F.; Tutuian, R.; Savarino, V.; et al. Gastroesophageal Reflux and Pulmonary Fibrosis in Scleroderma: A Study Using PH-Impedance Monitoring: A Study Using PH-Impedance Monitoring. *Am. J. Respir. Crit. Care Med.* **2009**, *179*, 408–413. [CrossRef]
211. Appel, J.Z., 3rd; Lee, S.M.; Hartwig, M.G.; Li, B.; Hsieh, C.-C.; Cantu, E., 3rd; Yoon, Y.; Lin, S.S.; Parker, W.; Davis, R.D. Characterization of the Innate Immune Response to Chronic Aspiration in a Novel Rodent Model. *Respir. Res.* **2007**, *8*, 87. [CrossRef] [PubMed]
212. Christmann, R.B.; Wells, A.U.; Capelozzi, V.L.; Silver, R.M. Gastroesophageal Reflux Incites Interstitial Lung Disease in Systemic Sclerosis: Clinical, Radiologic, Histopathologic, and Treatment Evidence. *Semin. Arthritis Rheum.* **2010**, *40*, 241–249. [CrossRef]
213. de Souza, R.B.C.; Borges, C.T.L.; Capelozzi, V.L.; Parra, E.R.; Jatene, F.B.; Kavakama, J.; Kairalla, R.A.; Bonfá, E. Centrilobular Fibrosis: An Underrecognized Pattern in Systemic Sclerosis. *Respiration* **2009**, *77*, 389–397. [CrossRef] [PubMed]
214. Venalis, P.; Kumánovics, G.; Schulze-Koops, H.; Distler, A.; Dees, C.; Zerr, P.; Palumbo-Zerr, K.; Czirják, L.; Mackevic, Z.; Lundberg, I.E.; et al. Cardiomyopathy in Murine Models of Systemic Sclerosis: Histopathologic Features of Cardiomyopathy in SSc. *Arthritis Rheumatol.* **2015**, *67*, 508–516. [CrossRef]
215. Allanore, Y.; Meune, C. Primary Myocardial Involvement in Systemic Sclerosis: Evidence for a Microvascular Origin. *Clin. Exp. Rheumatol.* **2010**, *28*, S48–S53.

216. Hachulla, A.-L.; Launay, D.; Gaxotte, V.; de Groote, P.; Lamblin, N.; Devos, P.; Hatron, P.-Y.; Beregi, J.-P.; Hachulla, E. Cardiac Magnetic Resonance Imaging in Systemic Sclerosis: A Cross-Sectional Observational Study of 52 Patients. *Ann. Rheum. Dis.* **2009**, *68*, 1878–1884. [CrossRef]
217. Hesselstrand, R.; Scheja, A.; Akesson, A. Mortality and Causes of Death in a Swedish Series of Systemic Sclerosis Patients. *Ann. Rheum. Dis.* **1998**, *57*, 682–686. [CrossRef] [PubMed]
218. Ioannidis, J.P.A.; Vlachoyiannopoulos, P.G.; Haidich, A.-B.; Medsger, T.A., Jr.; Lucas, M.; Michet, C.J.; Kuwana, M.; Yasuoka, H.; van den Hoogen, F.; Te Boome, L.; et al. Mortality in Systemic Sclerosis: An International Meta-Analysis of Individual Patient Data. *Am. J. Med.* **2005**, *118*, 2–10. [CrossRef]
219. Steen, V.D.; Medsger, T.A., Jr. Severe Organ Involvement in Systemic Sclerosis with Diffuse Scleroderma. *Arthritis Rheum.* **2000**, *43*, 2437–2444. [CrossRef]
220. Kahan, A.; Coghlan, G.; McLaughlin, V. Cardiac Complications of Systemic Sclerosis. *Rheumatology* **2009**, *48* (Suppl. S3), iii45–iii48. [CrossRef]
221. Allanore, Y.; Meune, C.; Kahan, A. Outcome Measures for Heart Involvement in Systemic Sclerosis. *Rheumatology* **2008**, *47* (Suppl. S5), v51–v53. [CrossRef] [PubMed]
222. Ferri, C.; Valentini, G.; Cozzi, F.; Sebastiani, M.; Michelassi, C.; La Montagna, G.; Bullo, A.; Cazzato, M.; Tirri, E.; Storino, F.; et al. Systemic Sclerosis: Demographic, Clinical, and Serologic Features and Survival in 1,012 Italian Patients. *Medicine* **2002**, *81*, 139–153. [CrossRef] [PubMed]
223. Purevsuren, M.; Uehara, M.; Ishizuka, M.; Suzuki, Y.; Shimbo, M.; Kakuda, N.; Ishii, S.; Sumida, H.; Miyazaki, M.; Yamashita, T.; et al. Native T1 Mapping in Early Diffuse and Limited Systemic Sclerosis, and Its Association with Diastolic Function. *J. Cardiol.* **2023**, *82*, 100–107. [CrossRef]
224. Bulkley, B.H.; Ridolfi, R.L.; Salyer, W.R.; Hutchins, G.M. Myocardial Lesions of Progressive Systemic Sclerosis. A Cause of Cardiac Dysfunction. *Circulation* **1976**, *53*, 483–490. [CrossRef] [PubMed]
225. Belloli, L.; Carlo-Stella, N.; Ciocia, G.; Chiti, A.; Massarotti, M.; Marasini, B. Myocardial Involvement in Systemic Sclerosis. *Rheumatology* **2008**, *47*, 1070–1072. [CrossRef]
226. Desai, C.S.; Lee, D.C.; Shah, S.J. Systemic Sclerosis and the Heart: Current Diagnosis and Management. *Curr. Opin. Rheumatol.* **2011**, *23*, 545–554. [CrossRef]
227. Tzelepis, G.E.; Kelekis, N.L.; Plastiras, S.C.; Mitseas, P.; Economopoulos, N.; Kampolis, C.; Gialafos, E.J.; Moyssakis, I.; Moutsopoulos, H.M. Pattern and Distribution of Myocardial Fibrosis in Systemic Sclerosis: A Delayed Enhanced Magnetic Resonance Imaging Study. *Arthritis Rheum.* **2007**, *56*, 3827–3836. [CrossRef]
228. Lekakis, J.; Mavrikakis, M.; Emmanuel, M.; Prassopoulos, V.; Papazoglou, S.; Papamichael, C.; Moulopoulou, D.; Kostamis, P.; Stamatelopoulos, S.; Moulopoulos, S. Cold-Induced Coronary Raynaud's Phenomenon in Patients with Systemic Sclerosis. *Clin. Exp. Rheumatol.* **1998**, *16*, 135–140.
229. Meune, C.; Allanore, Y.; Devaux, J.-Y.; Dessault, O.; Duboc, D.; Weber, S.; Kahan, A. High Prevalence of Right Ventricular Systolic Dysfunction in Early Systemic Sclerosis. *J. Rheumatol.* **2004**, *31*, 1941–1945.
230. Kahan, A.; Devaux, J.Y.; Amor, B.; Menkès, C.J.; Weber, S.; Venot, A.; Strauch, G. The Effect of Captopril on Thallium 201 Myocardial Perfusion in Systemic Sclerosis. *Clin. Pharmacol. Ther.* **1990**, *47*, 483–489. [CrossRef]
231. Duboc, D.; Kahan, A.; Maziere, B.; Loc'h, C.; Crouzel, C.; Menkès, C.J.; Amor, B.; Strauch, G.; Guérin, F.; Syrota, A. The Effect of Nifedipine on Myocardial Perfusion and Metabolism in Systemic Sclerosis. A Positron Emission Tomographic Study. *Arthritis Rheum.* **1991**, *34*, 198–203. [CrossRef] [PubMed]
232. Kahan, A.; Jy, D.; Amor, B.; Menkes, C.-J.; Weber, S.; Guerin, F.; Venot, A.; Strauch, G. Pharmacodynamic Effect of Nicardipine on Left Ventricular Function in Systemic Sclerosis. *J. Cardiovasc. Pharmacol.* **1990**, *15*, 249–253. [CrossRef] [PubMed]
233. Gigante, A.; Leodori, G.; Pellicano, C.; Villa, A.; Rosato, E. Assessment of Kidney Involvement in Systemic Sclerosis: From Scleroderma Renal Crisis to Subclinical Renal Vasculopathy. *Am. J. Med. Sci.* **2022**, *364*, 529–537. [CrossRef]
234. Lewandowski, B.; Domysławska, I.; Klimiuk, P.A.; Sierakowski, S. Kidney Crisis in Systemic Sclerosis. *Rocz. Akad. Med. Bialymst.* **2005**, *50* (Suppl. S1), 294–296.
235. Denton, C.P.; Lapadula, G.; Mouthon, L.; Müller-Ladner, U. Renal Complications and Scleroderma Renal Crisis. *Rheumatology* **2009**, *48* (Suppl. S3), iii32–iii35. [CrossRef]
236. Steen, V.D. Kidney Involvement in Systemic Sclerosis. *Presse Med.* **2014**, *43*, e305–e314. [CrossRef]
237. Cole, A.; Ong, V.H.; Denton, C.P. Renal Disease and Systemic Sclerosis: An Update on Scleroderma Renal Crisis. *Clin. Rev. Allergy Immunol.* **2023**, *64*, 378–391. [CrossRef] [PubMed]
238. Chang, M.; Wang, R.J.; Yangco, D.T.; Sharp, G.C.; Komatireddy, G.R.; Hoffman, R.W. Analysis of Autoantibodies against RNA Polymerases Using Immunoaffinity-Purifed RNA Polymerase I, II, and III Antigen in an Enzyme-Linked Immunosorbent Assay. *Clin. Immunol. Immunopathol.* **1998**, *89*, 71–78. [CrossRef]
239. Steen, V.D. Autoantibodies in Systemic Sclerosis. *Semin. Arthritis Rheum.* **2005**, *35*, 35–42. [CrossRef]

240. Santiago, M.; Baron, M.; Hudson, M.; Burlingame, R.W.; Fritzler, M.J. Antibodies to RNA Polymerase III in Systemic Sclerosis Detected by ELISA. *J. Rheumatol.* **2007**, *34*, 1528–1534.

241. Haviv, Y.S.; Safadi, R. Normotensive Scleroderma Renal Crisis: Case Report and Review of the Literature. *Ren. Fail.* **1998**, *20*, 733–736. [CrossRef] [PubMed]

242. Steen, V.D.; Medsger, T.A., Jr. Case-Control Study of Corticosteroids and Other Drugs That Either Precipitate or Protect from the Development of Scleroderma Renal Crisis. *Arthritis Rheum.* **1998**, *41*, 1613–1619. [CrossRef] [PubMed]

243. Sugimoto, T.; Soumura, M.; Danno, K.; Kaji, K.; Kondo, M.; Hirata, K.; Nakazawa, J.; Uzu, T.; Nishio, Y.; Kashiwagi, A. Scleroderma Renal Crisis in a Patient with Anticentromere Antibody-Positive Limited Cutaneous Systemic Sclerosis. *Mod. Rheumatol.* **2006**, *16*, 309–311. [CrossRef]

244. Sugimoto, T.; Sanada, M.; Kashiwagi, A. Is Scleroderma Renal Crisis with Anti-Centromere Antibody-Positive Limited Cutaneous Systemic Sclerosis Overlooked in Patients with Hypertension and/or Renal Dysfunction? *Nephrology* **2008**, *13*, 179–180. [CrossRef] [PubMed]

245. Batal, I.; Domsic, R.T.; Shafer, A.; Medsger, T.A., Jr.; Kiss, L.P.; Randhawa, P.; Bastacky, S. Renal Biopsy Findings Predicting Outcome in Scleroderma Renal Crisis. *Hum. Pathol.* **2009**, *40*, 332–340. [CrossRef]

246. Hudson, M.; Baron, M.; Tatibouet, S.; Furst, D.E.; Khanna, D.; International Scleroderma Renal Crisis Study Investigators. Exposure to ACE Inhibitors Prior to the Onset of Scleroderma Renal Crisis-Results from the International Scleroderma Renal Crisis Survey. *Semin. Arthritis Rheum.* **2014**, *43*, 666–672. [CrossRef]

247. Bose, N.; Chiesa-Vottero, A.; Chatterjee, S. Scleroderma Renal Crisis. *Semin. Arthritis Rheum.* **2015**, *44*, 687–694. [CrossRef]

248. Bütikofer, L.; Varisco, P.A.; Distler, O.; Kowal-Bielecka, O.; Allanore, Y.; Riemekasten, G.; Villiger, P.M.; Adler, S.; EUSTAR collaborators. ACE Inhibitors in SSc Patients Display a Risk Factor for Scleroderma Renal Crisis-a EUSTAR Analysis. *Arthritis Res. Ther.* **2020**, *22*, 59. [CrossRef]

249. Pope, J.E.; Denton, C.P.; Johnson, S.R.; Fernandez-Codina, A.; Hudson, M.; Nevskaya, T. State-of-the-Art Evidence in the Treatment of Systemic Sclerosis. *Nat. Rev. Rheumatol.* **2023**, *19*, 212–226. [CrossRef]

250. Campochiaro, C.; Allanore, Y. An Update on Targeted Therapies in Systemic Sclerosis Based on a Systematic Review from the Last 3 Years. *Arthritis Res. Ther.* **2021**, *23*, 155. [CrossRef]

251. Bukiri, H.; Volkmann, E.R. Current Advances in the Treatment of Systemic Sclerosis. *Curr. Opin. Pharmacol.* **2022**, *64*, 102211. [CrossRef] [PubMed]

252. Volkmann, E.R.; Andréasson, K.; Smith, V. Systemic Sclerosis. *Lancet* **2023**, *401*, 304–318. [CrossRef] [PubMed]

sclerosis

Review

Pathophysiology in Systemic Sclerosis: Current Insights and Future Perspectives

Suzan Al-Gburi [1,2,*], Pia Moinzadeh [1] and Thomas Krieg [1,2,3,4,*]

1 Department of Dermatology, University Hospital of Cologne, 50937 Cologne, Germany; pia.moinzadeh@uk-koeln.de
2 Translational Matrix Biology, Medical Faculty, University of Cologne, 50931 Cologne, Germany
3 Center for Molecular Medicine Cologne (CMMC), University of Cologne, 50931 Cologne, Germany
4 Cologne Excellence Cluster on Cellular Stress Responses in Ageing-Associated Diseases (CECAD), University of Cologne, 50931 Cologne, Germany
* Correspondence: suzan.al-gburi@uk-koeln.de (S.A.-G.); thomas.krieg@uni-koeln.de (T.K.)

Abstract: Background: Systemic sclerosis (SSc) is a rare connective tissue disease characterized by vasculopathy, autoimmunity, and fibrosis. Due to its low prevalence and heterogeneous clinical presentation, early diagnosis remains challenging, often delaying appropriate treatment. The disease progresses from microvascular dysfunction, manifesting as Raynaud's phenomenon, to systemic fibrosis affecting multiple organs, including the lungs, gastrointestinal tract, heart, and kidneys. There have been considerable advancements in understanding the pathophysiology of the disease during the last few years and this has already resulted in the improvement of the therapeutic approaches used to control organ-specific manifestations. However, the underlying cause of the disease still remains incompletely elucidated. **Methods:** Here, we summarize the current knowledge on the SSc pathogenesis. **Results:** The pathophysiology involves an interplay of chronic inflammation, impaired vascular function, and excessive extracellular matrix deposition, leading to progressive organ damage. Endothelial dysfunction in SSc is driven by immune-mediated injury, oxidative stress, and the imbalance of vasoconstrictors and vasodilators, leading to capillary loss and chronic hypoxia. Autoantibodies against endothelial cells or other toxic factors induce apoptosis and impair angiogenesis, further exacerbating vascular damage. Despite increased angiogenic factor levels, capillary repair mechanisms are defective, resulting in progressive ischemic damage. Dysregulated immune responses involving Th2 cytokines, B cells, and macrophages contribute to fibroblast activation and excessive collagen deposition. Transforming growth factor-beta (TGF-β) plays a central role in fibrotic progression, while fibroblasts resist apoptosis, perpetuating tissue scarring. The extracellular matrix in SSc is abnormally stiff, reinforcing fibroblast activation and creating a self-perpetuating fibrotic cycle. **Conclusions:** Advances in molecular and cellular understanding have facilitated targeted therapies, yet effective disease-modifying treatments remain limited. Future research should focus on precision medicine approaches, integrating biomarkers and novel therapeutics to improve patient outcomes.

Keywords: scleroderma; fibrosis; pathophysiology; extracellular matrix; inflammation; autoimmunity

1. Introduction

Systemic sclerosis (SSc) is a rare, complex connective tissue disease that presents significant challenges. Its low prevalence can often lead to delays in early diagnosis and the initiation of appropriate treatment [1]. Given the multi-organ complications, SSc patients require multidisciplinary management and continuous follow-up. Nonetheless, the pathomechanisms driving disease onset and progression remain incompletely understood.

Overall, SSc is uniquely defined by its combination of vasculopathy, autoimmunity, and fibrosis. However, vasculopathy is an early trigger, often manifesting as Raynaud's syndrome (Figure 1A), which can precede disease onset [2,3], serving as an early marker of microcirculatory dysfunction in the acral regions. As the disease progresses, digital ulceration (Figure 1B) may develop, sometimes leading to necrosis and eventual fingertip loss. Additionally, patients may experience extensive calcifications, severe pruritus, and prominent telangiectasias [2]. The clinical presentation of advanced SSc is highly characteristic and relatively easy to diagnose. However, early-stage cases are frequently overlooked, suggesting that the disease may be more prevalent than currently recognized [1]. Recent works by several groups have emphasized the need for the early detection of SSc and have developed the concept of VEDOSS (very early diagnoses of systemic sclerosis) [4]. In later stages or rapidly progressing subtypes, systemic involvement extends beyond the skin (Figure 1C), frequently affecting the internal organs. Pulmonary complications, particularly lung fibrosis and renal disease, are common. Gastrointestinal manifestations, such as reflux, gastric telangiectasia, and esophageal motility disorders, are observed in most patients, while musculoskeletal involvement is also frequent. Cardiac disease, though often underestimated, is likely more prevalent than previously thought [3,5–7]. Substantial progress in managing organ complications has led to an improved quality of life for many patients [8,9]. Nevertheless, developing disease-modifying therapies requires a deeper understanding of the pathophysiological events driving fibrosis and tissue damage [8,9].

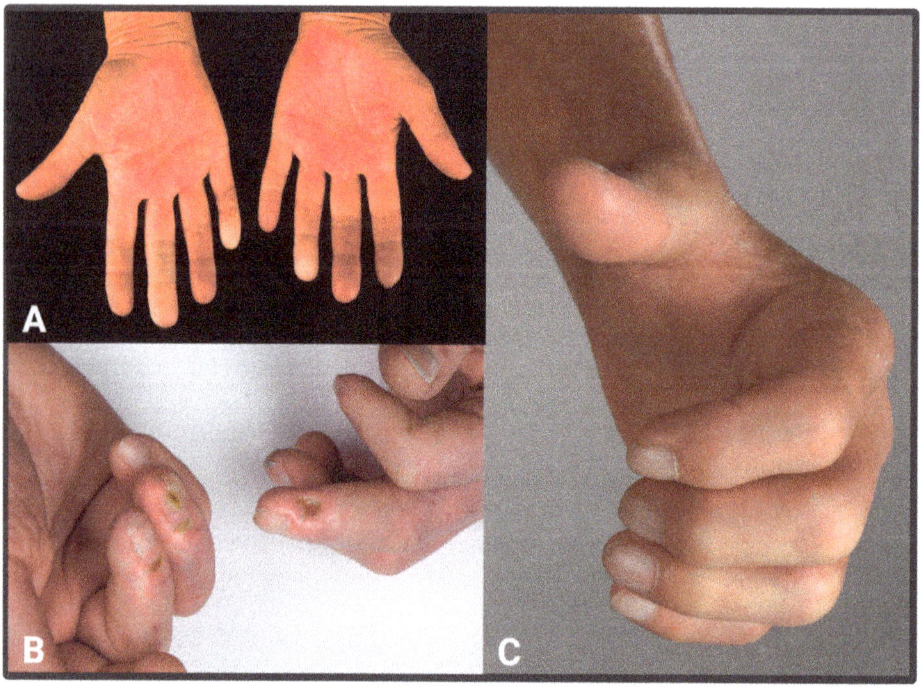

Figure 1. Clinical features of vasculopathy and fibrosis in SSc patients: (**A**) Raynaud's phenomenon; (**B**) digital ulcers; (**C**) severe stiffening of the skin leading to contractures.

In the following, we summarize the current knowledge on SSc pathogenesis and discuss how novel biomedical techniques have enhanced our understanding of fibrotic mechanisms.

2. Etiology and Risk Factors

Although the development of systemic sclerosis requires an (unknown) trigger, the involvement of genetic factors in the pathogenesis of SSc has been studied first in twin studies, analyzing human leucocyte antigen genes and more recently also in large multicenter genome-wide association studies. These have identified many genes (e.g., TNFSF4 (1q25.1), STAT4 (2q32.2-q32.3), DNASE1L3 (3p14.3), and IRF5-TNPO3 (7q32.1) or CD247) [10,11] that are involved in the control of vasculopathy and fibrosis and which are probably related to susceptibility to disease development. In addition, several environmental factors have been identified that lead to scleroderma or scleroderma-like conditions. Examples include silica dust, drugs, food contaminants, and others [12]. Although the exact mode of action of most compounds is still not understood, the data suggest that genetic susceptibility, together with external factors including potential viral infections [13], are crucial for the initial disease induction.

3. Vascular Alterations and Endothelial Damage in SSc

An interplay of autoimmune processes, vascular endothelial damage, and an overproduction of extracellular matrix (ECM) are crucial for pathophysiology and determine the clinical characteristics of this disease. In routine histology, the key stages of SSc pathogenesis can be detected: initial endothelial cell swelling followed by lympho-histiocytic inflammatory infiltration around affected blood vessels, and ultimately, dense extracellular matrix deposition with activated myofibroblasts and homogenized collagen bundles (Figure 2). Extensive research into the cellular and molecular alterations underlying these processes has facilitated the identification of novel therapeutic targets.

The Raynaud phenomenon (RP) usually manifests as a very characteristic and early clinical sign preceding sclerosis. Vascular changes can be easily detected clinically through nailfold microscopy [14], which can indicate vascular dysfunction even before the manifestation of fibrosis. These include early changes such as capillary ectasias, active patterns with megacapillaries and hemorrhages, and late changes that present as capillary bunching. The early inflammatory changes also appear histologically as prominent perivascular and periadnexial infiltrates [15,16].

Autopsy studies have shown widespread intimal proliferation affecting pulmonary, coronary, and renal arteries which is not inflammatory in nature. Early signs of vascular dysfunction include impaired permeability and tone, alongside an imbalance between vasoconstrictor endothelin (ET) [17] and vasodilator nitric oxide (NO) [18,19]. Platelet activation and coagulation abnormalities further contribute to the vasculopathy observed in SSc patients. The early stage of systemic sclerosis is also often clinically referred to as an edematous phase, as affected patients may experience swelling of the fingers ("puffy fingers") (Figure 1A) and milk glass opacities in the lungs, which are characteristic of alveolar or interstitial edema.

The exact cause of the initial vascular injury remains unclear, with potential contributors including infectious agents, cytotoxic T cells, and autoantibodies targeting endothelial cells [7,20]. Microcirculatory changes, such as capillary dropout and altered architecture, are prominent, alongside endothelial cell injury, which is central to the pathogenesis of SSc vasculopathy. It is hypothesized that chronic circulatory disturbance, with repetitive hypoxia and the release of Vascular Endothelial Growth Factor (VEGF) and TGF-β, increases vascular permeability. In addition, endothelial cell swelling and subsequent apoptosis occur (Figure 2), leading to the altered expression of adhesion molecules [2,21]. High levels of von Willebrand factor and ET-1 indicate endothelial damage, while conflicting reports exist regarding endothelial apoptosis [22]. As a result, fluid and blood extravasation occurs, along with the influx of immune cells. It remains unclear whether vascular leakage is the primary cause of immune cell infiltration or if the presence of inflammatory cells secondarily affects vascular permeability [23].

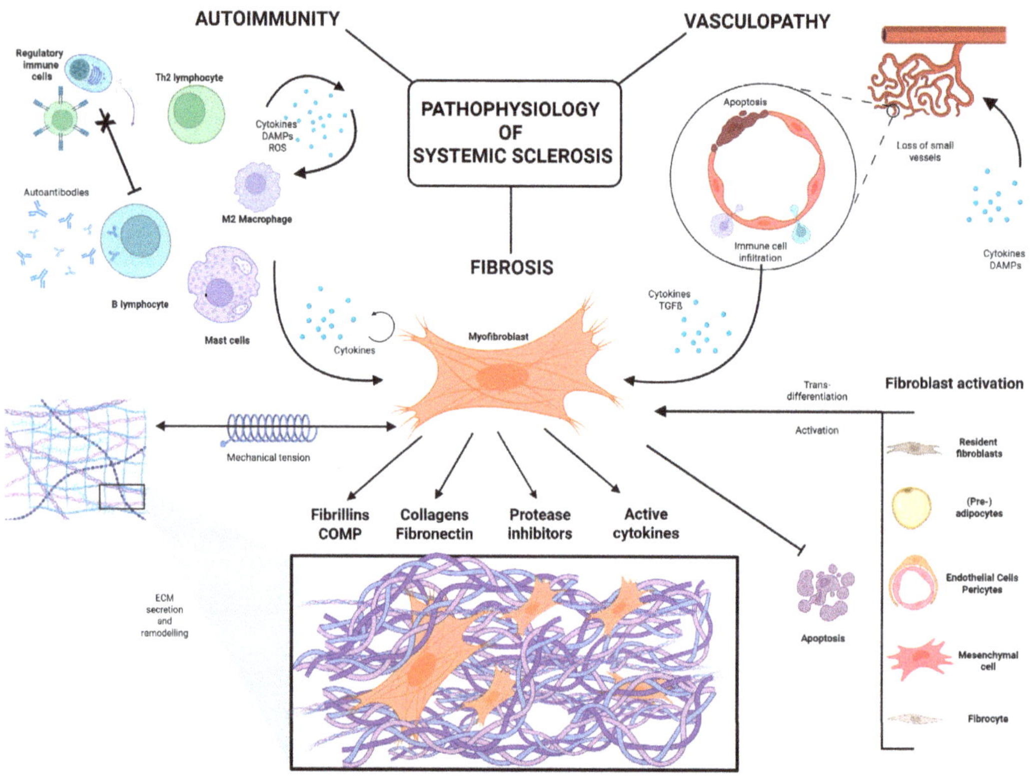

Figure 2. Pathophysiology in SSc: The pathogenesis of systemic sclerosis (SSc) involves a multifaceted interplay between vascular injury, immune dysregulation, and fibroblast activation, culminating in progressive fibrosis and organ dysfunction. Initial endothelial cell damage and immune cell infiltration lead to the loss of small vessels and the release of pro-inflammatory mediators, including cytokines, reactive oxygen species (ROS), and damage-associated molecular patterns (DAMPs). These activate both innate and adaptive immune cells such as Th2 lymphocytes, B cells, mast cells, and M2 macrophages. B cells generate pathogenic autoantibodies, while Th2 cytokines and TGF-β stimulate fibroblast activation and myofibroblast differentiation. Myofibroblasts, derived from multiple cellular sources including resident fibroblasts, (pre-)adipocytes, endothelial cells, and mesenchymal cells, excessively produce extracellular matrix (ECM) components such as collagens, fibronectin, and fibrillins. Mechanical tension within the ECM feeds back to further activate fibroblasts via integrin-mediated signaling. This positive feedback loop sustains a stiffened ECM environment, impairs fibroblast apoptosis, and perpetuates fibrosis. The figure illustrates the central role of myofibroblasts in ECM remodeling and the integration of immune, vascular, and fibrotic pathways in SSc progression. Created in BioRender. Al-Gburi, S. (2025) https://BioRender.com/hdz8tk7, accessed on 18 May 2025 [21].

Chronic inflammation promotes endothelial–mesenchymal transformation, which facilitates a profibrotic state (Figure 2). Endothelial cells play a key role in vasoregulation, tissue homeostasis, immune regulation, and platelet aggregation, as they act as "guards" between tissue and blood vessels, controlling various immunological processes. Endothelial dysfunction promotes a pro-inflammatory state [24]. Furthermore, many studies have shown that autoantibodies against endothelial cells (so-called anti-endothelial cell autoantibodies [AECAs]) can induce endothelial apoptosis [25]. These autoantibodies comprise a heterogeneous group of proteins that target various structures of endothelial cells and are found in approximately 22–86% of patients with systemic sclerosis. They stimulate the production of reactive oxygen species, the formation of PDGF (platelet-derived growth factor), and the expression of various adhesion molecules, such as VCAM-1, ICAM-1, and E-selectin, which facilitate leukocyte invasion [26]. Pericytes, which help stabilize blood vessels, may differentiate into various cell types and are involved in vascular changes in SSc [27].

Elevated levels of ET-1 have been linked to various SSc complications, promoting vasoconstriction and fibroblast activity [28]. Conversely, NO production is reduced, impairing vascular relaxation and contributing to enhanced platelet aggregation and oxidative injury [29].

Angiogenesis, the formation of new blood vessels [30,31], is disrupted in SSc, despite elevated levels of angiogenic factors like Vascular Endothelial Growth Factor (VEGF) [31]. This lack of response leads to significant capillary loss without significant new vessel formation. Additionally, vasculogenesis and the role of progenitor cells in vascular repair are not well understood, with conflicting evidence regarding their presence in SSc.

Altogether, endothelial dysfunction, particularly in microcirculation, appears to drive the early phases and progression of this disease. However, these vascular alterations can also be responsible for major clinical complications such as pulmonary arterial hypertension (PAH), digital ulcers, and renal crisis [32]. Conversely, vasoprotective or vasodilatory therapies, such as those with prostaglandin agonists, endothelin-1 receptor antagonists, and PDE5 inhibitors, positively influence vasculopathic complications [33].

4. Autoimmune Dysregulation in Systemic Sclerosis

Systemic sclerosis (SSc) is characterized by the dysregulated interplay between the innate and adaptive immune systems (Figure 2). Apoptotic and damaged endothelial cells release damage-associated molecular patterns (DAMPs), which recruit and activate immune cells [34]. This immune activation occurs even before overt endothelial cell damage is detectable and is driven by elevated levels of pro-inflammatory cytokines like interleukin (IL)-6 [35]. The interplay between vascular damage and immune activation perpetuates a self-sustaining cycle that exacerbates disease progression.

The adaptive immune system plays a crucial role in SSc pathogenesis (Figure 2), with type 2 helper T (Th2) cells being particularly active. These cells produce IL-4 and IL-13, which drive fibroblast proliferation, enhance extracellular matrix (ECM) production, and increase collagen synthesis. Additionally, IL-4 and IL-13 suppress matrix metalloproteinases (MMPs) [36], further contributing to ECM accumulation (Table 1). These cytokines stimulate the production of transforming growth factor-β (TGF-β), a central mediator of fibrosis that activates the SMAD and mitogen-activated protein kinase (MAPK) signaling pathways in fibroblasts [37]. This cascade promotes fibroblast proliferation and collagen deposition while inhibiting ECM degradation. Feedback loops involving TGF-β and Th2 cytokines sustain fibrosis in a vicious cycle.

B cells, including plasma cells and their precursors [38], significantly contribute to SSc by producing autoantibodies against DNA-topoisomerase 1, centromeres, endothelial cells, and other antigens [39]. Many of these autoantibodies are markers for disease development; other autoantibodies, e.g., targeting endothelial cells [25], PDGF receptors, and fibrillin-1, are thought to directly activate fibroblasts [40], stimulating collagen synthesis. Furthermore, B cells produce IL-6, which promotes Th2 differentiation (Table 1) and macrophage polarization toward the M2 phenotype. Dysregulated regulatory B cells (Bregs) exacerbate disease by reducing IL-10 production, which diminishes their immunosuppressive effects.

The innate immune system also plays a critical role in SSc (Figure 2). Macrophages, particularly M2 macrophages, contribute to both tissue repair and fibrosis by producing profibrotic cytokines, including TGF-β, IL-4, IL-13, and IL-6 [41–43]. These cytokines activate fibroblasts and drive ECM deposition (Table 1). Neutrophils contribute through the release of reactive oxygen species (ROS) [44] and neutrophil extracellular traps (NETs) [45,46], which liberate latent TGF-β from the ECM, amplifying fibrosis. Plasmacytoid dendritic cells (pDCs) further contribute by producing interferon-α (IFN-α) and chemokine CXCL4 [47], both of which sustain immune activation and chronic inflammation (Table 1). Enhanced Toll-like receptor-8 (TLR8) signaling in pDCs establishes a positive feedback loop that maintains this inflammatory state.

Mast cells play multifaceted roles in SSc, attracted to fibrotic lesions by local signals such as plasminogen activator inhibitor-1 (PAI-1). Upon activation, mast cells release profibrotic mediators, including TGF-β, PDGF [48], and fibronectin. Direct interactions between mast cells and fibroblasts via adhesion molecules like intercellular adhesion molecule-1 (ICAM-1) further contribute to ECM deposition [49]. However, studies suggest that fibrosis can progress independently of mast cells, highlighting the complexity of SSc pathogenesis [50].

The intricate interactions between immune cells and fibroblasts are central to SSc pathogenesis. Fibroblasts in affected tissues exhibit a profibrotic phenotype, producing excessive amounts of collagen and other ECM components. Cytokines like TGF-β, IL-4, and IL-13 [51] from immune cells reinforce this phenotype, perpetuating chronic inflammation and fibrosis (Table 1). Insights from animal models, such as tight-skin mice, have demonstrated that targeting these cytokines can reduce fibrosis [52]. Similarly, models of graft-versus-host disease (GVHD), which share features with SSc, have shown that inhibiting Th2 cytokines prevents fibrotic progression [53].

Taken together, SSc is driven by the complex interactions among endothelial dysfunction, immune dysregulation, and fibroblast activation. The crosstalk between immune cells and fibroblasts creates a self-perpetuating cycle of inflammation and fibrosis. The contributions of Th2 cells, B cells, macrophages, neutrophils, dendritic cells, and mast cells highlight the multifactorial nature of immune activation in SSc. Targeting key cytokines such as IL-4, IL-13, TGF-β, and IL-6 holds therapeutic potential (Table 1). Understanding these mechanisms provides crucial insights into developing targeted therapies aimed at modulating immune responses, reducing fibrosis, and improving vascular function in SSc patients.

Table 1. Cytokines, chemokines, and growth factors in systemic sclerosis.

Cytokines/chemokines/growth factors involved in vasculopathy		
Endothelin-1 (ET-1)	Potent vasoconstrictor; promotes vascular dysfunction, fibroblast activation, and is elevated in SSc patients. Involved in PAH and DU development.	[17,28]
Nitric Oxide (NO)	Vasodilator; its impaired production leads to vascular tone dysregulation, platelet aggregation, and oxidative injury.	[18,19,29]
Vascular Endothelial Growth Factor (VEGF)	Key factor for angiogenesis; elevated in SSc but ineffective, leading to defective capillary repair and progressive ischemia.	[30,31]
Platelet-Derived Growth Factor (PDGF)	Induces fibroblast proliferation, contributing to vascular remodeling and fibrosis; linked to vascular dysfunction in SSc.	[26,48]
CXCL4	Chemokine produced by plasmacytoid dendritic cells; amplifies immune activation, vascular injury, and fibrosis.	[47]
Interleukin-6 (IL-6)	Elevated early; drives endothelial activation, Th2 polarization, and chronic inflammation, and contributes to vascular damage.	[35,41]
Cytokines/chemokines/growth factors involved in fibrosis		
Transforming Growth Factor-β (TGF-β)	Master regulator of fibrosis; promotes fibroblast activation, ECM production, myofibroblast differentiation, and suppresses ECM degradation.	[37,54,55]
Interleukin-4 (IL-4)	Th2 cytokine; enhances fibroblast proliferation and collagen production, suppresses ECM degradation, and promotes fibrotic progression.	[36,51]
Interleukin-13 (IL-13)	Works alongside IL-4; boosts collagen synthesis and fibroblast proliferation; and sustains fibrotic cycles.	[36,51]
Interleukin-6 (IL-6)	In addition to vascular roles, promotes M2 macrophage polarization and enhances fibrotic signaling.	[41,43]
Interferon-α (IFN-α)	Produced by plasmacytoid dendritic cells; promotes immune activation and maintains fibrotic and inflammatory environments.	[47]
Oncostatin M	Produced by mononuclear cells; acts synergistically with IL-6 to stimulate fibroblast activation and fibrosis.	[41]
Connective Tissue Growth Factor (CTGF)	Acts downstream of TGF-β; critical in fibroblast activation and persistent ECM accumulation.	[56]
Osteopontin (OPN)	Pro-inflammatory glycoprotein promoting fibroblast activation, myofibroblast differentiation, ECM deposition, and chronic inflammation; linked to disease severity in SSc.	[57]
Interleukin-17 (IL-17)	Pro-inflammatory cytokine from Th17 cells; enhances fibroblast proliferation, collagen expression, and synergizes with TGF-β in fibrotic pathways.	[58,59]
Interleukin-11 (IL-11)	Promotes fibroblast activation, ECM production, and collagen deposition; implicated in lung and skin fibrosis. Revelant for cardiac and renal fibrosis.	[60,61]
Interleukin-31 (IL-31)	Associated with pruritus in SSc; emerging evidence suggests profibrotic roles via immune–fibroblast crosstalk.	[62,63]

5. Fibrosis and ECM Deposition in SSc

The excessive deposition of ECM molecules is a hallmark of scleroderma and is ultimately responsible for tissue damage with all the clinical implications (Figure 1C). The persistent activation of fibroblasts and their transformation into myofibroblasts play a critical role in this pathological process. Myofibroblasts are key mediators of ECM remodeling, and their sustained presence in SSc results in uncontrolled ECM synthesis, fibrosis, and ultimately, irreversible tissue damage (Figure 2).

5.1. Activation and Origin of Fibroblasts in SSc

The origins of activated fibroblasts in SSc remain a topic of extensive research [64,65]. They may arise from multiple sources, including circulating progenitor cells, subcutaneous layers, resident tissue fibroblasts, and transdifferentiated epithelial or endothelial cells (Figure 2). Once activated, fibroblasts acquire the characteristics of myofibroblasts, which are central to wound healing and scar formation. These cells exhibit contractile properties, express alpha-smooth muscle actin (α-SMA), and contribute to ECM production [66]. Under physiological conditions, myofibroblasts facilitate tissue repair and are subsequently eliminated through apoptosis [67]. However, in SSc, myofibroblasts are thought to persist due to a dysregulation in apoptotic pathways, leading to excessive ECM deposition. This results in increased tissue stiffness, reduced mechanical stability, and progressive fibrosis, ultimately impairing organ function [68–70] (Figure 2).

5.2. Fibroblast Survival and Resistance to Apoptosis

Myofibroblast survival in SSc is facilitated by an imbalance between pro-apoptotic and anti-apoptotic signals. Apoptosis, a crucial mechanism for eliminating excess myofibroblasts following tissue repair, is regulated by proteins such as BAX and BIM (pro-apoptotic) and BCL-2 family proteins (anti-apoptotic). In physiological wound healing, myofibroblasts undergo apoptosis when ECM stiffness decreases, reducing BCL-2 signaling and allowing BIM-mediated cell death [71–73].

In SSc, however, mechanotransduction pathways alter apoptotic signaling, increasing the expression of BIM while simultaneously upregulating BCL-XL, an anti-apoptotic protein that inhibits BIM activation. This allows myofibroblasts to evade apoptosis and continue producing ECM components. Experimental studies have shown that inhibiting BCL-XL can promote myofibroblast apoptosis [74].

Transforming growth factor-beta (TGFβ) is a key profibrotic cytokine implicated in SSc pathogenesis (Table 1). Elevated levels of TGFβ are observed in SSc skin and lung tissues, where it stimulates fibroblast activation, ECM synthesis, and myofibroblast differentiation [54,55]. TGFβ also influences apoptotic pathways by modulating sphingolipid metabolism, particularly through the downregulation of acid sphingomyelinase (ASMase), a critical enzyme in Fas-mediated apoptosis. Reduced ASMase levels in SSc fibroblasts are thought to promote apoptosis resistance and enhance fibrotic signaling [75]. MicroRNAs (miRNAs) further contribute to the apoptotic imbalance in SSc. miRNA-21, which is upregulated in SSc fibroblasts, binds to and degrades the mRNA of pro-apoptotic BAX, further suppressing myofibroblast apoptosis. This has been reported to create a pro-survival environment, perpetuating fibrosis and ECM accumulation [76].

In addition to reduced apoptosis, myofibroblast populations in SSc might expand due to increased transdifferentiation and activation. TGFβ, PDGF, and connective tissue growth factor (CTGF) drive fibroblast differentiation into myofibroblasts [56] (Table 1). However, circulating fibrocytes, epithelial–mesenchymal transition (EMT), endothelial-to-mesenchymal transition (EndoMT), and pericyte differentiation [77–79] might also contribute to this process (Figure 2).

A notable feature of SSc is the loss of subcutaneous adipose tissue. Adipocytes are increasingly recognized as contributors to fibrotic progression through adipocyte–myofibroblast transition (AMT). TGFβ stimulation of adipocytes inhibits adipogenesis and upregulates profibrotic genes, leading to the conversion of adipocytes into fibroblast-like cells. Both adipose-derived mesenchymal stem cells and mature adipocytes undergo this transition, contributing to the fibrosis seen in SSc patients (Figure 2).

Mechanical tension is a crucial regulator of fibroblast function and myofibroblast differentiation. In SSc, increased ECM stiffness enhances fibroblast activation via integrins and focal adhesion complexes. α11β1 integrin, in particular, plays a critical role in fibrosis by transducing the mechanical and biochemical signals that sustain myofibroblast activity. Depletion of α11β1 integrin has been shown to suppress fibrosis and impair fibroblast transdifferentiation. Increased mechanical tension also promotes TGFβ activation from its latent form in the ECM (Figure 2). TGFβ is sequestered within the ECM in an inactive state, but integrin-mediated tension releases active TGFβ, perpetuating fibroblast activation and ECM deposition. These findings highlight the interplay between mechanical and biochemical cues in fibrosis progression [80–84].

Fibroblasts are a heterogeneous population with distinct functional properties. Recent studies utilizing single-cell and bulk RNA sequencing have identified fibroblast subtypes that are enriched in SSc skin. Profibrotic fibroblasts expressing markers such as COMP, COL11A1, MYOC, CCL19, and SFRP4 are significantly increased, while antifibrotic fibroblasts marked by CXCL12 and PI16 are reduced. The balance between these fibroblast subsets correlates with disease severity. Increased levels of profibrotic fibroblasts are associated with progressive skin fibrosis, whereas higher proportions of CXCL12+ and PI16+ fibroblasts correlate with stable disease. Machine learning models incorporating fibroblast markers have improved the classification of progressive versus stable SSc cases, highlighting their potential as diagnostic and therapeutic targets [85].

5.3. The ECM in SSc

Fibrosis in SSc is characterized by the excessive deposition of collagen types I, III, V, and VI, as well as fibronectin, elastin, glycosaminoglycans, and proteoglycans. The ECM of SSc patients also contains increased levels of damage-associated molecular patterns (DAMPs), such as fibronectin-EDA and tenascin-C, which activate profibrotic pathways through toll-like receptor 4 (TLR4) signaling. Cartilage oligomeric matrix protein (COMP) is highly expressed in SSc and other fibrotic conditions. COMP regulates collagen fibrillogenesis and is essential for the ECM's structural integrity. It also facilitates collagen secretion, contributing to the excessive accumulation and altered macromolecular arrangement observed in fibrotic tissues [21].

Although the excessive deposition of different components of the ECM is characteristic for fibrotic processes, it also has to be noted that the stiffness of the tissue depends on the macromolecular organization of the collagens. This is determined by various factors. The so-called FACITs (fibril-associated collagens with interrupted triple helices) play a crucial role in controlling the macromolecular organization and the fibril diameter. In addition to their structural significance, these extracellular matrix (ECM) proteins can also have functional activities. It has been shown that collagen XII, a FACIT collagen in skin, significantly influences the number of myofibroblasts. Mechanistically, this can be attributed to the indirect communication between macrophages and fibroblasts, where collagen XII affects the release of fibrogenic cytokines by macrophages [86]. This is also true for other non-collagenous ECM proteins, such as COMP, which are induced during fibrotic processes [87]. All of these proteins have both structural and functional activities, alter the macromolecular organization and biomechanical properties of connective tissue, and regulate the function of fibroblasts, endothelial cells, and inflammatory cells in fibrotic processes (Figure 2).

6. Therapeutic Approaches for SSc Based on the Understanding of Its Pathophysiology

Understanding these mechanisms at a molecular level provides an insight into potential therapeutic strategies, including targeting apoptosis pathways, modulating TGFβ signaling, and disrupting mechanical tension-mediated fibroblast activation. Future research focusing on fibroblast heterogeneity and ECM dynamics will be crucial in developing effective treatments for SSc and related fibrotic diseases.

Recent technological breakthroughs and an improved understanding of disease mechanisms at the cellular and molecular levels have already led to better patient stratification and the development of novel therapeutic approaches. Clinical trials now benefit from molecular classification based on gene expression profiles in skin biopsies. While the predictive value of this classification is still being evaluated, it enhances patient selection for targeted therapies when combined with serum biomarkers and refined clinical criteria [88].

Therapeutic advancements have significantly improved the management of organ complications associated with SSc [89]. Mainly for diffuse cutaneous SSc patients, immunosuppressive agents such as mycophenolate mofetil, methotrexate, cyclophosphamide, rituximab, and tocilizumab are widely used [89–94], while patients with rapidly progressive disease may benefit from autologous hematopoietic stem cell transplantation [95]. Lung disease management has improved, with mycophenolate mofetil for SSc-ILD and antifibrotic agents like nintedanib [89,96] and possibly pirfenidone showing promise. PAH is commonly treated with combination therapy, including phosphodiesterase 5 inhibitors and endothelin receptor antagonists, sometimes supplemented with prostacyclin analogs. Most recently, sotatercept, a first-in-class activin-signaling inhibitor, has also been approved for the treatment of PAH [97]. Raynaud's phenomenon and digital ulcers are managed using calcium channel blockers, phosphodiesterase 5 inhibitors, and intravenous iloprost, with bosentan helping to prevent new ulcer formation [98–101]. However, more research is needed to optimize treatment strategies for other disease manifestations.

Novel compounds target the microvascular alterations, the immune response (e.g., JAK inhibitors, IL-4/IL-13 inhibitors, Belimumab), and also the different steps in the activation of myofibroblasts (e.g., TGFβ inhibitors, ROCK inhibitors, LPA inhibitors) [102].

Given the pivotal role of B cells in SSc pathogenesis, CD19-targeting chimeric antigen receptor (CAR) T cell therapy has emerged as a new approach for severe diffuse SSc in patients unresponsive to conventional treatments. Recent studies demonstrate that CAR T cell therapy can halt disease progression, improve key clinical features such as skin fibrosis and lung function, and reduce autoantibody levels.

Future research must assess the durability of these therapeutic effects and compare CAR T cell therapy with other advanced treatments, such as autologous stem cell transplantation and CD20-targeting therapies. All these new approaches have been developed based on a better understanding of the pathophysiology of this complex disease and mark a promising step toward more effective and potentially curative treatments for the benefit of patients with systemic sclerosis.

7. Conclusions

At the core of SSc pathogenesis lies a dynamic and self-reinforcing interplay between vascular injury, chronic immune activation, and fibroblast dysregulation. Early endothelial dysfunction—possibly triggered by genetic predisposition, environmental exposures, or infectious insults—leads to capillary dropout, impaired vasoregulation, and hypoxia. This vascular damage is compounded by the emergence of autoantibodies and the infiltration of various immune cells that further drive inflammation and fibrosis. Immune mediators, particularly Th2 cytokines (IL-4, IL-13), TGF-β, and IL-6 (Table 1), perpetuate fibroblast activation and ECM accumulation. Notably, fibroblasts in SSc not only become resistant to apoptosis but also exhibit enhanced mechanosensing capabilities that amplify fibrotic responses in the context of increased tissue stiffness.

Recent advances have further illuminated the cellular origins and heterogeneity of fibroblasts involved in SSc, uncovering key transcriptional and functional differences that correlate with disease activity and treatment response. Technologies such as single-cell RNA sequencing and machine learning models have identified distinct profibrotic and antifibrotic fibroblast populations, offering potential biomarkers for disease stratification and new targets for therapeutic intervention.

Therapeutically, while conventional immunosuppressive regimens remain standard in managing diffuse cutaneous disease and organ involvement, novel strategies are emerging from our improved understanding of disease biology. These include antifibrotic agents like nintedanib, biologics targeting cytokine pathways (e.g., IL-4/IL-13, IL-6) (Table 1), and cellular therapies such as autologous hematopoietic stem cell transplantation. In severe refractory cases, CAR T cell therapies targeting CD19+ B cells show early promise, demonstrating potential not only to halt disease progression but to reverse key pathological features.

However, despite these advancements, there is still no universally effective disease-modifying therapy for SSc. Many of the current interventions primarily address symptoms or specific organ manifestations without altering the fundamental disease trajectory. The variability in clinical course and treatment response among patients underscores the urgent need for precision medicine approaches. Integrating molecular classifications, serum biomarkers, and tissue-based gene expression profiles into clinical decision-making will be essential for tailoring therapy and improving long-term outcomes.

Funding: SA was funded by "Köln Fortune" [134/2023]. This research was funded by DFG [KR 558/17-1] and by Deutsche Forschungsgemeinschaft; Edith Busch Foundation.

Conflicts of Interest: P.M. reports lecture fees from Boehringer Ingelheim and Janssen, as well as advisory board fees of Almirall, unrelated to the present manuscript. T.K. and S.A.-G. declare no conflict of interest.

References

1. Volkmann, E.R.; Andréasson, K.; Smith, V. Systemic sclerosis. *Lancet* **2023**, *401*, 304–318. [CrossRef]
2. Gabrielli, A.; Avvedimento, E.V.; Krieg, T. Mechanisms of Disease Scleroderma. *N. Engl. J. Med.* **2009**, *360*, 1989–2003. [CrossRef]
3. Distler, J.H.W.; Györfi, A.-H.; Ramanujam, M.; Whitfield, M.L.; Königshoff, M.; Lafyatis, R. Shared and distinct mechanisms of fibrosis. *Nat. Rev. Rheumatol.* **2019**, *15*, 705–730. [CrossRef] [PubMed]
4. Ross, R.L.; Caballero-Ruiz, B.; Clarke, E.L.; Kakkar, V.; Wasson, C.W.; Mulipa, P.; De Lorenzis, E.; Merchant, W.; Di Donato, S.; Rindone, A.; et al. Biological hallmarks of systemic sclerosis are present in the skin and serum of patients with Very Early Diagnosis of Systemic Sclerosis (VEDOSS). *Rheumatology* **2024**, keae698, *ahead of print*. [CrossRef] [PubMed]
5. Varga, J.; Abraham, D. Systemic sclerosis: A prototypic multisystem fibrotic disorder. *J. Clin. Investigation.* **2007**, *117*, 557–567. [CrossRef] [PubMed]
6. Wynn, T.A.; Ramalingam, T.R. Mechanisms of fibrosis: Therapeutic translation for fibrotic disease. *Nat. Med.* **2012**, *18*, 1028–1040. [CrossRef]
7. Avouac, J.; Riemekasten, G.; Meune, C.; Ruiz, B.; Kahan, A.; Allanore, Y. Autoantibodies against endothelin 1 Type A receptor are strong predictors of digital ulcers in systemic sclerosis. *J. Rheumatol.* **2015**, *42*, 1801–1807. [CrossRef]
8. Lescoat, A.; Varga, J.; Matucci-Cerinic, M.; Khanna, D. New promising drugs for the treatment of systemic sclerosis: Pathogenic considerations, enhanced classifications, and personalized medicine. *Expert Opin. Investig. Drugs* **2021**, *30*, 635–652. [CrossRef]

9. Del Galdo, F.; Lescoat, A.; Conaghan, P.G.; Bertoldo, E.; Čolić, J.; Santiago, T.; Suliman, Y.A.; Matucci-Cerinic, M.; Gabrielli, A.; Distler, O.; et al. EULAR recommendations for the treatment of systemic sclerosis: 2023 update. *Ann. Rheum. Dis.* **2024**, *84*, 29–40. [CrossRef]
10. Broen, J.C.A.; Radstake, T.R.D.J.; Rossato, M. The role of genetics and epigenetics in the pathogenesis of systemic sclerosis. *Nat. Rev. Rheumatol.* **2014**, *10*, 671–681. [CrossRef]
11. López-Isac, E.; Acosta-Herrera, M.; Kerick, M.; Assassi, S.; Satpathy, A.T.; Granja, J.; Mumbach, M.R.; Beretta, L.; Simeón, C.P.; Carreira, P.; et al. GWAS for systemic sclerosis identifies multiple risk loci and highlights fibrotic and vasculopathy pathways. *Nat. Commun.* **2019**, *10*, 1–14. [CrossRef] [PubMed]
12. De Martinis, M.; Ciccarelli, F.; Sirufo, M.M.; Ginaldi, L. An overview of environmental risk factors in systemic sclerosis. *Expert Rev. Clin. Immunol.* **2016**, *12*, 465–478. [CrossRef]
13. Moroncini, G.; Svegliati, S.; Grieco, A.; Cuccioloni, M.; Mozzicafreddo, M.; Paolini, C.; Agarbati, S.; Spadoni, T.; Amoresano, A.; Pinto, G.; et al. Adeno-Associated Virus Type 5 Infection via PDGFRα Is Associated With Interstitial Lung Disease in Systemic Sclerosis and Generates Composite Peptides and Epitopes Recognized by the Agonistic Immunoglobulins Present in Patients With Systemic Sclerosis. *Arthritis Rheumatol.* **2024**, *76*, 620–630. [CrossRef]
14. Jung, P.; Trautinger, F. Kapillarmikroskopie. *JDDG-J. Ger. Soc. Dermatol.* **2013**, *11*, 731–736. [CrossRef]
15. Fieischmajer, R.; Perlish, J.S. Capillary Alterations in Scleroderma. *J. Am. Acad. Dermatol.* **1980**, *2*, 161–170. [CrossRef]
16. Smith, V.; Herrick, A.L.; Ingegnoli, F.; Damjanov, N.; De Angelis, R.; Denton, C.P.; Distler, O.; Espejo, K.; Foeldvari, I.; Frech, T.; et al. Standardisation of nailfold capillaroscopy for the assessment of patients with Raynaud's phenomenon and systemic sclerosis. *Autoimmun. Rev.* **2020**, *19*, 102458. [CrossRef] [PubMed]
17. Rokni, M.; Shaker, M.S.; Kavosi, H.; Shokoofi, S.; Mahmoudi, M.; Farhadi, E. The role of endothelin and RAS/ERK signaling in immunopathogenesis-related fibrosis in patients with systemic sclerosis: An updated review with therapeutic implications. *Arthritis Res. Ther.* **2022**, *24*, 1–13. [CrossRef] [PubMed]
18. Allanore, Y.; Borderie, D.; Hilliquin, P.; Hernvann, A.; Levacher, M.; Lemaréchal, H.; Ekindjian, O.G.; Kahan, A. Low Levels of Nitric Oxide (NO) in Systemic Sclerosis: Inducible NO Synthase Production Is Decreased in Cultured Peripheral Blood Monocyteumacrophage Cells. *Rheumatology* **2001**, *40*, 1089–1096. [CrossRef]
19. Hinz, B. The role of myofibroblasts in wound healing. *Curr. Res. Transl. Med.* **2016**, *64*, 171–177. [CrossRef] [PubMed]
20. Binda, M.; Moccaldi, B.; Civieri, G.; Cuberli, A.; Doria, A.; Tona, F.; Zanatta, E. Autoantibodies Targeting G-Protein-Coupled Receptors: Pathogenetic, Clinical and Therapeutic Implications in Systemic Sclerosis. *Int. J. Mol. Sci.* **2024**, *25*, 2299. [CrossRef]
21. Rosendahl, A.; Schönborn, K.; Krieg, T. Pathophysiology of systemic sclerosis (scleroderma). *Kaohsiung J. Med. Sci.* **2022**, *38*, 187–195. [CrossRef] [PubMed]
22. Su, J.; An, X.-R.; Li, Q.; Li, X.-X.; Cong, X.-D.; Xu, M. Improvement of vascular dysfunction by argirein through inhibiting endothelial cell apoptosis associated with ET-1/Nox4 signal pathway in diabetic rats. *Sci. Rep.* **2018**, *8*, 12620. [CrossRef] [PubMed]
23. Bruni, C.; Frech, T.; Manetti, M.; Rossi, F.W.; Furst, D.E.; De Paulis, A.; Rivellese, F.; Guiducci, S.; Matucci-Cerinic, M.; Bellando-Randone, S. Vascular leaking, a pivotal and early pathogenetic event in systemic sclerosis: Should the door be closed? *Front. Immunol.* **2018**, *9*, 2045. [CrossRef] [PubMed]
24. De Ciuceis, C.; Amiri, F.; Brassard, P.; Endemann, D.H.; Touyz, R.M.; Schiffrin, E.L. Reduced vascular remodeling, endothelial dysfunction, and oxidative stress in resistance arteries of angiotensin II-infused macrophage colony-stimulating factor-deficient mice: Evidence for a role in inflammation in angiotensin-induced vascular injury. *Arter. Thromb. Vasc. Biol.* **2005**, *25*, 2106–2113. [CrossRef]
25. Günther, J.; Rademacher, J.; van Laar, J.M.; Siegert, E.; Riemekasten, G. Functional autoantibodies in systemic sclerosis. *Semin. Immunopathol.* **2015**, *37*, 529–542. [CrossRef]
26. Sartori-Valinotti, J.C.; Tollefson, M.M.; Reed, A.M. Updates on morphea: Role of vascular injury and advances in treatment. *Autoimmune Dis.* **2013**, *2013*, 1–8. [CrossRef]
27. Talotta, R.; Atzeni, F.; Ditto, M.C.; Gerardi, M.C.; Batticciotto, A.; Bongiovanni, S.; Puttini, P.S. Certainties and uncertainties concerning the contribution of pericytes to the pathogenesis of systemic sclerosis. *J. Scleroderma Relat. Disord.* **2018**, *3*, 14–20. [CrossRef]
28. Cozzani, E.; Javor, S.; Laborai, E.; Drosera, M.; Parodi, A. Endothelin-1 Levels in Scleroderma Patients: A Pilot Study. *ISRN Dermatol.* **2013**, *2013*, 125632. [CrossRef]
29. Takagi, K.; Kawaguchi, Y.; Hara, M.; Sugiura, T.; Harigai, M.; Kamatani, N. Serum nitric oxide (NO) levels in systemic sclerosis patients: Correlation between NO levels and clinical features. *Clin. Exp. Immunol.* **2003**, *134*, 538–544. [CrossRef] [PubMed] [PubMed Central]
30. Cantatore, F.P.; Maruotti, N.; Corrado, A.; Ribatti, D. Angiogenesis Dysregulation in the Pathogenesis of Systemic Sclerosis. *Biomed Res. Int.* **2017**, *2017*, 5345673. [CrossRef]

31. Darby, I.A.; Laverdet, B.; Bonte, F.; Desmouliere, A. Fibroblasts and myofibroblasts in wound healing. *Clin. Cosmet. Investig. Dermatol.* **2014**, *7*, 301–311. [PubMed]
32. Hunzelmann, N.; Krieg, T. Sklerodermie. In *Braun-Falco's Dermatologie, Venerologie Und Allergologie*, 7th ed.; Plewig, G., Ruzicka, T., Kaufmann, R., Hertl, M., Eds.; Springer: Berlin/Heidelberg, Germany, 2018; pp. 919–936. [CrossRef]
33. Pattanaik, D.; Brown, M.; Postlethwaite, A.E. Vascular involvement in systemic sclerosis (scleroderma). *J. Inflamm. Res.* **2011**, *4*, 105–125. [CrossRef]
34. Roumm, A.D.; Whiteside, T.L.; Medsger, T.A.; Rodnan, G.P. Lymphocytes in the skin of patients with progressive systemic sclerosis. *Arthritis Rheum.* **1984**, *27*, 645–653. [CrossRef]
35. Hasegawa, M.; Sato, S.; Ihn, H.; Takehara, K. Enhanced Production of Interleukin-6 (IL-6), Oncostatin M and Soluble IL-6 Receptor by Cultured Peripheral Blood Mononuclear Cells from Patients with Systemic Sclerosis. *Rheumatology* **1999**, *38*, 612–617. [CrossRef] [PubMed]
36. Mori, R.; Shaw, T.J.; Martin, P. Molecular mechanisms linking wound inflammation and fibrosis: Knockdown of osteopontin leads to rapid repair and reduced scarring. *J. Investig. Dermatol.* **2008**, *128*, 1435–1447. [CrossRef] [PubMed]
37. Massagué, J. TGFβ signalling in context. *Nat. Rev. Mol. Cell Biol.* **2012**, *13*, 616–630. [CrossRef] [PubMed]
38. Agarbati, S.; Benfaremo, D.; Viola, N.; Paolini, C.; Baroni, S.S.; Funaro, A.; Moroncini, G.; Malavasi, F.; Gabrielli, A. Increased expression of the ectoenzyme CD38 in peripheral blood plasmablasts and plasma cells of patients with systemic sclerosis. *Front. Immunol.* **2022**, *13*, 1072462. [CrossRef]
39. Yoshizaki, A.; Fukasawa, T.; Ebata, S.; Yoshizaki-Ogawa, A.; Sato, S. Involvement of B cells in the development of systemic sclerosis. *Front. Immunol.* **2022**, *13*, 938785. [CrossRef]
40. Grassegger, A.; Pohla-Gubo, G.; Frauscher, M.; Hintner, H. Autoantibodies in systemic sclerosis (scleroderma): Clues for clinical evaluation, prognosis and pathogenesis. *Wien. Med. Wochenschr.* **2008**, *158*, 19–28. [CrossRef]
41. Higashi-Kuwata, N.; Jinnin, M.; Makino, T.; Fukushima, S.; Inoue, Y.; Muchemwa, F.C.; Yonemura, Y.; Komohara, Y.; Takeya, M.; Mitsuya, H.; et al. Characterization of Monocyte/Macrophage Subsets in the Skin and Peripheral Blood Derived from Patients with Systemic Sclerosis. *Arthritis Res. Ther.* **2010**, *12*, R128. [CrossRef]
42. Knipper, J.A.; Willenborg, S.; Brinckmann, J.; Bloch, W.; Maaß, T.; Wagener, R.; Krieg, T.; Sutherland, T.; Munitz, A.; Rothenberg, M.E.; et al. Interleukin-4 Receptor α Signaling in Myeloid Cells Controls Collagen Fibril Assembly in Skin Repair. *Immunity* **2015**, *43*, 803–816. [CrossRef] [PubMed]
43. Khalil, N.; Bereznayj, I.O.; Sporn, M.; Greenberg, A.H. Macrophage Production of Transforming Growth Factor r and Fibroblast Collagen Synthesis in Chronic Pulmonary Inflammation. *J. Exp. Med.* **1989**, *170*, 727–737. [CrossRef]
44. Vona, R.; Giovannetti, A.; Gambardella, L.; Malorni, W.; Pietraforte, D.; Straface, E. Oxidative stress in the pathogenesis of systemic scleroderma: An overview. *J. Cell Mol. Med.* **2018**, *22*, 3308–3314. [CrossRef]
45. Tecchio, C.; Micheletti, A.; Cassatella, M.A. Neutrophil-derived cytokines: Facts beyond expression. *Front. Immunol.* **2014**, *5*, 508. [CrossRef]
46. Thiam, H.R.; Wong, S.L.; Wagner, D.D.; Waterman, C.M. Cellular Mechanisms of NETosis. *Annu. Rev. Cell Dev. Biol.* **2020**, *36*, 191–218. [CrossRef] [PubMed] [PubMed Central]
47. Lande, R.; Lee, E.Y.; Palazzo, R.; Marinari, B.; Pietraforte, I.; Santos, G.S.; Mattenberger, Y.; Spadaro, F.; Stefanantoni, K.; Iannace, N.; et al. CXCL4 assembles DNA into liquid crystalline complexes to amplify TLR9-mediated interferon-α production in systemic sclerosis. *Nat. Commun.* **2019**, *10*, 1–14. [CrossRef] [PubMed]
48. Maugeri, N.; Capobianco, A.; Rovere-Querini, P.; Ramirez, G.A.; Tombetti, E.; Valle, P.D.; Monno, A.; D'Alberti, V.; Gasparri, A.M.; Franchini, S.; et al. Platelet Microparticles Sustain Autophagy-Associated Activation of Neutrophils in Systemic Sclerosis. *Sci. Transl. Med.* **2018**, *10*, 3089. [CrossRef] [PubMed]
49. Conti, P.; Caraffa, A.; Mastrangelo, F.; Tettamanti, L.; Ronconi, G.; Frydas, I.; Kritas, S.K.; Theoharides, T.C. Critical role of inflammatory mast cell in fibrosis: Potential therapeutic effect of IL-37. *Cell Prolif.* **2018**, *51*, e12475. [CrossRef]
50. Overed-Sayer, C.; Rapley, L.; Mustelin, T.; Clarke, D.L. Are mast cells instrumental for fibrotic diseases? *Front. Pharmacol. Front. Pharmacol.* **2014**, *4*, 174. [CrossRef]
51. Gasparini, G.; Cozzani, E.; Parodi, A. Interleukin-4 and interleukin-13 as possible therapeutic targets in systemic sclerosis. *Cytokine* **2020**, *125*, 154799. [CrossRef]
52. McGaha, T.; Saito, S.; Phelps, R.G.; Gordon, R.; Noben-Trauth, N.; Paul, W.E.; Bona, C. Lack of Skin Fibrosis in Tight Skin (TSK) Mice with Targeted Mutation in the Interleukin-4Ra and Transforming Growth Factor-b Genes. *J. Investig. Dermatol.* **2001**, *116*, 136–143. [CrossRef] [PubMed]
53. Foley, J.E.; Mariotti, J.; Ryan, K.; Eckhaus, M.; Fowler, D.H. Th2 Cell Therapy of Established Acute Graft-Versus-Host Disease Requires IL-4 and IL-10 and Is Abrogated by IL-2 or Host-Type Antigen-Presenting Cells. *Biol. Blood Marrow Transplant.* **2008**, *14*, 959–972. [CrossRef] [PubMed]
54. Kaliterna, D.M.; Petrić, M. Biomarkers of skin and lung fibrosis in systemic sclerosis. *Expert Rev. Clin. Immunol.* **2019**, *15*, 1215–1223. [CrossRef]

55. Lafyatis, R. Transforming growth factor β—At the centre of systemic sclerosis. *Nat. Rev. Rheumatol.* **2014**, *10*, 706–719. [CrossRef]
56. Yamakage, A.; Kikuchi, K.; Smith, E.A.; Leroy, E.C.; Trojanowska, M. Selective Upregulation of Platelet-Derived Growth Factor C~Receptors by Transforming Growth Factor/~ in Scleroder Fibroblasts. Available online: http://rupress.org/jem/article-pdf/175/5/1227/1673399/1227.pdf (accessed on 18 May 2025).
57. Lang, F.; Li, Y.; Yao, R.; Jiang, M. Osteopontin in Chronic Inflammatory Diseases: Mechanisms, Biomarker Potential, and Therapeutic Strategies. *Biology* **2025**, *14*, 428. [CrossRef] [PubMed]
58. Ahmed, S.; Misra, D.P.; Agarwal, V. Interleukin-17 pathways in systemic sclerosis-associated fibrosis. *Rheumatol. Int.* **2019**, *39*, 1135–1143. [CrossRef]
59. Chizzolini, C.; Dufour, A.M.; Brembilla, N.C. Is there a role for IL-17 in the pathogenesis of systemic sclerosis? *Immunol. Lett.* **2018**, *195*, 61–67. [CrossRef]
60. Tan, Y.; Mosallanejad, K.; Zhang, Q.; O'brien, S.; Clements, M.; Perper, S.; Wilson, S.; Chaulagain, S.; Wang, J.; Abdalla, M.; et al. IL11-mediated stromal cell activation may not be the master regulator of pro-fibrotic signaling downstream of TGFβ. *Front. Immunol.* **2024**, *15*, 1293883. [CrossRef]
61. O'Reilly, S. Interleukin-11 and its eminent role in tissue fibrosis: A possible therapeutic target. *Clin. Exp. Immunol.* **2023**, *214*, 154–161. [CrossRef]
62. Kuzumi, A.; Yoshizaki, A.; Matsuda, K.M.; Kotani, H.; Norimatsu, Y.; Fukayama, M.; Ebata, S.; Fukasawa, T.; Yoshizaki-Ogawa, A.; Asano, Y.; et al. Interleukin-31 promotes fibrosis and T helper 2 polarization in systemic sclerosis. *Nat. Commun.* **2021**, *12*, 1–18. [CrossRef]
63. Yaseen, B.; Lopez, H.; Taki, Z.; Zafar, S.; Rosario, H.; Abdi, B.A.; Vigneswaran, S.; Xing, F.; Arumalla, N.; Black, S.; et al. Interleukin-31 promotes pathogenic mechanisms underlying skin and lung fibrosis in scleroderma. *Rheumatology* **2020**, *59*, 2625–2636. [CrossRef] [PubMed]
64. Gabbiani, G.; Ryan, G.B.; Majno, G. Presence of modified fibroblasts in granulation tissue and their possible role in wound contraction. *Experientia* **1971**, *27*, 549–550. [CrossRef] [PubMed]
65. Gabbiani, G. 50 Years of Myofibroblasts: How the Myofibroblast Concept Evolved. In *Myofibroblasts: Methods and Protocols*; Hinz, B., Lagares, D., Eds.; Springer: New York, NY, USA, 2021; pp. 1–5. [CrossRef]
66. Hinz, B.; Phan, S.H.; Thannickal, V.J.; Galli, A.; Bochaton-Piallat, M.-L.; Gabbiani, G. The myofibroblast: One function, multiple origins. *Am. J. Pathol.* **2007**, *170*, 1807–1816. [CrossRef]
67. Schuster, R.; Younesi, F.; Ezzo, M.; Hinz, B. The Role of Myofibroblasts in Physiological and Pathological Tissue Repair. *Cold Spring Harb. Perspect. Biol.* **2022**, *15*, a041231. [CrossRef]
68. van Caam, A.; Vonk, M.; Hoogen, F.v.D.; van Lent, P.; van der Kraan, P. Unraveling SSc pathophysiology; The myofibroblast. *Front. Immunol.* **2018**, *9*, 2452. [CrossRef] [PubMed]
69. Ihn, H. Scleroderma, Fibroblasts, Signaling, and Excessive Extracellular Matrix. *Curr. Rheumatol. Rep.* **2005**, *7*, 156–162. [CrossRef]
70. Chadli, L.; Sotthewes, B.; Li, K.; Andersen, S.N.; Cahir-McFarland, E.; Cheung, M.; Cullen, P.; Dorjée, A.; de Vries-Bouwstra, J.K.; Huizinga, T.W.J.; et al. Identification of regulators of the myofibroblast phenotype of primary dermal fibroblasts from early diffuse systemic sclerosis patients. *Sci. Rep.* **2019**, *9*, 1–12. [CrossRef]
71. Hinz, B.; Lagares, D. Evasion of apoptosis by myofibroblasts: A hallmark of fibrotic diseases. *Nat. Rev. Rheumatol.* **2020**, *16*, 11–31. [CrossRef] [PubMed]
72. Santiago, B.; Galindo, M.; Rivero, M.; Pablos, J.L. Decreased susceptibility to Fas-induced apoptosis of systemic sclerosis dermal fibroblasts. *Arthritis Rheum.* **2001**, *44*, 1667–1676. [CrossRef] [PubMed]
73. Jelaska, A.; Korn, J.H. Role of apoptosis and transforming growth factor beta1 in fibroblast selection and activation in systemic sclerosis. *Arthritis Rheum.* **2000**, *43*, 2230–2239. [CrossRef] [PubMed]
74. Lagares, D.; Santos, A.; Grasberger, P.E.; Liu, F.; Probst, C.K.; Rahimi, R.A.; Sakai, N.; Kuehl, T.; Ryan, J.; Bhola, P.; et al. Targeted apoptosis of myofibroblasts with the BH3 mimetic ABT-263 reverses established fibrosis. *Sci. Transl. Med.* **2017**, *9*, eaal3765. [CrossRef] [PubMed] [PubMed Central]
75. Samuel, G.H.; Lenna, S.; Bujor, A.M.; Lafyatis, R.; Trojanowska, M. Acid sphingomyelinase deficiency contributes to resistance of scleroderma fibroblasts to Fas-mediated apoptosis. *J. Dermatol. Sci.* **2012**, *67*, 166–172. [CrossRef]
76. Jafarinejad-Farsangi, S.; Farazmand, A.; Gharibdoost, F.; Karimizadeh, E.; Noorbakhsh, F.; Faridani, H.; Mahmoudi, M.; Jamshidi, A.R. Inhibition of MicroRNA-21 induces apoptosis in dermal fibroblasts of patients with systemic sclerosis. *Int. J. Dermatol.* **2016**, *55*, 1259–1267. [CrossRef]
77. Rajkumar, V.S.; Sundberg, C.; Abraham, D.J.; Rubin, K.; Black, C.M. Activation of microvascular pericytes in autoimmune Raynaud's phenomenon and systemic sclerosis. *Arthritis Rheum.* **1999**, *42*, 930–941. [CrossRef]
78. Sonnylal, S.; Shi-Wen, X.; Leoni, P.; Naff, K.; Van Pelt, C.S.; Nakamura, H.; Leask, A.; Abraham, D.; Bou-Gharios, G.; de Crombrugghe, B. Selective expression of connective tissue growth factor in fibroblasts in vivo promotes systemic tissue fibrosis. *Arthritis Rheum.* **2010**, *62*, 1523–1532. [CrossRef]

79. Nikitorowicz-Buniak, J.; Denton, C.P.; Abraham, D.; Stratton, R. Partially evoked epithelial-mesenchymal transition (EMT) is associated with increased TGFβ signaling within lesional scleroderma skin. *PLoS ONE* **2015**, *10*, e0134092. [CrossRef] [PubMed]
80. Blumbach, K.; Zweers, M.C.; Brunner, G.; Peters, A.S.; Schmitz, M.; Schulz, J.-N.; Schild, A.; Denton, C.P.; Sakai, T.; Fässler, R.; et al. Defective granulation tissue formation in mice with specific ablation of integrin-linked kinase in fibroblasts—Role of TGFβ1 levels and RhoA activity. *J. Cell Sci.* **2010**, *123*, 3872–3883. [CrossRef]
81. Schulz, J.-N.; Zeltz, C.; Sørensen, I.W.; Barczyk, M.; Carracedo, S.; Hallinger, R.; Niehoff, A.; Eckes, B.; Gullberg, D. Reduced granulation tissue and wound strength in the absence of α11β1 integrin. *J. Investig. Dermatol.* **2015**, *135*, 1435–1444. [CrossRef] [PubMed]
82. Schulz, J.-N.; Plomann, M.; Sengle, G.; Gullberg, D.; Krieg, T.; Eckes, B. New developments on skin fibrosis—Essential signals emanating from the extracellular matrix for the control of myofibroblasts. *Matrix Biol.* **2018**, *68–69*, 522–532. [CrossRef]
83. Sawant, M.; Hinz, B.; Schönborn, K.; Zeinert, I.; Eckes, B.; Krieg, T.; Schuster, R. A story of fibers and stress: Matrix-embedded signals for fibroblast activation in the skin. *Wound Repair Regen.* **2021**, *29*, 515–530. [CrossRef]
84. Lagares, D.; Busnadiego, O.; García-Fernández, R.A.; Kapoor, M.; Liu, S.; Carter, D.E.; Abraham, D.; Shi-Wen, X.; Carreira, P.; Fontaine, B.A.; et al. Inhibition of focal adhesion kinase prevents experimental lung fibrosis and myofibroblast formation. *Arthritis Rheum.* **2012**, *64*, 1653–1664. [CrossRef] [PubMed]
85. Zhu, H.; Luo, H.; Skaug, B.; Tabib, T.; Li, Y.-N.; Tao, Y.; Matei, A.-E.; Lyons, M.A.; Schett, G.; Lafyatis, R.; et al. Fibroblast Subpopulations in Systemic Sclerosis: Functional Implications of Individual Subpopulations and Correlations with Clinical Features. *J. Investig. Dermatol.* **2024**, *144*, 1251–1261.e13. [CrossRef] [PubMed]
86. Schönborn, K.; Willenborg, S.; Schulz, J.-N.; Imhof, T.; Eming, S.A.; Quondamatteo, F.; Brinckmann, J.; Niehoff, A.; Paulsson, M.; Koch, M.; et al. Role of collagen XII in skin homeostasis and repair. *Matrix Biol.* **2020**, *94*, 57–76. [CrossRef] [PubMed]
87. Schulz, J.-N.; Nüchel, J.; Niehoff, A.; Bloch, W.; Schönborn, K.; Hayashi, S.; Kamper, M.; Brinckmann, J.; Plomann, M.; Paulsson, M.; et al. COMP-assisted collagen secretion—A novel intracellular function required for fibrosis. *J. Cell Sci.* **2016**, *129*, 706–716. [CrossRef]
88. Pope, J.E.; Denton, C.P.; Johnson, S.R.; Fernandez-Codina, A.; Hudson, M.; Nevskaya, T. State-of-the-art evidence in the treatment of systemic sclerosis. *Nat. Rev. Rheumatol.* **2023**, *19*, 212–226. [CrossRef]
89. Distler, O.; Highland, K.B.; Gahlemann, M.; Azuma, A.; Fischer, A.; Mayes, M.D.; Raghu, G.; Sauter, W.; Girard, M.; Alves, M.; et al. Nintedanib for Systemic Sclerosis–Associated Interstitial Lung Disease. *N. Engl. J. Med.* **2019**, *380*, 2518–2528. [CrossRef]
90. Stratton, R.J.; Wilson, H.; Black, C.M. Pilot Study of Anti-Thymocyte Globulin plus Mycophenolate Mofetil in Recent-Onset Diffuse Scleroderma. *Rheumatology* **2001**, *40*, 84–88. [CrossRef]
91. Franco-Fuquen, P.; Figueroa-Aguirre, J.; Martínez, D.A.; Moreno-Cortes, E.F.; Garcia-Robledo, J.E.; Vargas-Cely, F.; Castro-Martínez, D.A.; Almaini, M.; Castro, J.E. Cellular therapies in rheumatic and musculoskeletal diseases. *J. Transl. Autoimmun.* **2025**, *10*, 100264. [CrossRef]
92. Kuzumi, A.; Ebata, S.; Baron, M.; Sato, S.; Yoshizaki, A. Usefulness of rituximab for the treatment of systemic sclerosis-associated interstitial lung disease: Further analysis of the DESIRES trial. *J. Am. Acad. Dermatol.* **2025**, *92*, 1402–1404. [CrossRef]
93. Davis, J.S.; Ferreira, D.; Paige, E.; Gedye, C.; Boyle, M. Infectious complications of biological and small molecule targeted immunomodulatory therapies. *Clin. Microbiol. Rev.* **2020**, *33*, 1–117. [CrossRef]
94. Colussi, L.; Dagri, A.; Pastore, S.; Tommasini, A.; Pin, A.; Taddio, A. Effect of the Janus kinase inhibitor tofacitinib in the treatment of juvenile scleroderma: A single-center experience. *Int. J. Rheum. Dis.* **2024**, *27*, 15295. [CrossRef] [PubMed]
95. Zeng, L.; Liu, C.; Wu, Y.; Liu, S.; Zheng, Y.; Hao, W.; Wang, D.; Sun, L. Efficacy and safety of mesenchymal stromal cell transplantation in the treatment of autoimmune and rheumatic immune diseases: A systematic review and meta-analysis of randomized controlled trials. *Stem Cell Res. Ther.* **2025**, *16*, 65. [CrossRef] [PubMed]
96. Campochiaro, C.; De Luca, G.; Lazzaroni, M.-G.; Armentaro, G.; Spinella, A.; Vigone, B.; Ruaro, B.; Stanziola, A.; Benfaremo, D.; De Lorenzis, E.; et al. Real-life efficacy and safety of nintedanib in systemic sclerosis-interstitial lung disease: Data from an Italian multicentre study. *RMD Open* **2023**, *9*, e002850. [CrossRef] [PubMed]
97. Humbert, M.; McLaughlin, V.; Gibbs, J.S.R.; Gomberg-Maitland, M.; Hoeper, M.M.; Preston, I.R.; Souza, R.; Waxman, A.; Subias, P.E.; Feldman, J.; et al. Sotatercept for the Treatment of Pulmonary Arterial Hypertension. *N. Engl. J. Med.* **2021**, *384*, 1204–1215. [CrossRef]
98. Matucci-Cerinic, M.; Kahaleh, B.; Wigley, F.M. Review: Evidence that systemic sclerosis is a vascular disease. *Arthritis Rheum.* **2013**, *65*, 1953–1962. [CrossRef]
99. Rigau, A.R.; Li, Y.-N.; Matei, A.-E.; Györfi, A.-H.; Bruch, P.-M.; Koziel, S.; Devakumar, V.; Gabrielli, A.; Kreuter, A.; Wang, J.; et al. Characterization of Vascular Niche in Systemic Sclerosis by Spatial Proteomics. *Circ. Res.* **2024**, *134*, 875–891. [CrossRef]
100. Cutolo, M.; Sulli, A.; Smith, V. Assessing microvascular changes in systemic sclerosis diagnosis and management. *Nat. Rev. Rheumatol.* **2010**, *6*, 578–587. [CrossRef]
101. Lemmers, J.; Velauthapillai, A.; van Herwaarden, N.; Vonk, M. Change of the microvascularization in systemic sclerosis, a matter of air. *Best Pr. Res. Clin. Rheumatol.* **2021**, *35*, 101683. [CrossRef]

102. Allanore, Y.; Wung, P.; Soubrane, C.; Esperet, C.; Marrache, F.; Bejuit, R.; Lahmar, A.; Khanna, D.; Denton, C.P. A randomised, double-blind, placebo-controlled, 24-week, phase II, proof-of-concept study of romilkimab (SAR156597) in early diffuse cutaneous systemic sclerosis. *Ann. Rheum. Dis.* **2020**, *79*, 1600–1607. [CrossRef]

sclerosis

Review

Biomarkers in Systemic Sclerosis

Claudio Karsulovic [1,2,*] and Lia Hojman [2,3]

1 Rheumatology Section, Internal Medicine Department, Facultad de Medicina Clínica Alemana de Santiago, Universidad del Desarrollo, Santiago P.O. Box 7630000, Chile
2 Investigation in Dermatology and Autoimmunity—IDeA Lab, Instituto de Ciencias e Innovación en Medicina, Universidad del Desarrollo, Santiago P.O. Box 7630000, Chile; lhojman@alemana.cl
3 Dermatology Section, Surgery Department, Facultad de Medicina Clínica Alemana de Santiago, Universidad del Desarrollo, Santiago P.O. Box 7630000, Chile
* Correspondence: ckarsulovic@alemana.cl; Tel.: +562-22101111

Abstract: Systemic sclerosis (SSc) is a complex autoimmune disease characterized by vasculopathy, immune dysregulation, and progressive fibrosis affecting the skin and internal organs. Pulmonary complications, including interstitial lung disease (ILD) and pulmonary arterial hypertension (PAH), are major contributors to morbidity and mortality, while skin fibrosis remains a hallmark of disease heterogeneity. Despite advances in understanding SSc pathogenesis, early diagnosis and timely therapeutic intervention remain challenging due to the rapid progression of inflammation and the narrow window before irreversible fibrosis occurs. The identification of reliable biomarkers is crucial for improving diagnosis, monitoring disease activity, and guiding treatment decisions in SSc. While autoantibodies are well-established diagnostic tools, this review focused on non-autoantibody biomarkers, including soluble proteins, cytokines, chemokines, epigenetic modifiers, and oxidative stress indicators. These biomarkers reflect diverse pathogenic mechanisms such as endothelial injury, fibroblast activation, immune signaling, and extracellular matrix remodeling. By examining the available evidence across both clinical and preclinical studies, this review provides an updated overview of molecular markers involved in inflammation and fibrosis in SSc. Understanding their biological significance and therapeutic potential may improve risk stratification, guide targeted interventions, and ultimately contribute to the development of precision medicine strategies in systemic sclerosis.

Keywords: systemic sclerosis; biomarkers; KL-6; IL-6; skin

1. Introduction

Systemic sclerosis (SSc), commonly referred to as scleroderma, is a multifaceted autoimmune disease characterized by vasculopathy, immune system dysregulation, and progressive fibrosis affecting the skin and internal organs. Among the clinical manifestations, cutaneous and pulmonary involvement are the most prevalent and contribute significantly to the disease's morbidity and mortality. Pulmonary complications, such as interstitial lung disease (ILD) and pulmonary arterial hypertension (PAH), are the leading causes of death in SSc, while skin fibrosis remains a defining feature of the disease's heterogeneity and progression. Despite advances in understanding SSc pathogenesis, early diagnosis and timely therapeutic intervention remain challenging due to the rapid progression of the inflammatory phase and the limited window of opportunity before irreversible fibrosis sets in. The identification of reliable biomarkers is crucial for improving the early diagnosis, monitoring disease activity, and tailoring therapeutic interventions in SSc. Biomarkers can serve as indicators of pathological processes and provide insights into the mechanisms driving the disease. While autoantibodies, such as anti-Scl-70 and anti-centromere antibodies, have long been established as diagnostic tools and predictors of specific clinical phenotypes, this review focused on non-autoantibody biomarkers. Specifically, we examined soluble proteins, cytokines, chemokines, epigenetic regulators, and other molecular indicators derived from studies in patient populations and animal models. These biomarkers not only reflect pathophysiological changes but also hold promise as potential therapeutic targets. Established examples include Krebs von den Lungen-6 (KL-6), a mucin-like glycoprotein associated with ILD severity; soluble CD146 (sCD146), a marker of endothelial dysfunction and fibrosis; and galectin-3, a protein implicated in cardiac fibrosis and systemic inflammation. Other molecules, such as Gremlin-1, insulin-like growth factor binding protein-7 (IGFBP7), S100A6, periostin, and malondialdehyde (MDA), are also explored for their potential roles in reflecting fibrotic progression, vascular remodeling, oxidative stress, and immune activation. Many of these candidates are currently under investigation in preclinical models or observational cohorts, contributing to a growing body of evidence on their potential utility in clinical settings. The exclusion of autoantibodies as biomarkers in this review is deliberate, aiming to emphasize less-explored molecular players with both diagnostic and therapeutic potential. While autoantibodies have been instrumental in defining SSc subtypes and predicting organ involvement, they offer limited insight into the dynamic and multifactorial nature of the disease. By focusing on non-autoantibody biomarkers, this review seeks to highlight molecules that capture broader physiological alterations and represent viable targets for intervention in both early and advanced stages of the disease. This review synthesizes current knowledge on non-autoantibody biomarkers in SSc, integrating established findings with emerging data. By examining their clinical relevance, biological roles, and therapeutic potential, we aimed to improve diagnostic precision and contribute to innovation in systemic sclerosis management. The ultimate goal is to enhance early detection, guide treatment strategies, and identify meaningful targets to improve patient outcomes.

2. Biomarkers in Systemic Sclerosis

2.1. IL-6

Interleukin-6 (IL-6) is a multifunctional cytokine that plays a critical role in the pathogenesis of systemic sclerosis (SSc), a complex autoimmune disease characterized by fibrosis, vascular dysfunction, and immune dysregulation (Table 1) [1]. IL-6 is produced by various cell types, including fibroblasts, T cells, B cells, and macrophages, and is involved in both inflammatory responses and fibrotic processes [2]. In SSc, elevated levels of IL-6 have been associated with disease severity and progression since fibroblasts produce IL-6 in response to inflammatory stimuli, which in turn promotes further fibroblast activation and collagen production [3]. This autocrine loop contributes significantly to the fibrotic process characteristic of the disease. Additionally, IL-6 has been shown to stimulate the production of other profibrotic factors, such as platelet-derived growth factor (PDGF) and procollagen type I, further exacerbating the fibrotic response [3]. The role of IL-6 in SSc extends beyond fibroblast activation. It is also implicated in the regulation of immune responses, such as the differentiation and activation of T cells, particularly Th17 cells, which are associated with inflammation and tissue damage in autoimmune diseases [4]. The interplay between IL-6 and other cytokines in the inflammatory milieu of SSc underscores its importance in the disease's pathophysiology and its therapeutic benefits [5]. Tocilizumab, an anti-IL-6 receptor monoclonal antibody, has shown promise in clinical trials, leading to improvements in skin sclerosis and pulmonary fibrosis in SSc patients [6]. The blockade of IL-6 signaling not only reduces inflammation but also appears to reverse TGF-β activation, a key pathway involved in fibrosis [7,8]. This suggests that IL-6 plays a dual role in promoting both inflammation and fibrosis in SSc, making it a potential therapeutic target.

Table 1. Comprehensive list of markers studied in systemic sclerosis.

Biomarker	Protein Type	Biological Function	Possible Role in SSc
MCP-1 (CCL2)	Chemokine	Monocyte and macrophage recruitment	Inflammation and fibrosis in skin and lung
KL-6	Glycoprotein	Alveolar injury marker	Indicator of interstitial lung disease in SSc
TGF-β	Cytokine	Induces fibroblast differentiation	Key mediator of fibrosis in SSc
Serum amyloid A (SAA)	Acute-phase protein	Inflammatory response	Associated with ILD and PAH in SSc
Soluble CD146	Glycoprotein	Endothelial function and angiogenesis	Indicator of ILD and endothelial dysfunction
CXCL4	Chemokine	Inflammation and fibrosis	Associated with ILD and PAH in SSc
sST2	Soluble receptor	Modulates IL-33	Predicts progressive vascular fibrosis in SSc
Endothelin-1	Peptide	Vasoconstriction and fibrosis	Contributes to PAH and vascular dysfunction
PAI-1	Serine protease inhibitor	Inhibits fibrinolysis	Promotes fibrosis in skin and lung
SPARC	Matricellular protein	ECM remodeling	Activates TGF-β and promotes fibrosis
Fibronectin	Glycoprotein	Cell adhesion and ECM	Altered in SSc fibroblasts
Periostin	Matricellular protein	Collagen interaction	Indicator of fibrosis
Tenascin-C	Glycoprotein	ECM maintenance	Contributes to pulmonary fibrosis
TET2	Epigenetic regulator	DNA demethylation	Downregulated in SSc fibroblasts
Cytohesin-2	Nucleotide exchange factor	Fibroblast migration	Enhances focal adhesion in SSc
miR-21	MicroRNA	Post-transcriptional regulation	Activates TGF-β and promotes fibrosis
miR-29	MicroRNA	Collagen regulation	Downregulated in SSc, promoting fibrosis
STING	Adaptor protein	Innate immune response	Excessive activation in SSc
(94)IP-10 (CXCL10)	Chemokine	Th1 lymphocyte attraction	Associated with pulmonary fibrosis
CCL18	Chemokine	Fibroblast activation	Associated with ILD severity and mortality
CX3CL1	Chemokine	Monocyte recruitment	Promotes fibroblast activation
HSP47	Chaperone	Collagen maturation	Promotes ECM accumulation
TWEAK	Cytokine	Fibroblast proliferation	Enhances vascular damage

Table 1. *Cont.*

Biomarker	Protein Type	Biological Function	Possible Role in SSc
Angiopoietin-2	Growth factor	Vascular destabilization	Biomarker of PAH in SSc
VEGF	Growth factor	Angiogenesis	Elevated in SSc but ineffective
NOX4	Enzyme	ROS production	Drives fibrosis
8-Isoprostane	Oxidative stress marker	Lipid peroxidation	Elevated in SSc
Leptin	Hormone	Energy regulation	Promotes inflammatory activation
Adiponectin	Hormone	Anti-inflammatory effect	Elevated in severe fibrosis
Gremlin-1	Protein	BMP regulation	Enhances TGF-β-mediated fibrosis
IGFBP7	Protein	IGF modulation	Associated with pulmonary fibrosis
IGF-1	Growth factor	Fibroblast differentiation	Promotes fibrosis
Galectin-3	Lectin	Immune activation and fibrosis	Indicator of cardiac involvement
Osteopontin	Glycoprotein	Cell adhesion	Linked to PAH and fibrosis
S100A6	Protein	Cell migration	Associated with fibroblast proliferation
FSTL1	Glycoprotein	TGF-β enhancer	Promotes fibrosis
NETosis	Cellular process	Neutrophil extracellular traps release	Promotes endothelial damage
LRG1	Protein	Endothelial dysfunction modulator	Associated with vascular fibrosis

2.2. MCP-1

Monocyte Chemoattractant Protein-1 (MCP-1), also known as CCL2, is a chemokine that plays a significant role in the pathogenesis of SSc (Table 1). It is primarily involved in the recruitment of monocytes and macrophages to sites of inflammation, contributing to the inflammatory and fibrotic processes characteristic of the disease [9]. In SSc, elevated levels of MCP-1 have been associated with disease activity [10]. MCP-1 is produced by various cell types, including fibroblasts, endothelial cells, and macrophages, in response to inflammatory stimuli. This production is often upregulated in the skin and lungs of SSc patients, correlating with the extent of fibrosis and vascular damage [11]. Some studies have shown that MCP-1 levels are significantly higher in the serum of SSc patients compared with healthy controls, and these levels correlate with clinical manifestations such as skin thickening and pulmonary involvement [10]. The MCP-1/CCR2 signaling axis is crucial in mediating the recruitment of monocytes to inflamed tissues. Upon binding to its receptor CCR2, MCP-1 activates various intracellular signaling pathways that promote monocyte migration and activation, leading to the accumulation of inflammatory cells in affected tissues [12,13]. This process is particularly relevant in SSc, where the influx of monocytes contributes to the chronic inflammatory environment and subsequent fibrosis. For example, MCP-1 has been shown to stimulate collagen production by fibroblasts, enhancing the fibrotic response [14]. Moreover, MCP-1 is implicated in the development of vascular complications in SSc [10]. Elevated MCP-1 levels have been associated with pulmonary arterial hypertension (PAH), a severe complication of SSc characterized by increased blood pressure in the pulmonary arteries [10]. The recruitment of inflammatory cells to the pulmonary vasculature can lead to vascular remodeling and dysfunction, contributing to the pathogenesis of PAH in SSc patients [15,16]. These findings emphasize the importance of MCP-1 as a target for therapeutic intervention. Recent studies have explored the therapeutic potential of targeting the MCP-1/CCR2 pathway in SSc [17]. The signaling axis has shown promise in preclinical models, suggesting that blocking MCP-1 or its receptor could mitigate the inflammatory and fibrotic processes associated with SSc [18]. Such approaches may provide new avenues for treatment, particularly for patients with progressive disease.

2.3. *KL-6*

Krebs von den Lungen-6 is a mucin-like glycoprotein primarily expressed on the surface of type II alveolar epithelial cells. It has emerged as a significant biomarker for interstitial lung disease (ILD), particularly in the context of SSc (Table 1). The elevation of KL-6 levels in serum is indicative of lung injury and has been correlated with disease severity and progression in SSc-associated ILD [19]. Research has demonstrated that KL-6 concentrations correlate negatively with pulmonary function parameters such as forced vital capacity (FVC) and diffusing capacity of the lungs for carbon monoxide (DLCO) [20]. It has been reported that reduced FVC and DLCO were significantly associated with increased KL-6 levels in SSc patients with ILD ($r = -0.47$ and $r = -0.58$, respectively; both $p < 0.05$) [21]. Also found that serum KL-6 levels at diagnosis could serve as a predictive biomarker for progression to end-stage lung disease, further emphasizing its prognostic value [21]. KL-6 has been recognized for its role in the fibrotic process, as it is secreted in response to lung injury and is involved in the regulation of collagen expression and myofibroblast differentiation [22,23]. Kuwana et al. identified a baseline KL-6 level > 1273 U/mL as predictive of more severe lung lesions in early SSc and demonstrated that this cutoff could help stratify patients by ILD progression risk [24]. Similarly, Stock et al. showed that KL-6 levels exceeding 1472 U/mL were predictive of a $\geq$15% decline in DLCO over a 2-year period, highlighting KL-6 as a reliable predictor of functional decline in SSc-ILD [25]. Elevated KL-6 levels have been associated with the extent of lung fibrosis and disease progression in other connective tissue diseases, suggesting that it may serve as a useful biomarker for monitoring disease activity [26]. In a prospective study with a 2-year follow-up, KL-6 was identified as a predictor of early progression in SSc-related ILD, outperforming other biomarkers such as CCL-18 [27]. The utility of KL-6 extends beyond SSc, as it has been studied in various interstitial lung diseases, including idiopathic pulmonary fibrosis (IPF) and other connective tissue diseases. For example, KL-6 levels have been shown to correlate with high-resolution computed tomography (HRCT) scores in patients with ILD, indicating its potential as a diagnostic tool [28,29]. Furthermore, KL-6 has been suggested as a biomarker for distinguishing between ILD and other common lung diseases, enhancing its clinical relevance [27].

2.4. *TGF-β*

Transforming growth factor-beta is a pivotal cytokine that plays a central role in the pathogenesis of SSc. The TGF-β signaling pathway is notably overactive in SSc, contributing significantly to the fibrotic processes that define the disease [30] (Table 1). TGF-β induces the activation of fibroblasts, leading to their transformation into myofibroblasts, which are responsible for excessive collagen production and extracellular matrix (ECM) deposition [31]. This process is mediated through both canonical (Smad-dependent) and non-canonical (Smad-independent) signaling pathways. The canonical pathway involves the phosphorylation of Smad proteins, which translocate to the nucleus and regulate the expression of fibrotic genes, while the non-canonical pathways involve various signaling cascades, including those mediated by reactive oxygen species (ROS) and Wnt signaling [32,33]. Some studies have shown that TGF-β levels correlate with disease activity in SSc patients. Elevated TGF-β expression has been observed in the skin and lungs of individuals with SSc, and this elevation is associated with the severity of fibrosis [34]. Inhibition of the TGF-β pathway has been proposed as a therapeutic strategy for SSc, with studies showing that targeting TGF-β signaling can ameliorate fibrosis in experimental models of the disease [35]. In other connective tissue diseases, it has been shown to stimulate the production of connective tissue growth factor (CTGF), which further amplifies fibrotic responses and promotes ECM accumulation [36]. Moreover, TGF-β can induce endothelial-to-mesenchymal transition (EndMT), a process that contributes to vascular dysfunction and fibrosis in SSc [37,38]. The interplay between TGF-β and other signaling pathways is also critical in the context of SSc. For example, TGF-β has been shown to interact with Wnt signaling, enhancing its profibrotic effects [39]. Additionally, the reciprocal regulation between TGF-β and ROS suggests a feedback loop that perpetuates fibrogenesis, as ROS can activate TGF-β signaling, further driving fibrosis [40,41]. Recent studies have explored the therapeutic potential of targeting TGF-β signaling in SSc. Pharmacological agents that inhibit TGF-β receptor activity or downstream signaling pathways have demonstrated antifibrotic effects in preclinical models [41,42].

2.5. Serum Amyloid A

Serum amyloid A (SAA) is an acute-phase protein that plays a significant role in the inflammatory response and has been studied as a potential biomarker in various diseases, including SSc and its pulmonary manifestations (Table 1). Elevated levels of SAA have been associated with disease activity and organ involvement, particularly in patients with interstitial lung disease (ILD) and pulmonary arterial hypertension (PAH) [43]. SAA levels can reflect the extent of inflammation and tissue damage, showing that elevated SAA levels correlate with increased disease severity and can serve as a prognostic marker for pulmonary complications [43]. In this cohort of SSc patients, higher serum SAA concentrations were found to be associated with the presence of ILD, suggesting its utility in monitoring lung involvement [43]. Moreover, SAA has been implicated in the pathogenesis of ILD. It is believed that SAA may contribute to the fibrotic process by promoting the activation of fibroblasts and the deposition of extracellular matrix components. SAA has been studied in other forms of ILD. Elevated SAA levels have been observed in patients with idiopathic pulmonary fibrosis (IPF) and other connective tissue disease-associated lung diseases, indicating its broader relevance as a biomarker for lung injury [44]. The correlation between SAA levels and lung function parameters, such as forced vital capacity (FVC) and diffusing capacity of the lungs for carbon monoxide (DLCO), further supports its potential as a non-invasive marker for assessing lung involvement in various interstitial lung diseases [43]. Furthermore, SAA levels can be influenced by various factors, including systemic inflammation and comorbidities, which may complicate their interpretation in clinical practice [45]. Importantly, SAA is largely regulated by upstream IL-6 signaling, and its elevation may primarily reflect IL-6-driven inflammation rather than direct pathogenic activity. Indeed, IL-6 blockade with tocilizumab has been shown to reduce SAA levels and improve lung outcomes in SSc patients [46,47].

2.6. Soluble CD146

Soluble CD146 (sCD146) is a glycoprotein that has garnered attention as a potential biomarker in SSc, particularly in relation to lung involvement [48] (Table 1). CD146, also known as melanoma cell adhesion molecule (MCAM), is primarily expressed on endothelial cells and plays a crucial role in cell adhesion, migration, and angiogenesis. The soluble form of CD146 is released into circulation and has been implicated in various inflammatory and fibrotic processes associated with SSc [49]. Elevated levels of sCD146 have been correlated with disease activity and severity in SSc patients, particularly those with interstitial lung disease (ILD) [49]. This correlation suggests that sCD146 could be utilized to monitor disease progression and therapeutic responses in patients with SSc-related lung involvement. The generation of sCD146 can arise from both the shedding and alternative splicing of the primary transcript, with maybe distinct roles in the pathophysiology of SSc [50]. Moreover, the role of sCD146 extends beyond mere biomarker potential; it may also be involved in the fibrotic process itself since the protein has been shown to act as a growth factor in various angiogenic and inflammation-related pathologies, suggesting that it could contribute to the mechanisms driving fibrosis in SSc [51]. This dual role as both a biomarker and a participant in disease pathology makes sCD146 a compelling target for further research [52].

2.7. CXCL4

CXCL4, also known as platelet factor 4, is a chemokine that has emerged as a significant biomarker in SSc. Elevated levels of CXCL4 have been associated with various clinical manifestations of the disease, including interstitial lung disease (ILD) and pulmonary arterial hypertension (PAH) [53] (Table 1). CXCL4 has been shown to play a crucial role in pathogenesis by influencing inflammatory and fibrotic processes. Circulating CXCL4 levels are increased in SSc patients and correlate with the progression of heart and lung disease, suggesting its potential as a biomarker for monitoring disease activity [54]. Moreover, changes in plasma CXCL4 levels were associated with improvements in lung function in patients receiving immunosuppressive therapy for SSc-related ILD [55]. Such correlations highlight the utility of CXCL4 in assessing therapeutic responses and disease progression. Furthermore, CXCL4 has been implicated in the fibrotic phenomenon associated with SSc. It is known to promote fibroblast activation and collagen production, contributing to the excessive fibrosis seen in SSc patients [56]. The chemokine's ability to trigger monocytes and macrophages to produce platelet-derived growth factor (PDGF-BB) further underscores its role in the fibrotic cascade [56,57]. Additionally, CXCL4 has been shown to induce endothelial-to-mesenchymal transition, a process that facilitates fibrosis and vascular remodeling [56]. The immune-modulatory functions of CXCL4 extend beyond fibrosis; it also influences T-cell responses. CXCL4 drives CD4 T cells to produce interleukin-17 (IL-17), linking it to Th17-mediated inflammation, which is often observed in SSc [56]. This Th17 skewing is significant, as it is associated with the inflammatory milieu in SSc and contributes to the disease's progression. Moreover, CXCL4 has been identified as a potential marker for predicting disease prognosis since anti-CXCL4 antibodies are present in SSc patients and correlate with the type I interferon signature, which is characteristic of a subset of SSc patients with more severe disease [58].

2.8. sST2

Soluble suppression of tumorigenicity 2 (sST2) is a member of the interleukin-1 receptor family. It is primarily recognized for its role in inflammation and fibrosis, particularly in the context of cardiovascular and pulmonary complications associated with SSc [59] (Table 1). It has been shown that elevated levels of sST2 are associated with disease severity and progression in SSc patients, where sST2 levels were significantly higher in patients with limited cutaneous systemic sclerosis (lcSSc) after nine years of disease compared with those with stable disease, indicating its potential as a biomarker for progressive vascular fibrosis [60]. This correlation suggests that sST2 may reflect the underlying pathophysiological processes in SSc, particularly those related to vascular remodeling and fibrosis. The role of sST2 extends beyond mere correlation with disease severity; it is also involved in the inflammatory response. Elevated sST2 levels have been linked to increased activity of interleukin-33 (IL-33), a cytokine that plays a critical role in promoting inflammation and fibrosis in SSc. The interaction between IL-33 and sST2 is complex, as sST2 acts as a decoy receptor for IL-33, potentially modulating its effects on inflammation and fibrosis [61]. Beyond its implications for vascular and fibrotic processes, sST2 has been associated with cardiac involvement in SSc. Elevated sST2 levels have been correlated with adverse cardiovascular events, making it a potential prognostic marker for cardiac complications in SSc patients [62]. sST2 has been shown to predict mortality in patients with heart failure, which may be relevant for SSc patients who often experience cardiac manifestations [63]. Furthermore, sST2 has been shown to reflect hemodynamic stress and pulmonary congestion, indicating its broader relevance in assessing lung involvement. Also, increased sST2 levels have been associated with pulmonary hypertension, suggesting that it may serve as a biomarker for assessing pulmonary vascular health in SSc patients [64].

2.9. Endotelin-1

Endothelin-1 (ET-1) is a potent vasoconstrictor peptide. Elevated levels of ET-1 have been consistently observed in SSc patients, correlating with disease severity and the presence of vascular complications such as pulmonary arterial hypertension (PAH) and digital ulcers [65] (Table 1). The role of ET-1 in SSc extends beyond its vasoconstrictive properties. It is involved in promoting inflammation and fibrosis, contributing to the excessive accumulation of extracellular matrix (ECM) components characteristic of SSc since ET-1 stimulates fibroblast proliferation and collagen synthesis, thereby enhancing the fibrotic response [66]. This profibrotic effect is mediated through the activation of endothelin receptors, primarily the endothelin type A (ETA) receptor, which has been shown to be upregulated in SSc fibroblasts [67]. The interaction between ET-1 and its receptors leads to the activation of signaling pathways that promote myofibroblast differentiation, a key process in the development of fibrosis [68]. Clinical studies have demonstrated that antagonism of the endothelin pathway can have beneficial effects on SSc. Bosentan, an oral dual endothelin receptor antagonist, has been shown to reduce the incidence of new digital ulcers in patients with SSc, highlighting the therapeutic potential of targeting ET-1 signaling [69]. Additionally, bosentan has been associated with improvements in pulmonary function and a reduction in the progression of pulmonary hypertension in SSc patients [70]. However, the effects of endothelin receptor antagonists on skin fibrosis remain less clear, with some studies indicating limited efficacy in this regard [71]. The involvement of ET-1 in the pathogenesis of SSc is based also on the interaction with transforming growth factor-beta (TGF-β), another key cytokine in SSc, to enhance fibrotic processes [72]. This interaction suggests a complex network of signaling pathways that contribute to the disease's progression, where ET-1 not only acts as a vasoconstrictor but also as a mediator of fibrosis and inflammation. Moreover, the expression of ET-1 and its receptors has been observed in various cell types involved in SSc, including endothelial cells, fibroblasts, and immune cells [73].

3. Other Biomarkers in Systemic Sclerosis

3.1. Extracellular Matrix Biomarkers in Systemic Sclerosis

The extracellular matrix (ECM) plays a pivotal role in the pathogenesis of systemic sclerosis (SSc), where excessive fibrosis and abnormal tissue remodeling drive disease progression. Several ECM-related proteins have been implicated in SSc, including plasminogen activator inhibitor-1 (PAI-1), secreted protein acidic and rich in cysteine (SPARC), and various collagen-associated molecules. PAI-1 is a serine protease inhibitor that disrupts fibrinolysis by inhibiting tPA and uPA, leading to excessive ECM deposition and fibrosis [74]. Elevated PAI-1 levels have been observed in the epidermis and endothelium of SSc patients, suggesting a role in fibrosis and vascular abnormalities [75]. Additionally, increased PAI-1 expression has been linked to diminished lung function, indicating its involvement in pulmonary fibrosis [75]. These findings highlight the potential of PAI-1 as a biomarker for disease activity in SSc, particularly concerning skin and pulmonary involvement [76]. SPARC, also known as osteonectin, is a protein that regulates ECM remodeling and collagen turnover. Increased SPARC expression in SSc fibroblasts enhances TGF-β signaling, leading to myofibroblast differentiation and excessive collagen production [77]. Additionally, SPARC has been linked to macrophage activation and endothelial dysfunction, highlighting its role in both inflammation and fibrosis [78]. Beyond these, dysregulated ECM proteins such as fibronectin, periostin, and tenascin-C contribute to the fibrotic response by altering fibroblast signaling and ECM integrity [79,80]. Clinical studies suggest that targeting PAI-1 and SPARC signaling pathways could be promising strategies for reducing fibrosis and restoring ECM balance in SSc [81] (Table 1).

3.2. *Gene Activity Modifiers in Systemic Sclerosis*

Epigenetic modifications and post-transcriptional regulation play critical roles in the pathogenesis of SSc. Among the most relevant genetic modulators in SSc are TET2 (ten-eleven translocation 2), cytohesin-2, and various microRNAs (miRNAs). TET2 is an epigenetic regulator involved in DNA demethylation, and its downregulation in SSc fibroblasts has been associated with hypermethylation of antifibrotic genes, leading to excessive collagen deposition and myofibroblast activation [82]. Cytohesin-2, a guanine nucleotide exchange factor, plays a role in fibroblast migration and ECM remodeling through the activation of ARF (ADP-ribosylation factor) GTPases [83,84]. Increased cytohesin-2 expression in SSc fibroblasts promotes paxillin-mediated focal adhesion, reinforcing the profibrotic phenotype [85]. Additionally, several miRNAs have been identified as key regulators of fibrosis and immune activation in SSc. miR-21, for instance, enhances TGF-β-driven fibroblast activation [86], while miR-29, which is downregulated in SSc, acts as a negative regulator of collagen production [87,88]. Other studies have also highlighted the STING pathway, which amplifies type I interferon responses and contributes to fibrosis via NF-κB signaling [89] (Table 1).

3.3. *Cytokines and Chemokines in Systemic Sclerosis*

The inflammatory landscape of SSc is shaped by a complex network of cytokines and chemokines that drive immune dysregulation. IP-10 (CXCL10), a chemokine-induced by interferon-gamma, is a potent attractant for Th1 lymphocytes and contributes to chronic immune activation [90]. Increased serum levels of IP-10 have been linked to pulmonary fibrosis and digital ulcers, suggesting its potential as a biomarker for disease progression [91]. Similarly, CCL18 (pulmonary and activation-regulated chemokine, PARC) is overexpressed in alternatively activated macrophages in SSc, promoting fibroblast proliferation and collagen deposition [92]. Elevated CCL18 levels in SSc patients correlate with lung fibrosis severity and increased mortality, underscoring its prognostic significance [93]. In addition to these chemokines, the CX3CL1-CX3CR1 axis facilitates monocyte recruitment and fibroblast activation, exacerbating the fibrotic process [94,95]. Emerging evidence also suggests a role for HSP47, a collagen-specific chaperone, in SSc fibrosis by stabilizing procollagen molecules in the endoplasmic reticulum, reinforcing excessive ECM accumulation [96,97]. Finally, targeting pro-inflammatory cytokines such as TWEAK (TNF-like weak inducer of apoptosis), which enhances fibroblast proliferation and monocyte recruitment, may offer novel therapeutic avenues for reducing fibrosis and vascular damage in SSc [98] (Table 1).

3.4. Vascular Modulators in Systemic Sclerosis

Vascular dysfunction is a hallmark of SSc, together with endothelial damage, aberrant angiogenesis, and vasculopathy, which play roles in disease progression. Among the key regulators of vascular homeostasis in SSc are angiopoietin-2 (Ang-2), vascular endothelial growth factor (VEGF), and plasminogen activator inhibitor-1 (PAI-1). Ang-2, produced by endothelial cells, destabilizes vascular structures, promoting inflammation and fibrosis [99]. Elevated Ang-2 levels correlate with pulmonary arterial hypertension (PAH) severity in SSc patients, suggesting its potential as a biomarker [100]. Decreased Angiopoietin-1 (Ang1) levels and increased Angiopoietin-2 (Ang2) levels have been observed in SSc patients compared with healthy controls, supporting the hypothesis that an imbalance between these molecules contributes to aberrant angiogenesis and microvascular damage [101]. Conversely, VEGF, a crucial pro-angiogenic factor, is paradoxically increased in SSc but fails to compensate for the loss of microvasculature, leading to ineffective angiogenesis [102,103]. PAI-1, a major inhibitor of fibrinolysis, contributes to endothelial dysfunction by promoting pro-coagulant activity, further exacerbating vascular complications [104] (Table 1).

3.5. Oxidative Stress in Systemic Sclerosis

Increased reactive oxygen species (ROS) production by endothelial cells and activated fibroblasts promotes DNA damage, cytokine release, and fibroblast differentiation [105]. Among the most studied oxidative stress mediators in SSc is NADPH oxidase (NOX), particularly NOX4, which is overexpressed in fibroblasts and contributes to TGF-β-driven fibrosis [106]. Additionally, markers of oxidative damage, such as 8-isoprostane and advanced oxidation protein products (AOPP), have been found elevated in SSc [107]. Oxidative stress also impacts endothelial dysfunction by reducing nitric oxide (NO) bioavailability, leading to vasoconstriction and microvascular damage [108]. Antioxidant therapies targeting NOX4 inhibition, mitochondrial dysfunction, and ROS scavengers have shown promise in preclinical models, suggesting that counteracting oxidative stress could slow disease progression [109] (Table 1).

3.6. Hormones in Systemic Sclerosis

Leptin, an adipokine primarily produced by adipocytes, is involved in immune modulation, energy homeostasis, and fibrotic signaling. Elevated serum leptin levels have been observed in SSc patients, correlating with disease severity, pulmonary arterial hypertension (PAH), and skin fibrosis [110,111]. Leptin promotes macrophage activation and T-cell proliferation, leading to a pro-inflammatory environment that amplifies fibroblast activation and extracellular matrix (ECM) deposition in other connective tissue diseases [112]. It has been proposed that adiponectin may mitigate endothelial damage and fibroblast overactivation [113]. Another critical player is gremlin-1, a BMP (bone morphogenetic protein) antagonist that inhibits antifibrotic BMP-4 and BMP-7 signaling, thereby enhancing TGF-β-mediated fibrosis in SSc [114,115]. IGFBP7 (insulin-like growth factor binding protein 7) is another emerging biomarker in SSc, as its elevated levels are associated with fibroblast proliferation, endothelial dysfunction, and pulmonary fibrosis progression [116,117]. Also, IGF-1 (insulin-like growth factor 1) is upregulated in SSc and contributes to fibroblast differentiation and collagen production, further exacerbating fibrosis and inflammation in other models [118]. Studies suggest that targeting leptin, gremlin-1, or IGF-1 pathways could modulate fibrotic signaling with the potential to slow fibrotic progression in other diseases [118] (Table 1).

3.7. Other Modulators in Systemic Sclerosis

Galectin-3, a β-galactoside-binding lectin, has been implicated in immune activation and fibrosis in SSc. Studies have shown that elevated serum galectin-3 levels correlate with cardiac involvement, pulmonary fibrosis, and increased mortality [119,120]. Galectin-3 enhances fibroblast activation, promotes TGF-β signaling, and facilitates myofibroblast differentiation, reinforcing pathological ECM remodeling [121]. Osteopontin (OPN), a glycoprotein involved in cell adhesion and immune regulation, is also upregulated in SSc, driving monocyte recruitment, fibroblast activation, and collagen synthesis [122]. Some studies suggest that elevated OPN levels predict pulmonary arterial hypertension (PAH) and increased mortality in SSc patients [122]. Another emerging biomarker is S100A6 (calcyclin), a calcium-binding protein associated with fibroblast proliferation, inflammatory cell migration, and oxidative stress responses in SSc [123]. FSTL1 (follistatin-like 1), a secreted glycoprotein, has been identified as a potent TGF-β enhancer, exacerbating fibroblast activation and ECM accumulation [124]. In addition, NETosis, a process where neutrophils release extracellular traps (NETs) composed of chromatin and proteases, has been implicated in vascular injury and immune dysregulation in SSc [125]. Excessive NET formation promotes endothelial damage and amplifies the fibrotic response in other models [126]. Finally, LRG1 (leucine-rich alpha-2-glycoprotein 1) is emerging as a key regulator of endothelial dysfunction and fibroblast differentiation, with increased LRG1 levels being associated with other inflammatory vascular complications [127,128] (Table 1).

4. Discussion

Systemic sclerosis (SSc) presents unique challenges that necessitate the search for early biomarkers capable of aiding in diagnosis and predicting specific organ involvement. Defining "early" in this context is complex, as a diagnosis cannot precede clinical manifestations—a long-standing issue in rheumatology. SSc typically progresses through cyclical phases, transitioning from an inflammatory state to a fibrotic one, often within as little as a year. In some cases, these cycles occur only once, while in others, each episode triggers additional organ involvement. While cutaneous manifestations remain a primary diagnostic focus, the early identification of rapidly progressive forms, as well as pulmonary, pulmonary vascular, and fibrotic cardiac involvement, should be prioritized.

Several biomarkers have emerged from studies on pulmonary involvement in SSc. KL-6, cytokines that act as precursors to the inflammatory process, and molecules associated with extracellular matrix deposition and fibrotic activation have been highlighted as potential indicators of progressive and irreversible lung fibrosis in patients with interstitial lung disease (ILD). A crucial question that arises is whether identifying a biomarker that reflects the underlying pathophysiological process is sufficient to provide therapeutic targets for halting disease progression.

Recent literature reinforces the central role of inflammation- and fibrosis-related mediators in systemic sclerosis pathogenesis. Notably, TNF-α has been linked to both fibrotic progression and vascular injury, with elevated levels correlating with pulmonary fibrosis and PAH [129]. The modulation of TNF-α and downstream markers such as VEGF, IL-6, and type I/III collagen fragments through biologic therapy provides further support for their use as dynamic biomarkers. Parallel insights from the EUSTAR cohort highlight how racial background influences autoantibody profiles (ACA, ATA) and pulmonary parameters such as FVC and DLCO, underlining the relevance of stratifying biomarker analysis by patient ancestry [130].

As a research group, we suggest that organizing biomarker interpretation around their molecular function and temporal involvement in disease progression could enhance our ability to predict tissue damage in systemic sclerosis. A plausible strategy may involve first establishing an inflammatory signature at the time of diagnosis, regardless of clinical phenotype. This could then be complemented by the identification of markers reflecting early activation of damage-related pathways in target organs—such as endothelial dysfunction or cardiomyocyte stress—and, finally, by assessing proteins associated with fibrotic commitment or irreversible remodeling. In this framework, incorporating epigenetic biomarkers, including regulatory proteins and non-coding RNAs, may offer an additional layer of insight, helping to define a patient-specific molecular signature at baseline that could inform both prognosis and treatment planning. Furthermore, leveraging multidimensional data analysis, including dimensionality reduction techniques such as principal component analysis (PCA), could enable a more precise reclassification of SSc subtypes at the time of diagnosis. This approach may help identify patients at higher risk of developing severe disease phenotypes or specific organ complications, facilitating personalized therapeutic strategies.

5. Conclusions

In this review, we compiled a comprehensive list of biomarkers with potential involvement in inflammatory, fibrotic pathways observed in SSc. Some of these markers have been validated in animal models, while others have been extensively studied in patient cohorts with defined clinical outcomes. The greatest challenge remains in further investigating and understanding the inflammatory pathways that drive terminal fibrosis and its progression rate, particularly in rapidly progressive skin forms. Identifying reliable and specific biomarkers for these processes could, through the integration of multiple variables, help establish a predictive profile for preventing irreversible tissue damage in SSc patients. Future studies should prioritize multi-omic approaches to better define the temporal dynamics of biomarker expression and their predictive value in disease progression. Ultimately, translating these molecular insights into clinical practice will be essential for developing targeted therapies, improving patient outcomes, and advancing precision medicine in systemic sclerosis.

Author Contributions: Conceptualization: C.K., L.H.; data curation: C.K., L.H.; formal analysis: C.K., L.H; funding acquisition: C.K., L.H.; investigation: C.K., L.H; resources: C.K., L.H.; supervision: C.K., L.H.; writing—original draft preparation: C.K., L.H.; writing—review and editing: C.K., L.H. All authors have read and agreed to the published version of the manuscript.

Funding: This research received no external funding.

Data Availability Statement: All data generated or analyzed during this study are included in this published article.

Conflicts of Interest: The authors declared no conflicts of interest.

References

1. Cardoneanu, A.; Burlui, A.M.; Macovei, L.A.; Bratoiu, I.; Richter, P.; Rezus, E. Targeting Systemic Sclerosis from Pathogenic Mechanisms to Clinical Manifestations: Why IL-6? *Biomedicines* **2022**, *10*, 318. [CrossRef]
2. Li, Y.; Zhao, J.; Yin, Y.; Li, K.; Zhang, C.; Zheng, Y. The Role of IL-6 in Fibrotic Diseases: Molecular and Cellular Mechanisms. *Int. J. Biol. Sci.* **2022**, *18*, 5405–5414. [PubMed]
3. Muangchan, C.; Pope, J. Interleukin 6 in Systemic Sclerosis and Potential Implications for Targeted Therapy. *J. Rheumatol.* **2012**, *39*, 1120–1124. [PubMed]
4. Grunwald, C.; Krętowska-Grunwald, A.; Adamska-Patruno, E.; Kochanowicz, J.; Kułakowska, A.; Chorąży, M. The Role of Selected Interleukins in the Development and Progression of Multiple Sclerosis—A Systematic Review. *Int. J. Mol. Sci.* **2024**, *25*, 2589. [CrossRef] [PubMed]
5. Kitaba, S.; Murota, H.; Terao, M.; Azukizawa, H.; Terabe, F.; Shima, Y.; Fujimoto, M.; Tanaka, T.; Naka, T.; Kishimoto, T.; et al. Blockade of Interleukin-6 Receptor Alleviates Disease in Mouse Model of Scleroderma. *Am. J. Pathol.* **2012**, *180*, 165–176.

6. Shima, Y.; Kuwahara, Y.; Murota, H.; Kitaba, S.; Kawai, M.; Hirano, T.; Arimitsu, J.; Narazaki, M.; Hagihara, K.; Ogata, A.; et al. The Skin of Patients with Systemic Sclerosis Softened During the Treatment with Anti-Il-6 Receptor Antibody Tocilizumab. *Rheumatology* **2010**, *49*, 2408–2412.
7. Ventéjou, S.; Schwieger-Briel, A.; Nicolai, R.; Christen-Zaech, S.; Schnider, C.; Hofer, M.; Bogiatzi, S.; Hohl, D.; De Benedetti, F.; Morren, M.-A. Case Report: Pansclerotic Morphea Clinical Features, Differential Diagnoses and Modern Treatment Concepts. *Front. Immunol.* **2021**, *12*, 656407.
8. Denton, C.P.; Ong, V.H.; Xu, S.; Chen-Harris, H.; Modrusan, Z.; Lafyatis, R.; Khanna, D.; Jahreis, A.; Siegel, J.; Sornasse, T. Therapeutic interleukin-6 blockade reverses transforming growth factor-beta pathway activation in dermal fibroblasts: Insights from the faSScinate clinical trial in systemic sclerosis. *Ann. Rheum. Dis.* **2018**, *77*, 1362–1371.
9. Kirichenko, T.V.; Bogatyreva, A.I.; Gerasimova, E.V.; Popkova, T.V.; Markina, Y.V.; Markin, A.M.; Gerasimova, D.A.; Orekhov, A.N. Inflammatory Response of Monocytes/Macrophages in Patients with Systemic Sclerosis. *Front. Biosci.-Landmark* **2024**, *29*, 259.
10. Yalçinkaya, Y.; Çinar, S.; Artim-Esen, B.; Kamali, S.; Öcal, L.; Deniz, G.; Inanç, M. The relationship between vascular biomarkers and disease characteristics in systemic sclerosis: Elevated MCP-1 is predominantly associated with fibrotic manifestations. *Clin. Exp. Rheumatol.* **2016**, *34* (Suppl. S100), 110–114.
11. Hasegawa, M.; Sato, S.; Takehara, K. Augmented production of chemokines (monocyte chemotactic protein-1 (MCP-1), macrophage inflammatory protein-1α (MIP-1α) and MIP-1β) in patients with systemic sclerosis: MCP-1 and MIP-1α may be involved in the development of pulmonary fibrosis. *Clin. Exp. Immunol.* **2001**, *117*, 159–165. [CrossRef] [PubMed]
12. Ehrlich, D.; Pirchl, M.; Humpel, C. Effects of Long-Term Moderate Ethanol and Cholesterol on Cognition, Cholinergic Neurons, Inflammation, and Vascular Impairment in Rats. *Neuroscience* **2012**, *205*, 154–166. [CrossRef]
13. Abdullah, H.; Mahdi Al-Mussawi, K.A.H. Relationship Between Monocyte Chemoattractant Protein-1 (MCP-1) and Pathogenicity of Trichomonas Vaginalis. *J. Pharm. Negat. Results.* **2022**, *13*, 575–579. [CrossRef]
14. Arai, M.; Ikawa, Y.; Chujo, S.; Hamaguchi, Y.; Ishida, W.; Shirasaki, F.; Hasegawa, M.; Mukaida, N.; Fujimoto, M.; Takehara, K. Chemokine Receptors CCR2 and CX3CR1 Regulate Skin Fibrosis in the Mouse Model of Cytokine-Induced Systemic Sclerosis. *J. Dermatol. Sci.* **2013**, *69*, 250–258. [CrossRef]
15. Zhang, J.; Li, G.; Gao, S.; Yao, Y.; Pang, L.; Li, Y.; Wang, W.; Zhao, Q.; Kong, D.; Li, C. Monocyte Chemoattractant Protein-1 Released From Polycaprolactone/Chitosan Hybrid Membrane to Promote Angiogenesis in Vivo. *J. Bioact. Compat. Polym.* **2014**, *29*, 572–588. [CrossRef]
16. Le Pavec, J.; Humbert, M.; Mouthon, L.; Hassoun, P.M. Systemic Sclerosis-associated Pulmonary Arterial Hypertension. *Am. J. Respir. Crit. Care Med.* **2010**, *181*, 1285–1293. [CrossRef]
17. Minsaas, L.; Planagumà, J.; Madziva, M.T.; Krakstad, B.F.; Masià-Balagué, M.; Katz, A.A.; Aragay, A.M. Filamin a Binds to CCR2B and Regulates Its Internalization. *PLoS ONE* **2010**, *5*, e12212. [CrossRef]
18. Haub, J.; Roehrig, N.; Uhrin, P.; Schabbauer, G.; Eulberg, D.; Melchior, F.; Shahneh, F.; Probst, H.C.; Becker, C.; Steinbrink, K.; et al. Intervention of Inflammatory Monocyte Activity Limits Dermal Fibrosis. *J. Investig. Dermatol.* **2019**, *139*, 2144–2153. [CrossRef]
19. Jiang, Y.; Luo, Q.; Han, Q.; Huang, J.; Ou, Y.; Chen, M.; Wen, Y.; Mosha, S.S.; Deng, K.; Chen, R. Sequential changes of serum KL-6 predict the progression of interstitial lung disease. *J. Thorac. Dis.* **2018**, *10*, 4705–4714. [CrossRef]
20. Sieiro Santos, C.; Antolín, S.C.; Lorenzo, J.D.C.; Garay, C.L.; Morales, C.M.; de Miguel, E.B.; Guerrero, M.R.; Herránz, L.S.; Álvarez, E.D. KL6 and IL-18 levels are negatively correlated with respiratory function tests and ILD extent assessed on HRCT in patients with systemic sclerosis-related interstitial lung disease (SSc-ILD). *Semin. Arthritis Rheum.* **2024**, *65*, 152366. [CrossRef]
21. Cho, E.J.; Park, K.J.; Ko, D.H.; Koo, H.J.; Lee, S.M.; Song, J.W.; Lee, W.; Lee, H.K.; Do, K.-H.; Chun, S.; et al. Analytical and Clinical Performance of the Nanopia Krebs Von Den Lungen 6 Assay in Korean Patients with Interstitial Lung Diseases. *Ann. Lab. Med.* **2019**, *39*, 245–251. [PubMed]
22. Fields, A.; Potel, K.N.; Cabuhal, R.; Aziri, B.; Stewart, I.; Schock, B. Mediators of Systemic Sclerosis-Associated Interstitial Lung Disease (SSc-ILD): Systematic Review and Meta-Analyses. *Thorax* **2022**, *78*, 799–807. [PubMed]
23. Xu, L.; Yan, D.R.; Zhu, S.L.; Gu, J.; Bian, W.; Rong, Z.H.; Shen, C. KL-6 regulated the expression of HGF, collagen and myofibroblast differentiation. *Eur. Rev. Med. Pharmacol. Sci.* **2013**, *17*, 3073–3077.
24. Kuwana, M.; Shirai, Y.; Takeuchi, T. Elevated serum krebs von den lungen-6 in early disease predicts subsequent deterioration of pulmonary function in patients with systemic sclerosis and interstitial lung disease. *J. Rheumatol.* **2016**, *43*, 1825–1831. [PubMed]
25. Stock, C.J.W.; Hoyles, R.K.; Daccord, C.; Kokosi, M.; Visca, D.; De Lauretis, A.; Alfieri, V.; Kouranos, V.; Margaritopoulos, G.; George, P.M.; et al. Serum markers of pulmonary epithelial damage in systemic sclerosis-associated interstitial lung disease and disease progression. *Respirology* **2021**, *26*, 461–468.
26. Wang, Y.; Chen, S.; Lin, J.; Xie, X.; Hu, S.; Lin, Q.; Zheng, K.; Du, G.; Huang, X.; Zhang, G.; et al. Lung Ultrasound B-Lines and Serum KL-6 Correlate with the Severity of Idiopathic Inflammatory Myositis-Associated Interstitial Lung Disease. *Rheumatology* **2019**, *59*, 2024–2029.

27. Salazar, G.A.; Kuwana, M.; Wu, M.; Estrada-Y-Martin, R.M.; Jin, Y.; Charles, J.; Mayes, M.D.; Assassi, S. KL-6 but Not CCL-18 Is a Predictor of Early Progression in Systemic Sclerosis-Related Interstitial Lung Disease. *J. Rheumatol.* **2018**, *45*, 1153–1158. [PubMed]
28. Zou, W. Elevated Serum KL-6 Concentration as an Early Detection Biomarker of Rituximab-Related Interstitial Lung Disease. 2023.
29. Soccio, P.; Moriondo, G.; D'alessandro, M.; Scioscia, G.; Bergantini, L.; Gangi, S.; Tondo, P.; Barbaro, M.P.F.; Cameli, P.; Bargagli, E.; et al. Role of BAL and Serum Krebs Von Den Lungen-6 (KL-6) in Patients with Pulmonary Fibrosis. *Biomedicines* **2024**, *12*, 269. [CrossRef]
30. Lafyatis, R. Transforming growth factor β—At the centre of systemic sclerosis. *Nat. Rev. Rheumatol.* **2014**, *10*, 706–719.
31. Frangogiannis, N.G. Transforming growth factor–β in tissue fibrosis. *J. Exp. Med.* **2020**, *217*, e20190103.
32. Zhang, Y.E. Non-Smad pathways in TGF-β signaling. *Cell Res.* **2009**, *19*, 128–139. [CrossRef]
33. Clayton, S.W.; Ban, G.I.; Liu, C.; Serra, R. Canonical and noncanonical TGF-β signaling regulate fibrous tissue differentiation in the axial skeleton. *Sci. Rep.* **2020**, *10*, 21364. [CrossRef] [PubMed]
34. Lu, J.; Liu, Q.; Wang, L.; Tu, W.; Chu, H.; Ding, W.; Jiang, S.; Ma, Y.; Shi, X.; Pu, W.; et al. Increased expression of latent TGF-β-binding protein 4 affects the fibrotic process in scleroderma by TGF-β/SMAD signaling. *Lab. Investig.* **2017**, *97*, 591–601. [CrossRef] [PubMed]
35. Utsunomiya, A.; Chino, T.; Kasamatsu, H.; Hasegawa, T.; Utsunomiya, N.; Luong, V.H.; Matsushita, T.; Sasaki, Y.; Ogura, D.; Niwa, S.-I.; et al. The Compound LG283 Inhibits Bleomycin-Induced Skin Fibrosis via Antagonizing TGF-β Signaling. *Arthritis Res. Ther.* **2022**, *24*, 94. [PubMed]
36. Roh, J.S.; Jeong, H.; Lee, B.; Song, B.W.; Han, S.J.; Lee, S.G. Mirodenafil Ameliorates Skin Fibrosis in Bleomycin-Induced Mouse Model of Systemic Sclerosis. *Anim. Cells Syst.* **2021**, *25*, 387–395. [CrossRef]
37. Wermuth, P.J.; Li, Z.; Mendoza, F.A.; Jimenez, S.A. Stimulation of Transforming Growth Factor-B1-Induced Endothelial-to-Mesenchymal Transition and Tissue Fibrosis by Endothelin-1 (ET-1): A Novel Profibrotic Effect of ET-1. *PLoS ONE* **2016**, *11*, e0161988. [CrossRef]
38. Cipriani, P.; Di Benedetto, P.; Ruscitti, P.; Capece, D.; Zazzeroni, F.; Liakouli, V.; Pantano, I.; Berardicurti, O.; Carubbi, F.; Pecetti, G.; et al. The Endothelial-mesenchymal Transition in Systemic Sclerosis Is Induced by Endothelin-1 and Transforming Growth Factor-β and May Be Blocked by Macitentan, a Dual Endothelin-1 Receptor Antagonist. *J. Rheumatol.* **2015**, *42*, 1808–1816. [CrossRef]
39. Beyer, C.; Reichert, H.; Akan, H.; Mallano, T.; Schramm, A.; Dees, C.; Palumbo-Zerr, K.; Lin, N.Y.; Distler, A.; Gelse, K.; et al. Blockade of Canonical WNT Signalling Ameliorates Experimental Dermal Fibrosis. *Ann. Rheum. Dis.* **2013**, *72*, 1255–1258. [CrossRef]
40. Liu, R.M.; Desai, L.P. Reciprocal Regulation of TGF-β and Reactive Oxygen Species: A Perverse Cycle for Fibrosis. *Redox Biol.* **2015**, *6*, 565–577. [CrossRef]
41. Wermuth, P.J.; Mendoza, F.A.; Jimenez, S.A. Abrogation of Transforming Growth Factor-B-Induced Tissue Fibrosis in Mice with a Global Genetic Deletion of Nox4. *Lab. Investig.* **2019**, *99*, 470–482. [CrossRef]
42. Tomčík, M.; Zerr, P.; Pitkowski, J.; Palumbo-Zerr, K.; Avouac, J.; Distler, O.; Becvar, R.; Senolt, L.; Schett, G.; Distler, J.H. Heat Shock Protein 90 (Hsp90) Inhibition Targets Canonical TGF-β Signalling to Prevent Fibrosis. *Ann. Rheum. Dis.* **2013**, *73*, 1215–1222. [CrossRef]
43. Lis-Święty, A.; Widuchowska, M.; Brzezińska-Wcisło, L.; Kucharz, E. High acute phase protein levels correlate with pulmonary and skin involvement in patients with diffuse systemic sclerosis. *J. Int. Med. Res.* **2018**, *46*, 1634–1639. [CrossRef] [PubMed]
44. Clarke, D.L.; Carruthers, A.M.; Mustelin, T.; Murray, L.A. Matrix regulation of idiopathic pulmonary fibrosis: The role of enzymes. *Fibrogenesis Tissue Repair.* **2013**, *6*, 20.
45. Vietri, L.; Fui, A.; Bergantini, L.; d'Alessandro, M.; Cameli, P.; Sestini, P.; Rottoli, P.; Bargagli, E. Serum amyloid A: A potential biomarker of lung disorders. *Respir. Investig.* **2020**, *58*, 21–27.
46. Lakota, K.; Carns, M.; Podlusky, S.; Mrak-Poljsak, K.; Hinchcliff, M.; Lee, J.; Tomsic, M.; Sodin-Semrl, S.; Varga, J. Serum amyloid a is a marker for pulmonary involvement in systemic sclerosis. *PLoS ONE* **2015**, *10*, e0110820.
47. Ogata, A.; Tanaka, T. Tocilizumab for the treatment of rheumatoid arthritis and other systemic autoimmune diseases: Current perspectives and future directions. *Int. J. Rheumatol.* **2012**, *2012*, 946048. [CrossRef] [PubMed]
48. Ito, T.; Tamura, N.; Okuda, S.; Tada, K.; Matsushita, M.; Yamaji, K.; Kato, K.; Takasaki, Y. Elevated serum levels of soluble CD146 in patients with systemic sclerosis. *Clin. Rheumatol.* **2017**, *36*, 119–124. [CrossRef]
49. Heim, X.; Joshkon, A.; Bermudez, J.; Bachelier, R.; Dubrou, C.; Boucraut, J.; Foucault-Bertaud, A.; Leroyer, A.S.; Dignat-George, F.; Blot-Chabaud, M.; et al. CD146/sCD146 in the Pathogenesis and Monitoring of Angiogenic and Inflammatory Diseases. *Biomedicines* **2020**, *8*, 592. [CrossRef] [PubMed]
50. Nollet, M.; Bachelier, R.; Joshkon, A.; Traboulsi, W.; Mahieux, A.; Moyon, A.; Muller, A.; Somasundaram, I.; Simoncini, S.; Peiretti, F.; et al. Involvement of Multiple Variants of Soluble CD146 in Systemic Sclerosis: Identification of a Novel Profibrotic Factor. *Arthritis Rheumatol.* **2022**, *74*, 1027–1038. [CrossRef]

51. Heim, X.; Bermudez, J.; Joshkon, A.; Kaspi, E.; Bachelier, R.; Nollet, M.; Vélier, M.; Dou, L.; Brodovitch, A.; Foucault-Bertaud, A.; et al. CD146 at the Interface between Oxidative Stress and the Wnt Signaling Pathway in Systemic Sclerosis. *J. Investig. Dermatol.* **2022**, *142*, 3200–3210.e5. [CrossRef]
52. Zhang, L.; Luo, Y.; Teng, X.; Wu, Z.; Li, M.; Xu, D.; Wang, Q.; Wang, F.; Feng, J.; Zeng, X.; et al. CD146: A potential therapeutic target for systemic sclerosis. *Protein Cell.* **2018**, *9*, 1050–1054. [CrossRef] [PubMed]
53. Le Tallec, E.; Bellamri, N.; Lelong, M.; Morzadec, C.; Frenger, Q.; Ballerie, A.; Cazalets, C.; Lescoat, A.; Gros, F.; Lecureur, V.; et al. Efferocytosis dysfunction in CXCL4-induced M4 macrophages: Phenotypic insights in systemic sclerosis in vitro and in vivo. *Front. Immunol.* **2024**, *15*, 1468821. [CrossRef] [PubMed]
54. Parker, M.J.S.; Jee, A.S.; Hansen, D.; Proudman, S.; Youssef, P.; Kenna, T.J.; Stevens, W.; Nikpour, M.; Sahhar, J.; Corte, T.J. Multiple serum biomarkers associate with mortality and interstitial lung disease progression in systemic sclerosis. *Rheumatology* **2024**, *63*, 2981–2988. [CrossRef]
55. Volkmann, E.R.; Tashkin, D.P.; Roth, M.D.; Clements, P.J.; Khanna, D.; Fürst, D.E.; Mayes, M.; Charles, J.; Tseng, C.-H.; Elashoff, R.M.; et al. Changes in Plasma CXCL4 Levels Are Associated with Improvements in Lung Function in Patients Receiving Immunosuppressive Therapy for Systemic Sclerosis-Related Interstitial Lung Disease. *Arthritis Res. Ther.* **2016**, *18*, 305. [CrossRef]
56. Affandi, A.J.; Carvalheiro, T.; Ottria, A.; de Haan, J.J.; Brans, M.A.D.; Brandt, M.M.; Tieland, R.G.; Lopes, A.P.; Fernández, B.M.; Bekker, C.P.; et al. CXCL4 Drives Fibrosis by Promoting Several Key Cellular and Molecular Processes. *Cell Rep.* **2022**, *38*, 110189. [CrossRef]
57. van der Kroef, M.; Carvalheiro, T.; Rossato, M.; de Wit, F.; Cossu, M.; Chouri, E.; Wichers, C.G.; Bekker, C.P.; Beretta, L.; Vazirpanah, N.; et al. CXCL4 Triggers Monocytes and Macrophages to Produce PDGF-BB, Culminating in Fibroblast Activation: Implications for Systemic Sclerosis. *J. Autoimmun.* **2020**, *111*, 102444. [CrossRef] [PubMed]
58. Lande, R.; Mennella, A.; Palazzo, R.; Pietraforte, I.; Stefanantoni, K.; Iannace, N.; Butera, A.; Boirivant, M.; Pica, R.; Conrad, C.; et al. Anti-Cxcl4 Antibody Reactivity Is Present in Systemic Sclerosis (SSc) and Correlates with the SSc Type I Interferon Signature. *Int. J. Mol. Sci.* **2020**, *21*, 5102. [CrossRef]
59. Nihtyanova, S.I.; Schreiber, B.E.; Ong, V.H.; Rosenberg, D.; Moinzadeh, P.; Coghlan, J.G.; Wells, A.U.; Denton, C.P. Prediction of Pulmonary Complications and Long-Term Survival in Systemic Sclerosis. *Arthritis Rheumatol.* **2014**, *66*, 1625–1635. [CrossRef]
60. Iannazzo, F.; Pellicano, C.; Colalillo, A.; Ramaccini, C.; Romaniello, A.; Gigante, A.; Rosato, E. Interleukin-33 and Soluble Suppression of Tumorigenicity 2 in Scleroderma Cardiac Involvement. *Clin. Exp. Med.* **2022**, *23*, 897–903. [CrossRef]
61. Wagner, A.; Köhm, M.; Nordin, A.; Svenungsson, E.; Pfeilschifter, J.; Radeke, H.H. Increased Serum Levels of the IL-33 Neutralizing sST2 in Limited Cutaneous Systemic Sclerosis. *Scand. J. Immunol.* **2015**, *82*, 269–274. [CrossRef]
62. Chen, D.; Untaru, R.; Stavropoulou, G.; Assadi-Khansari, B.; Kelly, C.; Croft, A.J.; Sugito, S.; Collins, N.J.; Sverdlov, A.L.; Ngo, D.T.M. Elevated Soluble Suppressor of Tumorigenicity 2 Predict Hospital Admissions Due to Major Adverse Cardiovascular Events (MACE). *J. Clin. Med.* **2023**, *12*, 2790. [CrossRef] [PubMed]
63. Manzano-Fernández, S.; Mueller, T.; Pascual-Figal, D.A.; Truong, Q.A.; Januzzi, J.L. Usefulness of Soluble Concentrations of Interleukin Family Member ST2 as Predictor of Mortality in Patients with Acutely Decompensated Heart Failure Relative to Left Ventricular Ejection Fraction. *Am. J. Cardiol.* **2011**, *107*, 259–267.
64. Banaszkiewicz, M.; Pietrasik, A.; Darocha, S.; Piłka, M.; Florczyk, M.; Dobosiewicz, A.; Kędzierski, P.; Pędzich-Placha, E.; Kochman, J.; Opolski, G.; et al. Soluble ST2 Protein as a New Biomarker in Patientswith Precapillary Pulmonary Hypertension. *Arch. Med. Sci.* **2020**, *16*, 1442–1451.
65. Aghaei, M.; Gharibdost, F.; Zayeni, H.; Akhlaghi, M.; Sedighi, S.; Rostamian, A.; Aghdami, N.; Shojaa, M. Endothelin-1 in systemic sclerosis. *Indian Dermatol Online J.* **2012**, *3*, 14. [PubMed]
66. Kawaguchi, Y.; Suzuki, K.; Hara, M.; Hidaka, T.; Ishizuka, T.; Kawagoe, M.; Nakamura, H. Increased endothelin-1 production in fibroblasts derived from patients with systemic sclerosis. *Ann. Rheum. Dis.* **1994**, *53*, 506–510. [CrossRef]
67. Duangrat, R.; Parichatikanond, W.; Likitnukul, S.; Mangmool, S. Endothelin-1 Induces Cell Proliferation and Myofibroblast Differentiation through the ETAR/Gαq/ERK Signaling Pathway in Human Cardiac Fibroblasts. *Int. J. Mol. Sci.* **2023**, *24*, 4475. [CrossRef]
68. Jing, J.; Dou, T.; Yang, J.L.; Chen, X.B.; Cao, H.L.; Min, M.; Cai, S.; Zheng, M.; Man, X. Role of Endothelin-1 in the Skin Fibrosis of Systemic Sclerosis. *Eur. Cytokine Netw.* **2015**, *26*, 10–14.
69. Ture, H.Y.; Lee, N.Y.; Kim, N.R.; Nam, E.J. Raynaud's Phenomenon: A Current Update on Pathogenesis, Diagnostic Workup, and Treatment. *Vasc. Spec. Int.* **2024**, *40*, 26.
70. ya Kawashiri, S.; Ueki, Y.; Terada, K.; Yamasaki, S.; Aoyagi, K.; Kawakami, A. Improvement of plasma endothelin-1 and nitric oxide in patients with systemic sclerosis by bosentan therapy. *Rheumatol. Int.* **2014**, *34*, 221–225. [CrossRef]
71. Jordan, S.; Distler, J.H.; Maurer, B.; Walker, U.A.; Huscher, D.; Allanore, Y.; Riemekasten, G.; Distler, O. Effect of Endothelin-1 Receptor Antagonists on Skin Fibrosis in Scleroderma Patients From the EUSTAR Database. *J. Scleroderma Relat. Disord.* **2016**, *1*, 220–225.

72. Lagares, D.; García-Fernández, R.A.; Jiménez, C.L.; Magán-Marchal, N.; Busnadiego, Ó.; Lamas, S.; Rodríguez-Pascual, F. Endothelin 1 Contributes to the Effect of Transforming Growth Factor B1 on Wound Repair and Skin Fibrosis. *Arthritis Rheum.* **2010**, *62*, 878–889.
73. Tinazzi, E.; Puccetti, A.; Patuzzo, G.; Barbieri, A.; Argentino, G.; Federico, C.; Marzia, D.; Ruggero, B.; Giacomo, M.; Andrea, O.; et al. Endothelin Receptors Expressed by Immune Cells Are Involved in Modulation of Inflammation and in Fibrosis: Relevance to the Pathogenesis of Systemic Sclerosis. *J. Immunol. Res.* **2015**, *2015*, 147616.
74. Odler, B.; Foris, V.; Gungl, A.; Müller, V.; Hassoun, P.M.; Kwapiszewska, G.; Olschewski, H.; Kovacs, G. Biomarkers for Pulmonary Vascular Remodeling in Systemic Sclerosis: A Pathophysiological Approach. *Front. Physiol.* **2018**, *9*, 587. [CrossRef] [PubMed]
75. Iijima, H.; Fukutani, N.; Aoyama, T.; Fukumoto, T.; Uritani, D.; Kaneda, E.; Ota, K.; Kuroki, H.; Matsuda, S. Clinical Phenotype Classifications Based on Static Varus Alignment and Varus Thrust in Japanese Patients with Medial Knee Osteoarthritis. *Arthritis Rheumatol.* **2015**, *67*, 2354–2362. [PubMed]
76. Pincha, N.; Hajam, E.Y.; Badarinath, K.; Batta, S.P.R.; Masudi, T.; Dey, R.; Andreasen, P.; Kawakami, T.; Samuel, R.; George, R.; et al. PAI1 mediates fibroblast–mast cell interactions in skin fibrosis. *J. Clin. Investig.* **2018**, *128*, 1807–1819. [CrossRef] [PubMed]
77. Ham, S.M.; Song, M.J.; Yoon, H.S.; Lee, D.H.; Chung, J.H.; Lee, S.T. SPARC Is Highly Expressed in Young Skin and Promotes Extracellular Matrix Integrity in Fibroblasts via the TGF-β Signaling Pathway. *Int. J. Mol. Sci.* **2023**, *24*, 12179. [CrossRef]
78. Bradshaw, A.D. The role of secreted protein acidic and rich in cysteine (SPARC) in cardiac repair and fibrosis: Does expression of SPARC by macrophages influence outcomes? *J. Mol. Cell. Cardiol.* **2016**, *93*, 156–161.
79. Rudnik, M.; Hukara, A.; Kocherova, I.; Jordan, S.; Schniering, J.; Milleret, V.; Ehrbar, M.; Klingel, K.; Feghali-Bostwick, C.; Distler, O.; et al. Elevated Fibronectin Levels in Profibrotic CD14+ Monocytes and CD14+ Macrophages in Systemic Sclerosis. *Front. Immunol.* **2021**, *12*, 642891. [CrossRef]
80. Roblin, E.; Clark, K.E.N.; Beesley, C.; Ong, V.H.; Denton, C.P. Testing a candidate composite serum protein marker of skin severity in systemic sclerosis. *Rheumatol. Adv. Pract.* **2024**, *8*, rkae039. [CrossRef]
81. Bălănescu, P.; Balanescu, A.; Bălănescu, E.; Băicuș, C. Candidate Proteomic Biomarkers in Systemic Sclerosis Discovered Using Mass-Spectrometry: An Update of a Systematic Review (2014–2020). *Rom. J. Intern. Med.* **2021**, *59*, 101–111.
82. Ren, L.; Chang, Y.F.; Jiang, S.H.; Li, X.H.; Cheng, H.P. DNA methylation modification in Idiopathic pulmonary fibrosis. *Front. Cell Dev. Biol.* **2024**, *12*, 1416325. [CrossRef]
83. Torii, T.; Ohno, N.; Miyamoto, Y.; Kawahara, K.; Saitoh, Y.; Nakamura, K.; Takashima, S.; Sakagami, H.; Tanoue, A.; Yamauchi, J. Arf6 Guanine-Nucleotide Exchange Factor Cytohesin-2 Regulates Myelination in Nerves. *Biochem. Biophys. Res. Commun.* **2015**, *460*, 819–825. [CrossRef]
84. Wang, Y.; Çil, Ç.; Harnett, M.M.; Pineda, M.A. Cytohesin-2/ARNO: A Novel Bridge Between Cell Migration and Immunoregulation in Synovial Fibroblasts. *Front. Immunol.* **2022**, *12*, 809896. [CrossRef] [PubMed]
85. van den Bosch, M.; Poole, A.W.; Hers, I. Cytohesin-2 Phosphorylation by Protein Kinase C Relieves the Constitutive Suppression of Platelet Dense Granule Secretion by ADP-ribosylation Factor 6. *J. Thromb. Haemost.* **2014**, *12*, 726–735. [CrossRef] [PubMed]
86. Nikpour, M.; Hissaria, P.; Byron, J.; Sahhar, J.; Micallef, M.; Paspaliaris, W.; Roddy, J.; Nash, P.; Sturgess, A.; Proudman, S.; et al. Prevalence, Correlates and Clinical Usefulness of Antibodies to RNA Polymerase III in Systemic Sclerosis: A Cross-Sectional Analysis of Data From an Australian Cohort. *Arthritis Res. Ther.* **2011**, *13*, R211. [CrossRef] [PubMed]
87. Roderburg, C.; Urban, G.W.; Bettermann, K.; Vucur, M.; Zimmermann, H.W.; Schmidt, S.; Janssen, J.; Koppe, C.; Knolle, P.; Castoldi, M.; et al. Micro-Rna Profiling Reveals a Role for miR-29 in Human and Murine Liver Fibrosis. *Hepatology* **2011**, *53*, 209–218. [CrossRef]
88. Lauer, D.; Magnin, C.Y.; Kolly, L.R.; Wang, H.; Brunner, M.; Chabria, M.; Cereghetti, G.M.; Gabryś, H.S.; Tanadini-Lang, S.; Uldry, A.-C.; et al. Radioproteomics stratifies molecular response to antifibrotic treatment in pulmonary fibrosis. *JCI Insight.* **2024**, *9*, e181757. [CrossRef]
89. Hansen, A.L.; Buchan, G.; Rühl, M.; Mukai, K.; Salvatore, S.R.; Ogawa, E.; Andersen, S.D.; Iversen, M.B.; Thielke, A.L.; Gunderstofte, C.; et al. Nitro-Fatty Acids Are Formed in Response to Virus Infection and Are Potent Inhibitors of STING Palmitoylation and Signaling. *Proc. Natl. Acad. Sci. USA* **2018**, *115*, E7768–E7775. [CrossRef]
90. Gremmels, H.; Teraa, M.; de Jager, S.C.A.; Pasterkamp, G.; de Borst, G.J.; Verhaar, M.C. A Pro-Inflammatory Biomarker-Profile Predicts Amputation-Free Survival in Patients with Severe Limb Ischemia. *Sci. Rep.* **2019**, *9*, 10740. [CrossRef]
91. Magee, K.; Kelsey, C.; Kurzinski, K.L.; Ho, J.; Mlakar, L.; Feghali-Bostwick, C.; Torok, K.S. Interferon-Gamma Inducible Protein-10 as a Potential Biomarker in Localized Scleroderma. *Arthritis Res. Ther.* **2013**, *15*, R188. [CrossRef]
92. Oatis, D.; Herman, H.; Balta, C.; Ciceu, A.; Simon-Repolski, E.; Mihu, A.G.; Lepre, C.C.; Russo, M.; Trotta, M.C.; Gravina, A.G.; et al. Dynamic Shifts in Lung Cytokine Patterns in Post-Covid-19 Interstitial Lung Disease Patients: A Pilot Study. *Ther. Adv. Chronic Dis.* **2024**, *15*, 20406223241236257. [CrossRef] [PubMed]
93. Muñoz-Esquerre, M.; Aliagas, E.; López-Sánchez, M.; Escobar, I.; Huertas, D.; Penín, R.M.; Dorca, J.; Santos, S. Vascular Disease in COPD: Systemic and Pulmonary Expression of PARC (Pulmonary and Activation-Regulated Chemokine). *PLoS ONE* **2017**, *12*, e0177218. [CrossRef] [PubMed]

94. Aoyama, T.; Inokuchi, S.; Brenner, D.A.; Seki, E. CX3CL1-CX3CR1 Interaction Prevents Carbon Tetrachloride-Induced Liver Inflammation and Fibrosis in Mice. *Hepatology* **2010**, *52*, 1390–1400. [CrossRef]
95. Pezeshkian, F.; Shahriarirad, R.; Mahram, H. An overview of the role of chemokine CX3CL1 (Fractalkine) and CX3C chemokine receptor 1 in systemic sclerosis. *Immun. Inflamm. Dis.* **2024**, *12*, e70034. [CrossRef] [PubMed]
96. Chu, H.; Wu, T.; Wu, W.; Tu, W.; Jiang, S.; Chen, S.; Ma, Y.; Liu, Q.; Zhou, X.; Jin, L.; et al. Involvement of Collagen Binding Heat Shock Protein 47 in Scleroderma-Associated Fibrosis. *Protein Cell.* **2015**, *6*, 589–598. [CrossRef]
97. Artlett, C.M.; Connolly, L.M. TANGO1 Dances to Export of Procollagen from the Endoplasmic Reticulum. *Fibrosis* **2023**, *1*, 10008. [CrossRef]
98. Pehlıvan, Y.; Onat, A.M.; Ceylan, N.; Turkbeyler, I.H.; Buyukhatipoglu, H.; Comez, G.; Babacan, T.; Tarakcioglu, M. Serum Leptin, Resistin and TNF-α Levels in Patients with Systemic Sclerosis: The Role of Adipokines in Scleroderma. *Int. J. Rheum. Dis.* **2012**, *15*, 374–379. [CrossRef]
99. Didriksen, H.; Molberg, Ø.; Fretheim, H.; Gude, E.; Jordan, S.; Brunborg, C.; Palchevskiy, V.; Garen, T.; Midtvedt, Ø.; Andreassen, A.K.; et al. Association of Lymphangiogenic Factors with Pulmonary Arterial Hypertension in Systemic Sclerosis. *Arthritis Rheumatol.* **2021**, *73*, 1277–1287. [CrossRef]
100. Tsai, Y.; Lee, C.S.; Chiu, Y.; Kuo, H.C.; Lee, S.C.; Hwang, S.L.; Kuo, M.-C.; Chen, H.-C. Angiopoietin-2 as a Prognostic Biomarker of Major Adverse Cardiovascular Events and All-Cause Mortality in Chronic Kidney Disease. *PLoS ONE* **2015**, *10*, e0135181. [CrossRef]
101. Michalska-Jakubus, M.; Cutolo, M.; Smith, V.; Krasowska, D. Imbalanced serum levels of Ang1, Ang2 and VEGF in systemic sclerosis: Integrated effects on microvascular reactivity. *Microvasc. Res.* **2019**, *125*, 103881. [CrossRef]
102. Barile, R.; Rotondo, C.; Rella, V.; Trotta, A.; Cantatore, F.P.; Corrado, A. Fibrosis mechanisms in systemic sclerosis and new potential therapies. *Postgrad Med. J.* **2024**, *2024*, qgae169.
103. Papaioannou, A.I.; Zakynthinos, E.; Kostikas, K.; Kiropoulos, T.; Koutsokera, A.; Ziogas, A.; Koutroumpas, A.; Sakkas, L.; I Gourgoulianis, K.; Daniil, Z.D. Serum VEGF Levels Are Related to the Presence of Pulmonary Arterial Hypertension in Systemic Sclerosis. *BMC Pulm. Med.* **2009**, *9*, 18.
104. Apti Sengun, O.; Ergun, T.; Guctekin, T.; Alibaz Oner, F. Endothelial dysfunction, thrombophilia, and nailfold capillaroscopic features in livedoid vasculopathy. *Microvasc. Res.* **2023**, *150*, 104591.
105. Doridot, L.; Jeljeli, M.; Chêne, C.; Batteux, F. Implication of Oxidative Stress in the Pathogenesis of Systemic Sclerosis via Inflammation, Autoimmunity and Fibrosis. *Redox Biol.* **2019**, *25*, 101122. [CrossRef]
106. Piera-Velazquez, S.; Jimenez, S.A. Oxidative Stress Induced by Reactive Oxygen Species (ROS) and NADPH Oxidase 4 (NOX4) in the Pathogenesis of the Fibrotic Process in Systemic Sclerosis: A Promising Therapeutic Target. *J. Clin. Med.* **2021**, *10*, 4791. [CrossRef]
107. Chung, C.P.; Avalos, I.; Stein, C.M. Oxidative stress, microvascular dysfunction, and scleroderma: An association with potential therapeutic implications, a commentary on "Postocclusive reactive hyperemia inversely correlates with urinary 15-F2t-isoprostane levels in systemic sclerosis. " *Free. Radic. Biol. Med.* **2006**, *40*, 1698–1699. [PubMed]
108. Zanin-Silva, D.C.; Santana-Gonçalves, M.; Kawashima-Vasconcelos, M.Y.; Oliveira, M.C. Management of Endothelial Dysfunction in Systemic Sclerosis: Current and Developing Strategies. *Front. Med.* **2021**, *8*, 788250.
109. de Andrade, J.A.; Thannickal, V.J. Innovative approaches to the therapy of fibrosis. *Curr. Opin. Rheumatol.* **2009**, *21*, 649–655.
110. Lakota, K.; Wei, J.; Carns, M.; Hinchcliff, M.; Lee, J.H.; Whitfield, M.L.; Sodin-Semrl, S.; Varga, J. Levels of Adiponectin, a Marker for PPAR-gamma Activity, Correlate with Skin Fibrosis in Systemic Sclerosis: Potential Utility as Biomarker? *Arthritis Res Ther.* **2012**, *14*, R102.
111. Sebestyén, V.; Ujvárosy, D.; Ratku, B.; Lőrincz, H.; Csiha, S.; Tari, D.; Majai, G.; Somodi, S.; Szűcs, G.; Harangi, M.; et al. Inflammatory Biomarkers and Lipid Parameters May Predict an Increased Risk for Atrial Arrhythmias in Patients with Systemic Sclerosis. *Biomedicines* **2025**, *13*, 220. [CrossRef]
112. Lee, Y.H.; Song, G.G. Association of Circulating Resistin, Leptin, Adiponectin and Visfatin Levels with Behçet Disease: A Meta-Analysis. *Clin. Exp. Dermatol.* **2018**, *43*, 536–545. [PubMed]
113. Górska-Ciebiada, M.; Saryusz-Wolska, M.; Borkowska, A.; Ciebiada, M.; Loba, J. Adiponectin, Leptin and IL-1 B in Elderly Diabetic Patients with Mild Cognitive Impairment. *Metab. Brain Dis.* **2015**, *31*, 257–266.
114. Chatterjee, M.; Behrendt, A.; Schmid, M.; Beck, S.; Schneider, M.; Mack, A.F.; Müller, I.; Geisler, T.; Gawaz, M. Platelets as a Novel Source of Gremlin-1: Implications for Thromboinflammation. *Thromb. Haemost.* **2017**, *117*, 311–324. [PubMed]
115. Lofaro, F.D.; Giuggioli, D.; Bonacorsi, S.; Orlandi, M.; Spinella, A.; De Pinto, M.; Secchi, O.; Ferri, C.; Boraldi, F. BMP-4 and fetuin A in systemic sclerosis patients with or without calcinosis. *Front. Immunol.* **2024**, *15*, 1502324.
116. Torres, G.; Lancaster, A.C.; Yang, J.; Griffiths, M.; Brandal, S.; Damico, R.; Vaidya, D.; Simpson, C.E.; Martin, L.J.; Pauciulo, M.W.; et al. Low-affinity Insulin-like Growth Factor Binding Protein 7 and Its Association with Pulmonary Arterial Hypertension Severity and Survival. *Pulm. Circ.* **2023**, *13*, e12284.

117. Yan, Y.M.; Zheng, J.N.; Li, Y.; Yang, Q.; Shao, W.; Wang, Q. Insulin-Like Growth Factor Binding Protein 7 as a Candidate Biomarker for Systemic Sclerosis. *Clin. Exp. Rheumatol.* **2021**, *39*, 66–76. [PubMed]
118. Costales, J.L.; Kolevzon, A. The Therapeutic Potential of Insulin-Like Growth Factor-1 in Central Nervous System Disorders. *Neurosci. Biobehav. Rev.* **2016**, *63*, 207–222.
119. Agachi, S.; Groppa, L.; Rotaru, L.; Deseatnicova, E.; Chișlari, L.; Russu, E. Novel Biomarkers in Systemic Sclerosis. *Mold. J. Health Sci.* **2022**, *28*, 57–67.
120. Vértes, V.; Porpáczy, A.; Nógrádi, Á.; Tőkés-Füzesi, M.; Hajdu, M.; Czirják, L.; Komócsi, A.; Faludi, R. Galectin-3 and sST2: Associations to the Echocardiographic Markers of the Myocardial Mechanics in Systemic Sclerosis—A Pilot Study. *Cardiovasc. Ultrasound* **2022**, *20*, 1–10.
121. Zhao, C.N.; Mao, Y.M.; Liu, L.; Wu, Q.; Dan, Y.L.; Pan, H. Plasma Galectin-3 Levels Do Not Differ in Systemic Lupus Erythematosus Patients. *Int. J. Rheum. Dis.* **2019**, *22*, 1820–1824.
122. Bellan, M.; Piccinino, C.; Tonello, S.; Minisini, R.; Giubertoni, A.; Sola, D.; Pedrazzoli, R.; Gagliardi, I.; Zecca, E.; Calzaducca, E.; et al. Role of Osteopontin as a Potential Biomarker of Pulmonary Arterial Hypertension in Patients with Systemic Sclerosis and Other Connective Tissue Diseases (CTDs). *Pharmaceuticals* **2021**, *14*, 394. [CrossRef] [PubMed]
123. Bălănescu, P.; Bălănescu, E.; Băicuș, C.; Balanescu, A. S100A6, Calumenin and Cytohesin 2 as Biomarkers for Cutaneous Involvement in Systemic Sclerosis Patients: A Case Control Study. *J. Pers. Med.* **2021**, *11*, 368. [CrossRef]
124. Prieto-Echagüe, V.; Lodh, S.; Colman, L.; Bobba, N.; Santos, L.; Katsanis, N.; Escande, C.; Zaghloul, N.A.; Badano, J.L. BBS4 Regulates the Expression and Secretion of FSTL1, a Protein That Participates in Ciliogenesis and the Differentiation of 3t3-L1. *Sci Rep.* **2017**, *7*, 9765.
125. Kortam, N.; Liang, W.; Shiple, C.; Huang, S.; Gedert, R.; Clair, J.S.; Sarosh, C.; Foster, C.; Tsou, P.-S.; Varga, J.; et al. Elevated neutrophil extracellular traps in systemic sclerosis-associated vasculopathy and suppression by a synthetic prostacyclin analog. *Arthritis Res. Ther.* **2024**, *26*, 139. [PubMed]
126. Otake, S.; Saito, K.; Chiba, Y.; Yamada, A.; Fukumoto, S. S100a6 Knockdown Promotes the Differentiation of Dental Epithelial Cells Toward the Epidermal Lineage Instead of the Odontogenic Lineage. *FASEB J.* **2024**, *38*, e23608.
127. Yanagimachi, M.; Fukuda, S.; Tanaka, F.; Iwamoto, M.; Takao, C.; Oba, K.; Suzuki, N.; Kiyohara, K.; Kuranobu, D.; Tada, N.; et al. Leucine-Rich Alpha-2-Glycoprotein 1 and Angiotensinogen as Diagnostic Biomarkers for Kawasaki Disease. *PLoS ONE* **2021**, *16*, e0257138.
128. Wang, J.; Wang, J.; Zhong, J.; Liu, H.; Li, W.; Chen, M.; Xu, L.; Zhang, W.; Zhang, Z.; Wei, Z.; et al. LRG1 promotes atherosclerosis by inducing macrophage M1-like polarization. *Proc. Natl. Acad. Sci. USA* **2024**, *121*, e2405845121.
129. Jaeger, V.K.; Tikly, M.; Xu, D.; Siegert, E.; Hachulla, E.; Airò, P.; Valentini, G.; Cerinic, M.M.; Distler, O.; Cozzi, F.; et al. Racial differences in systemic sclerosis disease presentation: A European Scleroderma Trials and Research group study. *Rheumatology* **2020**, *59*, 1684–1694.
130. Murdaca, G.; Spanò, F.; Contatore, M.; Guastalla, A.; Puppo, F. Potential use of TNF-α inhibitors in systemic sclerosis. *Immunotherapy* **2014**, *6*, 283–289. [CrossRef]

sclerosis

Review

B-Cell-Depleting Immune Therapies as Potential New Treatment Options for Systemic Sclerosis

Gerhard Zugmaier [1,*], Matthias Klinger [1], Marion Subklewe [2], Faraz Zaman [3] and Franco Locatelli [4]

1 Amgen Research (Munich) GmbH, 81477 Munich, Germany
2 Department of Medicine III & Gene Center, University Hospital Munich, Ludwig-Maximilians-Universität, 81377 Munich, Germany; marion.subklewe@med.uni-muenchen.de
3 Amgen Inc., Thousand Oaks, CA 91320, USA; fzaman01@amgen.com
4 IRCCS Ospedale Pediatrico Bambino Gesù, Catholic University of the Sacred Heart, 00163 Rome, Italy; franco.locatelli@opbg.net
* Correspondence: gerhardz@amgen.com

Abstract: Background: Systemic sclerosis (SSc), also known as scleroderma, is a complex, chronic autoimmune disease characterized by fibrosis of the skin and internal organs, vasculopathy, and immune system dysregulation. The treatment of SSc has historically focused on symptom management and slowing down disease progression through conventional immune-suppressive agents. New therapeutic approaches have been emerging due to advances in understanding of the disease mechanisms, particularly in the areas of fibrosis, vascular involvement, and immune dysregulation. Methods: In this review of the literature, we discuss the current stage of development of B-cell-depleting immune therapies in SSc. Results: B-cell depletion therapy has become an area of growing interest in the treatment of SSc due to the role played by B cells in the pathogenesis of the disease. There is increasing evidence that B cells contribute to disease progression through multiple mechanisms. B cells in SSc are implicated in autoantibody production, cytokine production, and fibroblast activation. B cells are responsible for producing autoantibodies, such as anti-topoisomerase I (Scl-70) and anti-centromere antibodies, which are hallmarks of SSc. B cells release pro-inflammatory cytokines (such as interleukin-6 [IL-6] and transforming growth factor β [TGF-β]), which promote fibrosis and inflammation, they also contribute to the activation of fibroblasts, the cells responsible for excessive collagen production and fibrosis, a key feature of SSc. Conclusions: In light of these findings, therapies that target B cells are being investigated for their potential to modify the disease course in SSc, particularly by reducing autoantibody production, inflammation, and fibrosis.

Keywords: systemic sclerosis; autoimmunity; blinatumomab; B-cell depletion therapy

1. Introduction

Systemic sclerosis (SSc), also known as scleroderma, is a rare, chronic autoimmune connective tissue disorder characterized by fibrosis (thickening) of the skin and internal organs, vasculopathy (blood vessel dysfunction), and immune dysregulation. It primarily affects the skin, but can also involve various internal organs, including the heart, lungs, kidneys, and gastrointestinal tract. Systemic sclerosis has a broad spectrum of clinical manifestations, ranging from mild skin involvement to severe, life-threatening organ dysfunction. Systemic sclerosis is a rare disease, with an estimated prevalence of 50–300 cases per million people worldwide. The female-to-male ratio is approximately 4:1. Disease incidence peaks between 30 and 50 years [1].

Systemic sclerosis is classified into two major subtypes based on the extent of skin involvement. In limited cutaneous SSc, skin involvement is restricted to the hands, face, forearms, and feet. Commonly associated with a subtype called CREST syndrome, which includes Calcinosis, Raynaud's phenomenon, Esophageal dysmotility, Sclerodactyly, and Telangiectasias, internal organ involvement is generally less severe, but can still occur, particularly leading to pulmonary hypertension.

In diffuse cutaneous SSc, skin thickening extends beyond the hands and face, involving the trunk and proximal limbs, and is more likely to involve internal organs, including the lungs (interstitial lung disease [ILD]), heart, kidneys, and gastrointestinal system, with early and rapid visceral progression [1].

Systemic sclerosis holds a substantial risk of premature death. Mortality rates can be up to eightfold higher as compared with the general population [1].

The underlying mechanisms of SSc involve a complex interplay of immune system activation, vascular injury, and excessive fibrosis. The immune system attacks the body's tissues, resulting in chronic inflammation. A hallmark feature is the presence of specific autoantibodies, such as anti-centromere antibodies (common in limited cutaneous SSc) and anti-topoisomerase I (Scl-70) antibodies (associated with diffuse cutaneous SSc) [2]. Autoantibodies exacerbate endothelial dysfunction, which is central to vascular abnormalities in SSc (e.g., Raynaud's phenomenon and digital ulcers). Raynaud's phenomenon is defined by episodes of vasospasm in response to cold or stress, causing the fingers and toes to turn white, blue, or red [3]. Persistent presence of autoantibodies contributes to chronic immune dysregulation and fibrosis. Fibroblast-directed antibodies promote inflammation and fibrosis, amplifying tissue damage [4]. An overproduction of collagen and other extracellular matrix components leads to the thickening and hardening of the skin and internal organs. Skin thickening and hardening starting with swelling in the fingers is called sclerodactyly. Hyperpigmentation or hypopigmentation occurs in affected areas, and telangiectasias can be observed on the skin's surface. Esophageal dysmotility leads to acid reflux and difficulty in swallowing. Small bowel involvement can cause malabsorption, bloating, diarrhea, and, in most severe forms, paralytic ileus.

Interstitial lung disease and pulmonary arterial hypertension are major causes of morbidity and mortality. Symptoms include dyspnea, cough, and reduced exercise tolerance. Renal involvement can lead to scleroderma renal crisis, a potentially life-threatening condition characterized by a sudden onset of hypertension and renal failure. Cardiac involvement includes arrhythmias, heart failure, and pericarditis. The diagnosis of SSc is based on clinical features, autoantibody testing, and imaging studies [1].

2. Standard Treatment

The treatment of SSc is primarily focused on managing the specific symptoms and complications of the disease, as, at least so far, there is no known cure. Treatment approaches depend on whether the patient has limited cutaneous SSc or diffuse cutaneous SSc, as well as on the severity and type of organ involvement (e.g., pulmonary, renal, gastrointestinal).

Recommendations for the treatment of patients with SSc have been recently published by the European Alliance of Associations for Rheumatology (EULAR) in their updated guidelines [5]. The drugs usually employed depend on the organs involved and on the severity of the clinical manifestations, ranging from classical immune-suppressive drugs (including steroids, mofetil mycophenolate, methotrexate, and rituximab) to vascular-active agents (including phosphodiesterase 5 [PDE5] inhibitors, such as sildenafil, tadalafil, and vardenafil, or endothelin receptor antagonists (ERAs), such as bosentan and ambrisentan) in patients with ILD. Considering the poor prognosis of patients with lung involvement, the anti-interleukin-6 (IL-6) monoclonal antibody tocilizumab and the tyrosine-kinase inhibitor nintedanib are also considered for preventing the progression of SSc-associated ILD. For a more detailed overview of the different treatment options for patients with SSc, please refer to the recent EULAR recommendations [5].

In brief synthesis, treatment of skin and soft tissue involvement includes topical treatments, immune-suppressive drugs, and physical therapy. Topical treatments can, for example, include moisturizers and emollients, which can improve dryness of the skin. Immune-suppressive medications, such as methotrexate, mycophenolate mofetil, and cyclophosphamide, are administered against progressive skin thickening and fibrosis at early stages of diffuse cutaneous SSc. Physical therapy is applied to prevent contractures and stiffness. In some cases, phototherapy has improved skin symptoms in SSc [6].

Treatment of Raynaud's phenomenon includes calcium channel blockers (e.g., nifedipine or amlodipine), PDE5 inhibitors (e.g., sildenafil, tadalafil), endothelin receptor antagonists (e.g., bosentan), or iloprost (intravenous prostacyclin analog). Calcium channel blockers are also used as a first-line treatment to induce vasodilation.

For ILD, mycophenolate mofetil and cyclophosphamide are commonly administered as immune-suppressive agents. Nintedanib is an antifibrotic agent, while rituximab, an anti-cluster of differentiation 20 (anti-CD20) monoclonal antibody, is used as a B-cell-depleting agent. For pulmonary arterial hypertension, endothelin receptor antagonists (e.g., bosentan, ambrisentan) are administered to reduce vascular resistance in the lungs. Phosphodiesterase-5 inhibitors (e.g., sildenafil, tadalafil) improve vasodilation and exercise capacity. Prostacyclin analogs (e.g., epoprostenol, treprostinil, iloprost) are reserved for more advanced cases. Soluble guanylate cyclase stimulators (e.g., riociguat) are applied for increasing nitric oxide signaling and reducing pulmonary pressure [6].

Scleroderma renal crisis is a life-threatening complication, usually presenting with abrupt onset of severe hypertension and renal failure. Angiotensin-converting enzyme (ACE) inhibitors (e.g., captopril, enalapril) are the first-line choices of treatment.

Proton-pump inhibitors (e.g., omeprazole, lansoprazole) are widely used to treat gastroesophageal reflux disease, which is common in SSc. Prokinetic agents (e.g., metoclopramide, domperidone) are used to improve gastric emptying and reduce dysphagia and bloating. Antibiotics (e.g., rifaximin, tetracyclines) may be needed for treating bacterial overgrowth in the small intestine. Special diets (low-fiber, small frequent meals) may be recommended, and in severe cases, total parenteral nutrition may become necessary [6].

Immune-suppressive therapy (e.g., cyclophosphamide or mycophenolate mofetil) is applied to manage myocardial inflammation. Anti-arrhythmic drugs (e.g., amiodarone, beta-blockers) may be needed to control arrhythmias. Heart failure medications (e.g., diuretics, ACE inhibitors, beta-blockers) are used in cases of systolic or diastolic heart failure.

Immunomodulatory and anti-fibrotic therapies include a heterogeneous group of compounds. Cyclophosphamide is often used for severe skin disease and pulmonary involvement. It is typically given in cases of rapidly progressing diffuse cutaneous SSc with organ involvement. Mycophenolate mofetil is used as alternative to cyclophosphamide. Rituximab is studied for its role in reducing disease progression. Tocilizumab, an IL-6 receptor antagonist, has been studied for its potential role in reducing the progression of skin fibrosis. Autologous hematopoietic stem cell transplantation (HSCT), as an experimental therapy, has shown promise in selected patients with severe and rapidly progressing diffuse cutaneous SSc, offering the potential to reset the immune system [6–8].

3. B-Cell-Depleting Therapies as New Approach

In SSc, the excessive activation of the immune system contributes to fibrosis, vasculopathy, and tissue damage, raising the possibility that therapies aimed at reprogramming or depleting specific immune cells might help mitigate disease progression. B cells are involved in the autoimmune processes of SSc by producing autoantibodies, contributing to immune activation, and promoting fibrosis through the release of pro-fibrotic cytokines. Autoantibodies, such as anti-topoisomerase I (anti-Scl-70) and anti-centromere antibodies, are commonly associated with SSc, reflecting B-cell dysregulation. Recent evidence suggests that B cells play a key role in many autoimmune diseases by producing autoantibodies, including those that are commonly found in SSc [9].

4. Remodeling of the B-Cell Compartment

B-cell depletion, a therapeutic strategy employed in various autoimmune diseases and B-cell malignancies, induces significant changes within the immune system, commonly referred to as immune system remodeling. This process involves a series of adaptive responses that modify the composition, function, and interactions of immune cells, ultimately aiming to restore immune homeostasis while preserving the essential components of immune defense [10].

Surface antigens like CD19, CD20, and B-cell maturation antigen (BCMA) are targeted by therapies designed to eliminate autoreactive B cells. Food and Drug Administration (FDA)-approved T-cell engagers and chimeric antigen receptor T-cell (CAR-T) products have shown unprecedented efficacy in treating B-cell malignancies, such as acute lymphoblastic leukemia (ALL), non-Hodgkin lymphoma (NHL), and multiple myeloma (MM) [11–14]. These therapies work by selectively depleting B cells expressing specific markers, leading to profound changes in the immune landscape.

B-cell depletion therapies, particularly those targeting CD19, CD20, and BCMA, employ mechanisms such as antibody-mediated cell death, immune cell-mediated cytotoxicity, and CAR-T cell-induced apoptosis (see also Table 1) [15]. These interventions result in the elimination of both malignant and autoreactive B cells, thereby reducing pathogenic immune responses.

CD19 is a transmembrane glycoprotein expressed across various stages of B-cell development, from B-cell precursors to plasmablasts. Therapies targeting CD19, such as blinatumomab and CAR-T cell treatments, have demonstrated significant B-cell depletion, leading to long-term remissions in B-cell malignancies [12,13] and autoimmune diseases [16]. Notably, CD19 is absent on long-lived plasma cells, preserving these cells and maintaining antibody production and protective immunity against pathogens [15].

CD20 is predominantly expressed on mature B cells and absent on early progenitors and plasma cells. Anti-CD20 therapies effectively deplete mature B cells, but may not comprehensively eliminate autoreactive cells across all developmental stages [17]. Despite this limitation, these therapies contribute to the remodeling of the B-cell compartment by reducing the number of mature B cells and altering the immune environment [18].

BCMA is highly expressed on plasma cells and certain mature B cells, particularly in MM. Targeting BCMA primarily impacts plasma cells, leading to their depletion. This selective targeting spares other B-cell populations, limiting broader immune system remodeling, but offering substantial benefits in treating MM [19]. Targeting CD19 offers the advantage of preserving long-lived plasma cells, which are vital for maintaining protective immunity against widespread micro-organisms. This preservation ensures that the body retains its ability to respond to previously encountered pathogens, reducing the risk of infections post-treatment [15].

The primary goal of B-cell depletion in autoimmune diseases is to reduce the population of autoreactive B cells responsible for pathogenic antibody production. By eliminating these cells, therapies help mitigate autoimmune responses and promote immune tolerance [10]. Following B-cell depletion, the immune system undergoes a reconstitution phase where new B cells are generated from progenitor cells. This process can lead to the development of a more balanced and less autoreactive B-cell repertoire, contributing to sustained disease remission and reduced relapse rates.

B-cell depletion therapies induce significant immune system remodeling, characterized by the reduction in autoreactive B cells, reconstitution of B-cell populations, and maintenance of protective immunity. These adaptive responses aim to restore immune balance while preserving essential immune functions. As our understanding of these processes deepens, targeted B-cell therapies continue to evolve, offering promising prospects for the treatment of autoimmune diseases and B-cell malignancies [12,15].

Table 1. A comparison of rituximab with B-cell-depleting blinatumomab and CAR-T cell therapies.

Feature	Rituximab	Blinatumomab	CD19 CAR-T Cell Therapy
Mechanism of Action	Naked monoclonal antibody targeting CD20 on B cells. It acts mainly through complement-dependent cytotoxicity (CDC) and antibody-dependent cellular cytotoxicity (ADCC)	Bispecific T-cell engager (BiTE) targeting CD19 and CD3, linking T cells to cells expressing CD19	Autologous T cells genetically modified to express a chimeric antigen receptor (CAR) for targeting antigens, such as CD19
Indications	Non-Hodgkin lymphoma, chronic lymphocytic leukemia, rheumatoid arthritis, and other B-cell-mediated diseases	B-cell precursor acute lymphocytic leukemia (ALL)	ALL and other B-cell malignancies, non-Hodgkin lymphoma, and chronic lymphocytic leukemia (varies by CAR type)
Administration	Intravenous infusion	Continuous intravenous infusion over several days	Single infusion after T-cell harvesting, modification, and expansion
Onset of Action	Gradual (weeks to months for therapeutic effect)	Rapid (days to weeks)	Rapid, but dependent on the expansion and persistence of CAR-T cells
Side Effects	Infusion reactions, infections, and hypogammaglobulinemia	Cytokine release syndrome (CRS), neurological toxicities, and infections	CRS, neurotoxicity, hemophagocytic lymphohistiocytosis, infections, and prolonged B-cell aplasia
Durability	Requires multiple administrations/cycles; a substantial proportion of patients may relapse	Short-term responses with potential for relapse; maintenance may be needed	Long-term remissions in some cases; risk of relapse if CAR-T cells are exhausted or there is loss of the target on the surface of cells (antigen escape)
Cost	Relatively lower compared with newer therapies	Moderately high	Extremely high (hundreds of thousands of dollars)
FDA Approvals	Approved for B-cell malignancies (1997 onward)	Approved for B-cell precursor ALL (2014)	Multiple approvals (e.g., Kymriah, Yescarta for specific B-cell malignancies)
Challenges	Resistance due to loss of CD20 expression; not expressed in plasmablasts	Limited durability, logistical challenges of continuous infusion	High cost, manufacturing complexity, severe toxicities in some patients
References	[20,21]	[22,23]	[12,24]

5. Chimeric Antigen Receptor T-Cell (CAR-T)

CAR-T cell therapy is a novel immunotherapy primarily developed for treating hematologic cancers such as leukemia, lymphoma, and myeloma. It involves a genetic modification of patient's own T cells to express receptors that can redirect them to target specific antigens on cancer cells. Recently, there has been a growing interest in exploring the potential of CAR-T cell therapy for autoimmune diseases, including SSc, although it remains experimental in this context [25]. The idea behind using CAR-T cells in autoimmune diseases is to target and eliminate the specific immune cells that drive the aberrant immune responses and inflammation characteristic of these diseases. CAR-T cells can be engineered to specifically target and eliminate B cells secreting autoantibodies, thereby reducing the immune attack on the body's own tissues. One potential approach under investigation involves targeting CD19. Anti-CD19 CAR-T cell therapy, already used for B-cell malignancies, could theoretically be used to eliminate pathogenic B cells involved in the autoimmune process of SSc. In SSc, dysregulated immune responses contribute to fibrosis in the skin and internal organs. By depleting autoreactive immune cells, CAR-T cell therapy could potentially reduce inflammation and the progression of fibrosis. CAR-T cell therapy is being studied in various autoimmune diseases, such as systemic lupus erythematosus, inflammatory myopathies, myasthenia gravis, and optical neuromyelitis, where B-cell depletion has shown promise. The success in these diseases provides a foundation for exploring CAR-T cell therapy as a treatment for SSc [26].

6. Clinical Experience with CAR-T

The group of Erlangen treated six patients with severe diffuse SSc who had experienced an insufficient response to at least two treatments and were given CAR-T cells targeting CD19. In this study, it was clearly shown that CD19-targeting CAR T-cell therapy prevented further progression of fibrotic disease in patients with SSc. In addition, CAR T-cell treatment allowed for a reduction in and discontinuation of all immunosuppressive and antifibrotic treatment [25]. A longer follow-up period is needed to assess whether disease progression in SSc is blocked in a sustained manner. A case report on a 38-year-old female patient with ILD due to SSc describes treatment with CAR-T cells in addition to a pre-existing therapy with mycophenolate/nintedanib. Skin fibrosis improved. Also, dyspnea regressed. According to CT scans, pulmonary findings improved dramatically, including indices of ground glass opacification and fibrosis [27].

While the potential for CAR-T cell therapy in SSc is promising, research is still in its early stages, and there have been no large-scale clinical trials published specifically addressing its use in SSc [28].

CAR-T cell therapy carries risks of serious side effects, such as cytokine release syndrome and neurotoxicity. These side effects are well-documented in cancer treatments but need to be carefully studied in the context of autoimmune diseases, where the burden of CD19+ cells is certainly lower than that found in B-cell malignancies. In addition, the occurrence of secondary T-cell malignancies has been reported in patients with cancer treated with CAR-T cells based on a review reporting that 20–25 cases of T-cell malignancies have been documented in more than 34.000 patients that received autologous CAR-T cells in the United States [29].

In summary, while CAR-T cell therapy offers a novel potential approach for treating SSc, it remains in an experimental stage, and further research is needed to establish its efficacy and safety in this context.

7. Blinatumomab

Blinatumomab is a bispecific T-cell engager (BiTE) molecule that targets CD19 on B cells and engages CD3 on T cells to stimulate T-cell-mediated destruction of CD19-positive cells. It has been used primarily in the treatment of B cell ALL (B-ALL), where it has shown significant efficacy [30].

Given that B cells play a significant role in the pathogenesis of several autoimmune diseases, including SSc, the rationale behind using blinatumomab lies in targeting and depleting pathogenic B cells that contribute to disease progression. Depleting B cells may reduce the production of pathogenic autoantibodies and dampen immune activation, potentially halting or slowing disease progression in SSc. Blinatumomab's ability to engage T cells for more direct B-cell cytotoxicity offers a different mechanism of action compared with rituximab, which relies on complement-dependent cytotoxicity and antibody-dependent cellular cytotoxicity (Table 1). By depleting B cells, blinatumomab may reduce levels of pathogenic autoantibodies that drive disease progression in SSc [31].

There is ample evidence of pronounced B-cell depletion starting at a minimum efficacious blinatumomab dose of 9 μg/day [32–35].

Blinatumomab could help reset the immune system by eliminating B cells that present antigens and activate T cells, potentially leading to an overall decrease in autoimmune activity. Although the link between B-cell activity and fibrosis in SSc is indirect, reducing immune system activation could theoretically slow or reverse fibrotic processes in affected tissues, particularly the skin and lungs.

8. Clinical Experience with Blinatumomab

The use of blinatumomab in SSc has been demonstrated in a case report. This was also the first report worldwide of the application of blinatumomab in autoimmune disease as B-cell-depleting therapy. It was demonstrated that blinatumomab was safe and effective in a patient with severe, rapidly progressing SSc, resulting in significant B-cell depletion. Blinatumomab was well tolerated in patients with severe SSc, without increased susceptibility to infections. Clinically, the treatment with blinatumomab resulted in accelerated improvement of symptoms, indicating that depletion of B cells had an immediate anti-inflammatory effect during active SSc, and that lymphocytic infiltration (at the time of initiating therapy) may be a potential factor leading to tightness and stiffness of the skin. An improvement in acral perfusion was also observed, potentially indicating that B-cell depletion led to an improvement in fibrosis in SSc [36].

The second indication of autoimmune disease treated with blinatumomab was rheumatoid arthritis. Six patients with multidrug-resistant rheumatoid arthritis were treated with blinatumomab. Treatment was well tolerated and safe, with a transient increase in fever. Blinatumomab led to a rapid improvement of symptoms in all patients [37].

However, the role of blinatumomab in SSc is still exploratory, as it has not been approved or systematically studied in the context of autoimmune diseases. There have been no clinical trials directly investigating the use of blinatumomab in SSc; thus, its safety, efficacy, and optimal dosing in this population are only known from anecdotical evidence, and any use would be considered off-label and experimental.

As with CAR-T cell therapy, blinatumomab is known to cause cytokine release syndrome, a potentially life-threatening inflammatory reaction resulting from the activation of T cells (Table 1). Cytokine release syndrome could be particularly concerning in patients who already have compromised organ systems. B-cell depletion increases the risk of infections, especially in patients who may already be immunosuppressed due to SSc or its treatment. Blinatumomab's potent immune activation could exacerbate this risk. SSc patients may be more susceptible to the toxic effects of immune-modulating drugs due to existing organ damage (e.g., pulmonary fibrosis, cardiac involvement), and blinatumomab's side effects could worsen pre-existing conditions.

There is a general interest in using B-cell-depleting therapies in autoimmune diseases, but whether blinatumomab offers an advantage over current B-cell-targeting therapies like rituximab remains to be demonstrated. Further research is needed to explore whether blinatumomab, or similar BiTE therapies, could provide a benefit to patients with SSc. Preclinical studies focusing on the mechanism of B-cell depletion and its impact on fibrosis and autoimmunity in SSc would be an important first step. The immune-modulating and B-cell-depleting properties of blinatumomab offer a rationale for exploration in autoimmune diseases such as SSc, but much more research is needed before it can be considered a consolidated and standard therapeutic option for this condition. The optimal dose of blinatumomab to be used, and the recommended number of treatment cycles is also still to be defined. The respective capacity of blinatumomab and anti-CD19 CAR-T cells to effectively eliminate tissue-resident autoreactive B-cell clones in lymph-nodes and other secondary lymphoid tissues also remains to be evaluated. Depleting B cells in tissues eliminates any autoantibody-producing plasmablasts and abrogates antigen-presentation to B cells and subsequent B-cell-mediated cytokine production, thereby altering the local tissue composition.

9. Conclusions

Both blinatumomab and CAR T-cell therapy are attractive options for patients with SSc, being able to reset the B-cell compartment of the immune system and to induce durable patient benefits (Table 1). Ongoing studies in the future will clarify the respective advantages and limitations of either of the two approaches. For the time being, we can certainly conclude that the therapeutic array of patients with SSc is now enriched by these novel, promising, potentially curative options.

Author Contributions: All authors contributed to the writing of the manuscript. All authors have read and agreed to the published version of the manuscript.

Funding: The study received no funding.

Acknowledgments: We thank Kevin Doty from Amgen Inc. for writing support. Divyaanka Iyer, from Cactus Lifesciences Pvt. Ltd. (part of Cactus Communications) provided editorial assistance.

Conflicts of Interest: Gerhard Zugmaier, Faraz Zaman and Matthias Klinger are employed by Amgen. The remaining authors declare that the research was conducted in the absence of any commercial or financial relationships that could be construed as potential conflicts of interest.

References

1. Varga, J. Systemic Sclerosis and Related Disorders. In *Harrison's Principles of Internal Medicine*, 21st ed.; McGraw-Hill Education: New York, NY, USA, 2022.
2. Gabrielli, A.; Avvedimento, E.V.; Krieg, T. Scleroderma. *N. Engl. J. Med.* **2009**, *360*, 1989–2003. [CrossRef] [PubMed]
3. Koenig, M.; Joyal, F.; Fritzler, M.J.; Roussin, A.; Abrahamowicz, M.; Boire, G.; Goulet, J.R.; Rich, E.; Grodzicky, T.; Raymond, Y.; et al. Autoantibodies and microvascular damage are independent predictive factors for the progression of Raynaud's phenomenon to systemic sclerosis: A twenty-year prospective study of 586 patients, with validation of proposed criteria for early systemic sclerosis. *Arthritis Rheum.* **2008**, *58*, 3902–3912. [CrossRef] [PubMed]
4. Varga, J.; Abraham, D. Systemic sclerosis: A prototypic multisystem fibrotic disorder. *J. Clin. Investig.* **2007**, *117*, 557–567. [CrossRef] [PubMed]
5. Del Galdo, F.; Lescoat, A.; Conaghan, P.G.; Bertoldo, E.; Colic, J.; Santiago, T.; Suliman, Y.A.; Matucci-Cerinic, M.; Gabrielli, A.; Distler, O.; et al. EULAR recommendations for the treatment of systemic sclerosis: 2023 update. *Ann. Rheum. Dis.* **2024**. [CrossRef]

6. Kowal-Bielecka, O.; Fransen, J.; Avouac, J.; Becker, M.; Kulak, A.; Allanore, Y.; Distler, O.; Clements, P.; Cutolo, M.; Czirjak, L.; et al. Update of EULAR recommendations for the treatment of systemic sclerosis. *Ann. Rheum. Dis.* **2017**, *76*, 1327–1339. [CrossRef]
7. Bruera, S.; Sidanmat, H.; Molony, D.A.; Mayes, M.D.; Suarez-Almazor, M.E.; Krause, K.; Lopez-Olivo, M.A. Stem cell transplantation for systemic sclerosis. *Cochrane Database Syst. Rev.* **2022**, *7*, Cd011819. [CrossRef]
8. Keret, S.; Henig, I.; Zuckerman, T.; Kaly, L.; Shouval, A.; Awisat, A.; Rosner, I.; Rozenbaum, M.; Boulman, N.; Dortort Lazar, A.; et al. Outcomes in progressive systemic sclerosis treated with autologous hematopoietic stem cell transplantation compared with combination therapy. *Rheumatology* **2023**, *63*, 1534–1538. [CrossRef]
9. Yoshizaki, A.; Fukasawa, T.; Ebata, S.; Yoshizaki-Ogawa, A.; Sato, S. Involvement of B cells in the development of systemic sclerosis. *Front. Immunol.* **2022**, *13*, 938785. [CrossRef]
10. Clatworthy, M.R. Targeting B cells and antibody in transplantation. *Am. J. Transplant.* **2011**, *11*, 1359–1367. [CrossRef]
11. Ali, S.A.; Shi, V.; Maric, I.; Wang, M.; Stroncek, D.F.; Rose, J.J.; Brudno, J.N.; Stetler-Stevenson, M.; Feldman, S.A.; Hansen, B.G.; et al. T cells expressing an anti-B-cell maturation antigen chimeric antigen receptor cause remissions of multiple myeloma. *Blood* **2016**, *128*, 1688–1700. [CrossRef] [PubMed]
12. Maude, S.L.; Laetsch, T.W.; Buechner, J.; Rives, S.; Boyer, M.; Bittencourt, H.; Bader, P.; Verneris, M.R.; Stefanski, H.E.; Myers, G.D.; et al. Tisagenlecleucel in children and young adults with B-cell lymphoblastic leukemia. *N. Engl. J. Med.* **2018**, *378*, 439–448. [CrossRef] [PubMed]
13. Khvorost, D.; Kendall, B.; Jazirehi, A.R. Immunotherapy of hematological malignancies of human B-cell origin with CD19 CAR T lymphocytes. *Cells* **2024**, *13*, 662. [CrossRef] [PubMed]
14. Brudno, J.N.; Maus, M.V.; Hinrichs, C.S. CAR T cells and T-cell therapies for cancer: A translational science review. *JAMA* **2024**, *332*, 1924–1935. [CrossRef]
15. Muller, F.; Taubmann, J.; Bucci, L.; Wilhelm, A.; Bergmann, C.; Volkl, S.; Aigner, M.; Rothe, T.; Minopoulou, I.; Tur, C.; et al. CD19 CAR T-Cell Therapy in Autoimmune Disease-A Case Series with Follow-up. *N. Engl. J. Med.* **2024**, *390*, 687–700. [CrossRef]
16. Schett, G.; Müller, F.; Taubmann, J.; Mackensen, A.; Wang, W.; Furie, R.A.; Gold, R.; Haghikia, A.; Merkel, P.A.; Caricchio, R.; et al. Advancements and challenges in CAR T cell therapy in autoimmune diseases. *Nat. Rev. Rheumatol.* **2024**, *20*, 531–544. [CrossRef] [PubMed]
17. Beers, S.A.; French, R.R.; Chan, H.T.; Lim, S.H.; Jarrett, T.C.; Vidal, R.M.; Wijayaweera, S.S.; Dixon, S.V.; Kim, H.; Cox, K.L.; et al. Antigenic modulation limits the efficacy of anti-CD20 antibodies: Implications for antibody selection. *Blood* **2010**, *115*, 5191–5201. [CrossRef]
18. Tedder, T.F.; Inaoki, M.; Sato, S. The CD19-CD21 complex regulates signal transduction thresholds governing humoral immunity and autoimmunity. *Immunity* **1997**, *6*, 107–118. [CrossRef] [PubMed]
19. Carpenter, R.O.; Evbuomwan, M.O.; Pittaluga, S.; Rose, J.J.; Raffeld, M.; Yang, S.; Gress, R.E.; Hakim, F.T.; Kochenderfer, J.N. B-cell maturation antigen is a promising target for adoptive T-cell therapy of multiple myeloma. *Clin. Cancer Res.* **2013**, *19*, 2048–2060. [CrossRef]
20. Maloney, D.G.; Grillo-Lopez, A.J.; White, C.A.; Bodkin, D.; Schilder, R.J.; Neidhart, J.A.; Janakiraman, N.; Foon, K.A.; Liles, T.M.; Dallaire, B.K.; et al. IDEC-C2B8 (Rituximab) anti-CD20 monoclonal antibody therapy in patients with relapsed low-grade non-Hodgkin's lymphoma. *Blood* **1997**, *90*, 2188–2195. [CrossRef]
21. Coiffier, B.; Lepage, E.; Briere, J.; Herbrecht, R.; Tilly, H.; Bouabdallah, R.; Morel, P.; Van Den Neste, E.; Salles, G.; Gaulard, P.; et al. CHOP chemotherapy plus rituximab compared with CHOP alone in elderly patients with diffuse large-B-cell lymphoma. *N. Engl. J. Med.* **2002**, *346*, 235–242. [CrossRef] [PubMed]
22. Topp, M.S.; Gokbuget, N.; Stein, A.S.; Zugmaier, G.; O'Brien, S.; Bargou, R.C.; Dombret, H.; Fielding, A.K.; Heffner, L.; Larson, R.A.; et al. Safety and activity of blinatumomab for adult patients with relapsed or refractory B-precursor acute lymphoblastic leukaemia: A multicentre, single-arm, phase 2 study. *Lancet Oncol.* **2015**, *16*, 57–66. [CrossRef] [PubMed]
23. Kantarjian, H.; Stein, A.; Gokbuget, N.; Fielding, A.K.; Schuh, A.C.; Ribera, J.M.; Wei, A.; Dombret, H.; Foa, R.; Bassan, R.; et al. Blinatumomab versus Chemotherapy for Advanced Acute Lymphoblastic Leukemia. *N. Engl. J. Med.* **2017**, *376*, 836–847. [CrossRef] [PubMed]
24. June, C.H.; Sadelain, M. Chimeric Antigen Receptor Therapy. *N. Engl. J. Med.* **2018**, *379*, 64–73. [CrossRef]
25. Auth, J.; Muller, F.; Volkl, S.; Bayerl, N.; Distler, J.H.W.; Tur, C.; Raimondo, M.G.; Chenguiti Fakhouri, S.; Atzinger, A.; Coppers, B.; et al. CD19-targeting CAR T-cell therapy in patients with diffuse systemic sclerosis: A case series. *Lancet Rheumatol.* **2024**. [CrossRef] [PubMed]
26. Blache, U.; Tretbar, S.; Koehl, U.; Mougiakakos, D.; Fricke, S. CAR T cells for treating autoimmune diseases. *RMD Open* **2023**, *9*, e002907. [CrossRef] [PubMed]
27. Merkt, W.; Freitag, M.; Claus, M.; Kolb, P.; Falcone, V.; Röhrich, M.; Rodon, L.; Deicher, F.; Andreeva, I.; Tretter, T.; et al. Third-generation CD19.CAR-T cell-containing combination therapy in Scl70+ systemic sclerosis. *Ann. Rheum. Dis.* **2024**, *83*, 543–546. [CrossRef] [PubMed]

28. Bhandari, S.; Bhandari, S.; Bhandari, S. Chimeric antigen receptor T cell therapy for the treatment of systemic rheumatic diseases: A comprehensive review of recent literature. *Ann. Med. Surg.* **2023**, *85*, 3512–3518. [CrossRef] [PubMed]
29. Hamilton, M.P.; Sugio, T.; Noordenbos, T.; Shi, S.; Bulterys, P.L.; Liu, C.L.; Kang, X.; Olsen, M.N.; Good, Z.; Dahiya, S.; et al. Risk of second tumors and T-cell lymphoma after CAR T-cell therapy. *N. Engl. J. Med.* **2024**, *390*, 2047–2060. [CrossRef]
30. Litzow, M.R.; Sun, Z.; Mattison, R.J.; Paietta, E.M.; Roberts, K.G.; Zhang, Y.; Racevskis, J.; Lazarus, H.M.; Rowe, J.M.; Arber, D.A.; et al. Blinatumomab for MRD-negative acute lymphoblastic leukemia in adults. *N. Engl. J. Med.* **2024**, *391*, 320–333. [CrossRef]
31. Einsele, H.; Borghaei, H.; Orlowski, R.Z.; Subklewe, M.; Roboz, G.J.; Zugmaier, G.; Kufer, P.; Iskander, K.; Kantarjian, H.M. The BiTE (bispecific T-cell engager) platform: Development and future potential of a targeted immuno-oncology therapy across tumor types. *Cancer* **2020**, *126*, 3192–3201. [CrossRef] [PubMed]
32. Bargou, R.; Leo, E.; Zugmaier, G.; Klinger, M.; Goebeler, M.; Knop, S.; Noppeney, R.; Viardot, A.; Hess, G.; Schuler, M.; et al. Tumor regression in cancer patients by very low doses of a T cell-engaging antibody. *Science* **2008**, *321*, 974–977. [CrossRef]
33. Zugmaier, G.; Topp, M.S.; Alekar, S.; Viardot, A.; Horst, H.A.; Neumann, S.; Stelljes, M.; Bargou, R.C.; Goebeler, M.; Wessiepe, D.; et al. Long-term follow-up of serum immunoglobulin levels in blinatumomab-treated patients with minimal residual disease-positive B-precursor acute lymphoblastic leukemia. *Blood Cancer J.* **2014**, *4*, 244. [CrossRef] [PubMed]
34. Zugmaier, G.; Gökbuget, N.; Klinger, M.; Viardot, A.; Stelljes, M.; Neumann, S.; Horst, H.A.; Marks, R.; Faul, C.; Diedrich, H.; et al. Long-term survival and T-cell kinetics in relapsed/refractory ALL patients who achieved MRD response after blinatumomab treatment. *Blood* **2015**, *126*, 2578–2584. [CrossRef]
35. Nägele, V.; Zugmaier, G.; Goebeler, M.E.; Viardot, A.; Bargou, R.; Kufer, P.; Klinger, M. Relationship of T- and B-cell kinetics to clinical response in patients with relapsed/refractory non-Hodgkin lymphoma treated with blinatumomab. *Exp. Hematol.* **2021**, *100*, 32–36. [CrossRef]
36. Subklewe, M.; Magno, G.; Gebhardt, C.; Bücklein, V.; Szelinski, F.; Arévalo, H.J.R.; Hänel, G.; Dörner, T.; Zugmaier, G.; von Bergwelt-Baildon, M.; et al. Application of blinatumomab, a bispecific anti-CD3/CD19 T-cell engager, in treating severe systemic sclerosis: A case study. *Eur. J. Cancer* **2024**, *204*, 114071. [CrossRef]
37. Bucci, L.; Hagen, M.; Rothe, T.; Raimondo, M.G.; Fagni, F.; Tur, C.; Wirsching, A.; Wacker, J.; Wilhelm, A.; Auger, J.P.; et al. Bispecific T cell engager therapy for refractory rheumatoid arthritis. *Nat. Med.* **2024**, *30*, 1593–1601. [CrossRef]

sclerosis

Review

Preclinical and Clinical Data on Current Therapeutic Options for Micro- and Macrovascular Abnormalities in Systemic Sclerosis

Konstantina Bakopoulou [1], Issa El Kaouri [1], Elina Siliogka [2], Periklis Siliogkas [3], Russka Shumnalieva [4,5] and Tsvetelina Velikova [4,*]

1 Faculty of Medicine, Medical University Sofia, Boulevard 'Akademik Ivan Evstratiev Geshov' 15, 1431 Sofia, Bulgaria; 104170@students.mu-sofia.bg (K.B.); 104166@students.mu-sofia.bg (I.E.K.)
2 Faculty of Medicine, National and Kapodistrian University of Athens, Mikras Asias 75, 11527 Athens, Greece; elinasiliogka@gmail.com
3 General Hospital of Athens Korgialeneio—Benakeio Hellenic Red Cross, Athanasaki 11, 11526 Athens, Greece; periaek1@gmail.com
4 Medical Faculty, Sofia University St. Kliment Ohridski, 1407 Sofia, Bulgaria; rshumnalieva@yahoo.com
5 Department of Rheumatology, Clinic of Rheumatology, University Hospital St. Ivan Rilski, Faculty of Medicine, Medical University Sofia, 1612 Sofia, Bulgaria
* Correspondence: tsvelikova@medfac.mu-sofia.bg

Abstract: Background: Systemic sclerosis (SSc) represents a multidimensional disease affecting various organs and systems, with the common denominator being the vascular pathology encountered in the micro- and macrocirculation of SSc patients. Recently, much progress has been made toward understanding the molecular basis of endothelial injury and subsequent fibroblast activation, thus paving the way for specific therapy that can target and counteract these processes. **Aim:** In this review, we examined the latest preclinical and clinical data on therapeutic options to address vascular abnormalities in SSc. **Results:** We discuss the efficacy of current treatments, including pharmacological agents and emerging therapies, in mitigating vascular damage and improving patient outcomes based on preclinical models and clinical trials that offer evidence of their safety and effectiveness. **Conclusions:** Although promising therapeutic strategies emerge, optimizing the management of vascular abnormalities in SSc requires further research.

Keywords: systemic sclerosis; SSc; microvascular abnormalities; macrovascular abnormalities; vascular therapy; autoimmune disease; pharmacological agents; biologics; clinical trials; preclinical models; therapeutic options

1. Introduction

Systemic sclerosis (SSc) is a chronic autoimmune disease of the connective tissue with an unknown and complex pathogenesis [1]. It is primarily characterized by widespread damage, immune dysregulation, and extensive fibrosis of the skin and internal organs [2]. Based on the extent of skin involvement, it is classified into two main subtypes: limited cutaneous SSc (lcSSc) and diffuse cutaneous SSc (scSSc). lcSSc, typically, involves the skin of the face, neck, and distal extremities, whereas dcSSc affects more extensive skin areas, including the trunk and proximal limbs, and is associated with severe internal organ involvement [2].

The epidemiology of SSc varies geographically, with an estimated incidence of 1–2 cases per 100,000 persons per year and a prevalence of 10–30 cases per 100,000 persons [3]. The disease predominantly affects women, with a female-to-male ratio of approximately 5:1. SSc usually manifests between the ages of 30 and 50, though it can occur at any age [4].

According to the 2013 ACR/EULAR classification criteria [2], the diagnosis of SSc requires a combination of clinical features, including skin thickening, specific autoantibodies, and characteristic capillary changes visible via nail fold capillaroscopy. A study by

Araujo et al. (2017) found that 53% of patients with early SSc exhibited Raynaud's phenomenon (RP), abnormal capillaroscopy, and autoantibodies specific to SSc, underscoring the importance of these criteria in early disease detection [3]. Vascular abnormalities are fundamental in the pathogenesis and progression of SSc. Early in the disease, endothelial cell injury leads to chronic inflammation and subsequent fibrosis, contributing to both skin thickening and internal organ involvement. Microvascular damage is a crucial driver of clinical manifestations such as RP, digital ulcers (DUs), and pulmonary arterial hypertension (PAH) [5]. An increasing number of studies link epigenetic abnormalities—including particular changes affecting the immune cells, endothelial cells, and fibroblasts—to the pathophysiology of SSc, i.e., the function of non-coding RNAs, histone modifications, and DNA methylation, as well as how these epigenetic changes impact clinical manifestations of the disease [6].

The clinical significance of these abnormalities extends beyond localized tissue damage, contributing to systemic complications such as PAH, renal crisis, and increased cardiovascular risk, which significantly impact patient outcomes and quality of life. They are crucial in determining disease severity, progression, and overall prognosis. Therefore, effective monitoring and treating vascular involvement are essential for improving clinical outcomes and quality of life in those affected by SSc [5].

This review aims to summarize the new insights into the pathogenetic treatment of SSc by explaining the mechanisms, clinical features, and diagnostic approach applied in various SSc-specific vascular complications, including RP, DUs, PAH, and the involvement of mesenteric and peripheral arteries.

2. Pathogenesis of Vascular Abnormalities in SSc

2.1. Role of Autoantibodies in Immunopathogenesis of SSc

It has long been postulated that autoantibodies constitute a triggering event in the pathogenesis of SSc. Raschi et al. [7] successfully illustrated that some SSc-specific autoantibodies (anti-Scl70, anti-centromere, and anti-Th/To), when embedded in immune complexes, were essential in causing endothelial damage and vasculopathy.

Many autoantibodies have been associated with different phenotypes of vascular manifestations and/or the risk of vascular involvement. For instance, anti-RNA polymerase III antibodies confer a higher risk of gastroesophageal vascular ectasia, PAH, and renal crisis. Accordingly, anti-centromere, anti-Th/To, and anti-ribonucleoprotein (RNP) antibodies increase the risk of PAH. Digital infarcts and PAH have been associated with the presence of anti-endothelial cell antibodies [8].

2.2. Immune Cell Involvement in SSc

One of the mechanisms implicated in the pathogenesis of SSc is impaired T-cell homeostasis, which is associated with a decrease in the population of regulatory T cells (Tregs), as evidenced by blood and skin lesion analysis in SSc patients [9]. This is partially attributed to Treg conversion into the profibrotic Th2 and Th17 cell populations. Increasing evidence suggests that T-cell proliferation and cytokine secretion play a significant role in initiating SSc, indicating that T lymphocyte colonies, mainly Th2 and Th17, contribute to disease pathogenesis and fibrosis. Th2 cells produce IL-4, IL-5, IL-10, and IL-13—these are described as anti-inflammatory and profibrotic due to their pathognomonic actions as initiators of extracellular matrix (ECM) production and inhibition of Th1 cell function as noted by Bellando et al. [10].

Different phases of immune polarization have also been proposed, with Th2 polarization correlating with disease exacerbation, whereas a Th2-to-Th1 shift was shown to predict disease duration. Th2 response involves the secretion of IL-4 and IL-13, while antifibrotic IFN-γ mediates Th1 action. Indeed, polymorphisms in the IFN-γ gene have been found to confer an increased risk of SSc, especially associated with skin involvement [9]. IL-4 induces Th2 cell lineage and is further propagated by a positive feedback loop. Kurizinski et al. [11] propose the theory of skin fibrosis and damage due to the imbalance of Th1/Th2.

In addition, Ko et al. [12] highlight that disease progression is closely linked to Th2 immune polarization, while disease duration is often associated with shifts from Th2 to Th1 cells.

Th17 cells—characterized by their production of IL-17A, IL-17F, IL-21 and IL-22—are elevated in SSc patients with skin manifestations, in contrast to controls of healthy patients [13]. Th17 cells are elevated in the peripheral blood of SSc patients, accumulating at disease sites and participating in several physiological manifestations, including remodeling of the ECM, collagen deposition, and neutrophil recruitment. Bălănescu et al. [14] emphasized the critical role of Th17 in autoimmune tissue injury induction, leading to the characteristic finding of skin manifestations in SSc. Therapeutic targets covering Th17 may be utilized for SSc intervention, providing further insights into SSc pathogenesis [15]. The profibrotic Th2 response is further reinforced by the release of IL-6 by various cells and appears to be the putative cause of endothelial cell (EC) activation and apoptosis [8]. IL-6 is another important mediator of fibrotic processes leading to upregulated collagen transcription, although the exact mechanism has yet to be elucidated. This was further supported by an in vitro analysis conducted on dermal fibroblasts by O'Reilly et al. [16]. Their data demonstrated that the effect of IL-6 is highly dependent on the action of STAT3 and indirectly mediated by the TGF-β signaling pathway and SMAD3. Indeed, following the deletion of the IL-6 gene in animal models with lung fibrosis, the fibrotic processes were diminished. Consistent with this, in a culture of dermal fibroblasts from SSc patients, phospho-STAT3 was found to be increased. Finally, it was also demonstrated that Gremlin (a bone morphogenetic protein antagonist) is induced by IL-6 and mediated by canonical TGf-β signaling. Thus, Gremlin was concluded to be profibrotic, likely promoting vascular remodeling and pulmonary hypertension [16].

Cultures from dermal fibroblasts in SSc patients have demonstrated elevated IL-6 levels, correlated with earlier disease, increased mortality risk, unfavorable skin involvement, and accelerated decline in pulmonary function. Furthermore, these fibroblasts, when compared to normal fibroblasts, were noted to express higher levels of collagen alpha 1 (Col1), alpha-smooth muscle actin (αSMA), and connective tissue growth factor (CTGF). The complex nature of trans-signaling mechanisms involving IL-6 and TGF-β pathways results in cardiac, skin, and lung fibrosis, highlighting the significance of tocilizumab therapy and its effectiveness in limiting fibrosis [17,18].

Another recently described mediator of fibrosis is interleukin-11 (IL-11), a profibrotic cytokine exerting its action under the influence of TGF-β1. Its levels were noted to be increased in early dcSSc and patients with interstitial lung disease (ILD). It has been implicated in fibrotic processes not only in the skin but also in the heart and lungs. Additionally, Steadman et al. discovered that IL-11 influences the release of IL-33 (alarmin) at the early stage in fibroblasts, potentially promoting an inflammatory response, whereas at a later time, the influence ceases and fibrotic processes predominate [19]. Ye et al. suggested that the profibrotic effect of IL-11 might be controlled by blocking the IL-11 trans-signaling pathway through JAK2/STAT3 and sgp130Fc interference [20].

2.3. *Mechanisms of Endothelial Dysfunction and Injury in SSc*

The initiating stimulus of vascular injury in SSc can be secondary to various precipitants, including idiopathic, environmental, and infectious factors, autoantibody-mediated mechanisms, or oxidative stress caused by reactive oxygen species (ROS) [21]. Repeated cycles of endothelial injury propagate a vicious cycle of apoptosis and cell detachment, impairing vessel integrity. Acting synergistically with this, an imbalance between vasoconstricting (e.g., ET-1) and vasodilating mediators (e.g., NO and prostacyclin) is observed, leading to continuous and prolonged alterations in the vessel tone [9]. After von Willebrand Factor (vWF) release, platelet activation and aggregation result in hypercoagulability, thromboxane secretion (a potent vasoconstrictor), and fibrin deposition [22].

These processes culminate in terminal vessel damage, malfunctioning endothelial junctions with increased permeability of the microvasculature and vessel leak, evidenced by the formation of microvascular hemorrhages and localized edema [22]. The increased permeability and leaky cell junctions permit the recruitment of macrophages, Th2, Th17, and mast cells, resulting in a perivascular infiltration of pro-inflammatory cells [9].

It was recently reported that senescence of endothelial cells contributed to fibrosis through endothelial-to-mesenchymal transition [23]. Furthermore, cellular senescence is involved in overall SSc pathogenesis via direct alteration of cellular functions or indirect promotion of defective immune surveillance [24]. Chiu et al. confirmed these observations in their studies of skin biopsies of fibrotic lesions of SSc patients [25].

2.4. *Biomarkers of Endothelial Damage*

Muruganandam et al. concluded that the SSc-associated damage in ECs is evidenced by upregulated expression of E-selectin, vascular cell adhesion protein 1 (VCAM-1) and Intercellular Adhesion Molecule 1 (ICAM-1), vWF, tissue factor, and tissue thrombin. On the other hand, lower levels of thrombomodulin, fibrinolysis, and platelet count were observed in association with vasculopathy and DUs [22]. Angiopoietins (Ang-1 and Ang-2) are responsible for the modulation of EC activation and vessel modeling and growth through their interaction with the Tie2 tyrosine kinase receptor. Imbalance in Ang-1 and Ang-2 levels may have a causative role in vascular destruction and abnormal angiogenesis [26].

The same author suggested that increased levels of metalloproteinase tissue inhibitors, such as TIMP-4, correlated with cardiopulmonary vascular involvement. Additionally, neuropilins (NRP1-2) found on ECs were also flagged as potential predictors of PAH, Dus, and abnormalities in nail fold capillaries. Similarly, circulating levels of IL-18 binding protein were associated with PAH, whereas IL-33 and ST2 had predictive value in DUs and PAH. The levels of slit glycoproteins (Slit1-3) and sirtuin (SIRT1-7) molecules with regulatory function in angiogenesis were also elevated in SSc patients with microvascular involvement [22].

2.5. *Fibrotic Processes and Remodeling Affecting Blood Vessels*

The nature of the lesions observed in SSc vasculopathy can be destructive (capillary loss) or proliferative (thickening of the vessel wall). Underlying this, a vicious cycle is established with ECM deposition worsening hypoxia and, in turn, reduced oxygen tension, which activates the fibrotic processes [27]. Chronic inflammation prompts fibroblasts to commit to a myofibroblast transition under the influence of ET-1, leading to the intima's hypertrophy, the lumen's narrowing, and eventually vessel obliteration. These changes favor chronic ischemia and endothelial cell and capillary loss [21,27].

Additionally, the endothelial cells undergoing the endothelial-to-mesenchymal transition (EndoMT) following downregulation of their markers, such as CD31 and VE-cadherin, transform into a myofibroblast phenotype associated with increased expression of α-SMA, further reinforcing the fibrotic processes [21].

Dysfunction and/or a decreased number of endothelial progenitor cells (EPCs) hinder new angiogenesis, which, combined with the dysregulated function of the VEGF/VEGFR pathway, contributes to vasculopathy. More specifically, elevated levels of VEGF have been noted in SSc patients, which is associated with a robust angiogenic response and results in chaotic vessel patterns. Conversely, there is also increased expression of VEGF-165, an isoform with anti-angiogenic properties [21]. Pericytes seem to have a double role by directly inhibiting the angiogenic processes and simultaneously enhancing ECM deposition.

Another source of myofibroblast cell transformation occurs under the influence of the proliferator-activated receptor γ (PPAR-γ) pathway. Downregulation of this response promotes adipocyte differentiation into myofibroblasts [8]. Conversely, upregulation of the PPAR-γ pathway inhibits the TGF-β-mediated transdifferentiation of fibroblasts into myofibroblasts, therefore possessing both anti-inflammatory and antifibrogenic properties, preventing collagen and ECM deposition [22].

Subendothelial collagen exposure following injury results in platelet activation, which responds with the release of profibrotic cytokines such as TGF-β and serotonin. Serotonin, through interactions with TGF-β, has been demonstrated to promote ECM deposition.

Platelet-derived microparticles (PMPs) have also been implicated in the fibrotic processes encountered in SSc [8].

2.6. Molecular Mediators of Fibrosis

Many cytokines have been associated with a profibrotic/fibrogenic effect. However, in SSc, the main culprits appear to be TGF-β, IL-4, and IL-13, released mainly by Th2 cells [28]. As already discussed, platelet-derived mediators also have a putative role in fibrotic processes, including platelet-derived growth factor (PDGF), PMPs, and serotonin.

PDGF, specifically, signals through Ras to MAP kinase pathways and influences the activity of NADPH oxidases, resulting in the transcription of factors that increase ECM synthesis [28]. SSc is characterized by an enhanced endogenous potential and expression of thrombin, which, in turn, activates ECs and fibroblasts, inducing collagen synthesis, interfering with the action of matrix metalloproteinases and culminating in enhanced ECM production [22].

2.7. Genetic Markers Associated with Vascular Abnormalities in SSc

Great effort has been put into identifying potential susceptibility genes for SSc-associated vascular involvement. GWAS studies have located an SNP that is found upstream of the gene for the PPAR-γ pathway as a possible target [29,30]. Other less studied genes with, as of yet, unclear functions (incl. DDX6, DGKQ, and NAB1) were flagged in a meta-GWAS study. Dysfunction in the gene encoding caveolin 1 interferes with the TGF-β pathway to suppress fibrosis, which has also been suspected [30].

Dense microsatellite analysis in Japanese SSc patients harboring the risk haplotype HLA-DPB1*13:01 demonstrated a probable association between a retinoid X receptor-beta (RXRB) variant and anti-topo I antibody. RXRB interferes with the fibrotic processes by suppressing them [31]. Recently, Shumnalieva et al. demonstrated deregulation of miR-21 and miR-29a in the serum of patients with SSc, which have pro- and antifibrotic effects, respectively [32]. It was confirmed that altered miRNA expression in the circulation or tissues is related to immune activation, vasculopathy, and fibrosis development in SSc patients.

2.8. Key Signaling Pathways Involved in Vascular Abnormalities

As has already been highlighted, vascular dysfunction in SSc focuses on the imbalance between the action of vasoconstrictors—most notably ET-1 and vasodilators, e.g., NO. Indeed, ET-1 appears to be increased in the skin, vasculature, kidneys, and lungs of SSc patients [8]. On the other hand, lower levels of NO are encountered in the vessels of SSc patients. TGF-β1 plays a pivotal regulatory role in this pathway, activating noncanonical (Smad-independent) pathways promoting myofibroblast activation, ECM synthesis, and ET-1 elevation [33]. As Ko et al. hypothesized, ET-1 appears to have an amplifying role in the bidirectional pathway of fibrosis and vasculopathy [8].

Conversely, a transcription factor expressed in ECs, known as Friend leukemia virus integration 1 (FLI1), seems to regulate skin fibrosis negatively. CXCL4 released by platelets suppresses the FLI1 pathway. Lower levels of FLI1 are associated with impaired vessel formation, fibrosis, and abnormal immune responses. Additionally, CXCL4 upregulates the expression of thrombospondin 1 expression and diminishes the action of VEGF [33].

Caveolin-1 forms invaginations resulting in the internalization of the TGF-β1 receptor and blocking TGF-β1-dependent signaling. Studies in mice have demonstrated that deletion of caveolin-1 results in impaired vascular tone regulation, the induction of spontaneous EndoMT, and skin and lung fibrosis. VEGF-A is also elevated in mesenchymal cells in the case of caveolin-1 deficiency [34].

A key element of fibrosis is EndoMT. This, in turn, is regulated through the action of various pathways, such as β-catenin, Wnt, Akt, Notch, phosphoinositide 3-kinase (PI3K), NF-kB, Sp1, and bone morphogenetic protein 4 (BMP-4) [8].

3. Microvascular Abnormalities in SSc

The microvasculature is part of the circulatory system composed of vessels <300 µm diameter, including arterioles, capillaries, and venules. Microvascular pathologies can manifest as vasculopathies or vasculitides. Vasculopathy generally refers to non-inflammatory vascular lesions (including those caused by immune complex deposition or intravascular thrombosis). At the same time, vasculitis is characterized by leukocytic infiltration (polymorphonuclear or mononuclear) and fibrinoid changes of the vascular wall. In SSc, microvascular abnormalities are typically noticed in the form of vasculopathy [1].

3.1. Microvascular Abnormalities Mechanisms

SSc microvascular disease is characterized by microvasculopathy, vasospasm, a procoagulant state with thrombosis and fibrin deposition, and defective angiogenesis. Endothelial cell injury is thought to be the initial event in developing vascular disease in SSc [35]. Factors involved in this injury include autoantibodies, infections (e.g., CMV), cytotoxic T-cells, and reactive oxygen species. Affected endothelial cells demonstrate endothelial cell activation with increased leukocyte adhesion molecules, cytoplasmic vacuolization, ballooning, cytoskeletal rearrangement, loosening of tight junctions, and apoptotic changes [35]. Histologically, affected vessels are characterized by neointimal lesions (proliferation of endothelial and smooth muscle cells and collagen deposition in the intima layer), adventitial fibrosis, perivascular mononuclear cell infiltration, and pericyte activation. The characteristic neointimal lesion likely results from an aberrant endothelial cell repair [36].

These altered microvascular endothelial cells have decreased expression of endothelial NO-synthase with reduced NO and increased ET-1 production. NO is a potent vasodilator, which inhibits platelet aggregation, smooth muscle cell proliferation, and cytokine-induced endothelial activation [37]. On the other hand, ET-1 is a vasoconstrictive factor that mediates smooth muscle cell proliferation, fibrosis, and inflammation. These alterations lead to a vasoconstrictive and procoagulant state. Chronic tissue hypoxia caused by this microvasculopathy, vasoconstriction, and microthrombosis triggers angiogenesis, which is, however, dysregulated due to differential expression of proangiogenic and angiogenic factors [36]. These new vessels are not well structured and are easily destroyed, leading to reduced capillaries in a given tissue area (capillary rarefaction) and capillary loss. Collectively, these mechanisms lead to significant microvascular damage and organ dysfunction [37].

3.2. Clinical Manifestations of Microvascular Abnormalities in Systemic Sclerosis

Raynaud phenomenon (RP) is a primary clinical manifestation of microvascular abnormalities and is present in most patients with SSc. RP in SSc is associated with structural abnormalities of the microvasculature and immune response. It is characterized by episodic vasospasm of the digital arteries in response to cold or emotional stress [38]. Distal body areas (fingers, toes, and occasionally the nose and ears) are the most affected and are more exposed to ambient temperature changes. This vasospasm leads to a distinctive sequence of color changes in the skin: pallor (due to ischemia), blue (due to hypoxia/deoxygenation), and red (due to reperfusion). These episodes are often accompanied by pain, tingling and numbness in the affected areas. Chronic and severe RP can result in persistent ischemia, leading to tissue damage and complications [38].

DUs and pitting scars are typical in SSc. DUs are a common and debilitating consequence of chronic microvascular compromise, particularly in SSc. They are defined as a denuded tissue area with a well-demarcated border involving loss of both the dermis and epidermis. These painful sores, typically located at the fingertips, result from prolonged ischemia and are difficult to heal. They are prone to infection, further complicating treatment and recovery, and they have the possibility of resulting in irreversible tissue loss, as well as other significant complications, including osteomyelitis, gangrene, and amputation. Pitting scars are another result of chronic ischemia and the healing of digital ulcers. These small depressions in the DUs and pitting scars highlight the severe impact of microvascular abnormalities on daily living and long-term health outcomes [38].

3.3. Diagnostic Techniques for Microvascular Abnormalities

Nailfold capillaroscopy (NC) is a non-invasive diagnostic tool that evaluates the morphology of capillaries using an optical magnification system, which is used primarily in connective tissue diseases like SSc [39]. This technique involves the microscopic examination of the capillaries at the nail fold bed. Abnormal capillaroscopic findings include enlarged capillaries, avascular areas, microhemorrhages, and capillary loss. These patterns provide insight into the severity and progression of microvascular damage. NC is particularly useful for diagnosing and monitoring SSc, offering a window into the extent of microvascular involvement and guiding therapeutic decisions [39].

Laser Doppler imaging and other modalities are useful in vascular abnormalities associated with SSc detection. Laser techniques are non-invasive tools that assess skin capillary perfusion, including laser Doppler flowmetry, Doppler imaging, and laser speckle contrast imaging. Laser Doppler imaging (LDI) measures blood flow by detecting the Doppler shift induced by laser light scattering of moving red blood cells [40]. LDI produces detailed maps of blood flow distribution, highlighting areas with reduced perfusion. This is especially useful for assessing the severity and extent of conditions like Raynaud's phenomenon and other microvascular disorders. The advantage of laser Doppler techniques is that they not only provide information about morphology but also on the dynamic behavior of microcirculation with different stimuli. This unique feature of LDI constitutes a promising approach, and more studies must be carried out to investigate its utility in clinical practice. Other modalities include laser speckle contrast imaging (LSCI), which measures the fluctuating granular pattern produced by laser light reflected on moving red blood cells. LSCI is a less time-consuming technique than NC and can be used to evaluate perfusion in the cutaneous microcirculation. However, more studies are needed to validate LSCI in SSc [40].

4. Macrovascular Abnormalities

4.1. Mechanisms of Macrovascular Involvement and Damage in SSc

While small vessel involvement (microvasculopathy) is often regarded as the hallmark of SSc, large vessels can also be widely impacted (macrovasculopathy) [41]. Over the past decade, a growing amount of evidence regarding the involvement of large vessels has been published [42]. Bertolino et al. further emphasize that several studies have demonstrated a greater macrovascular involvement in SSc compared to control subjects with similar cardiovascular risk factors [43].

Matucci-Cerinic et al. define large vessels as those with an internal diameter greater than 100 microns and note that involvement of the microvasculature often occurs in conjunction with distal pathology of the small vessels [44]. The involvement of both elastic arteries (i.e., carotid artery and aorta) and muscular arteries (i.e., brachial and ulnar arteries) are characteristic of SSc [42]. Lescoat et al. suggest that a similar mechanism may contribute to both micro- and macrovascular vasculopathy [45]. The mechanism of macrovascular involvement remains unknown and is likely multifactorial. Accelerated atherosclerosis and endothelial dysfunction are believed to be critical components in the pathogenesis [43].

Figure 1 presents the main pathophysiological mechanisms of vascular impairment in SSc patients.

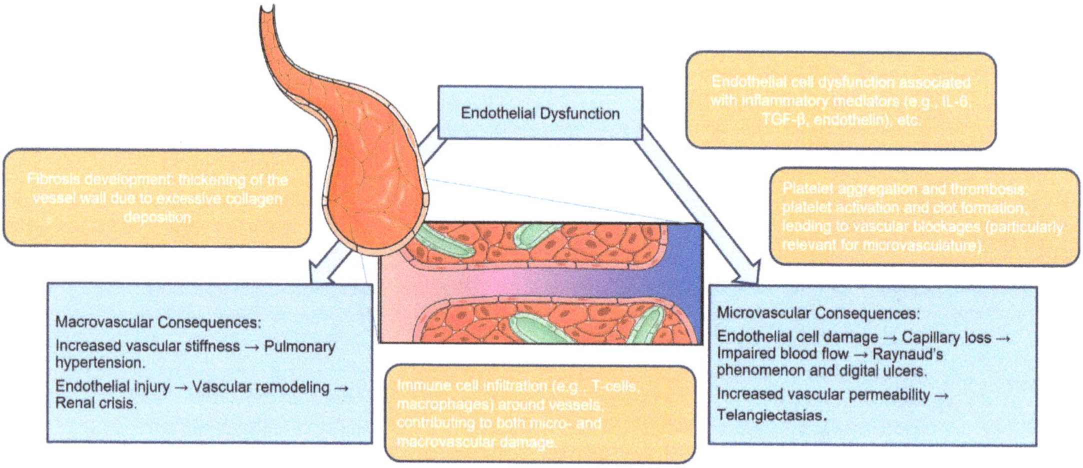

Figure 1. Pathophysiological mechanisms in micro- and macrovascular abnormalities in SSc patients. Parts of the figure were drawn by using pictures from Servier Medical Art. Servier Medical Art by Servier is licensed under a Creative Commons BY 4.0 (https://creativecommons.org/licenses/by/4.0/ (accessed on 10 September 2024)).

4.2. Clinical Manifestations of Macrovascular Abnormalities

Pulmonary arterial hypertension (PAH) is a common manifestation in patients with SSc [46], occurring in up to 12% of cases, and is often associated with severe complications [47], leading to significant morbidity and mortality [46]. This is further evidenced by Coghlan et al., who underline a considerable decrease in survival rates in SSc patients with PAH (56%), compared to (94%) in those without PAH [48]. This may partially be explained by the long asymptomatic period at the early disease phase and the non-specific symptoms of dyspnea and fatigue [47]. PAH comprises the two hallmarks of SSc, fibrogenesis and vasculopathy in the medium-sized pulmonary arteries, thus leading to obstruction of blood flow [41] and elevation of pulmonary artery pressure with subsequent right heart failure [49].

Ulnar artery occlusion (UAO) is considered an underestimated macrovascular manifestation of SSc, considering its eventual implication in DUs [50]. Supporting data on this is a study conducted by D'Alessandro et al., who assessed the macrovascular involvement in SSc using the resistance index (RI) and peak systolic velocity (PV) of ulnar and radial arteries by color Doppler sonography (CDUS) with spectral wave analysis (SWA). In total, 28% of those examined presented signs of UAOs [41]. Moreover, 83% of those with UAOs presented with DUs. D'Alessandro et al. emphasize the importance of UAO as a predictive indicator of DUs, considering the burden placed on patients. The radial artery is often spared in SSc vasculopathy, which is rather surprising considering the frequent implication of the ulnar artery [41].

Scleroderma renal crisis (SRC) is another form of SSc vascular disease. SRC affects around 5% of patients and is characterized by the sudden onset of severe hypertension due to the high renin state triggered by vascular injury. This may potentially be followed by acute renal failure [45].

4.3. Diagnostic Techniques for Macrovascular Abnormalities

The macrovascular involvement in SSc can be evaluated using various imaging techniques, as shown by D'Alessandro et al. One effective method is to measure the RI and PV of the radial and ulnar arteries using CDUS with SWA at the Guyon's canal of both wrists using a high-frequency probe in a controlled environment. The resistance index is defined as [(peak systolic velocity—peak diastolic velocity)/peak systolic velocity] [41].

Previous studies indicate that an RI greater than 0.70 may predict new DU development in SSc patients. However, findings suggest that healthy controls also exhibit an RI greater than 0.70, indicating that this parameter alone is insufficient for predicting DUs. Cut-off values of ulnar RI $\leq$ 0.82 and radial RI $\leq$ 0.88 classified 94% of healthy controls, underscoring the need for combined diagnostic approaches [41].

Recent research by Schioppo et al. highlights the utility of Power Doppler Ultrasound (PDUS) in assessing both macro- and microvascular involvement. PDUS can identify UAO and reduced blood flow in the finger pulp, which are associated with capillary loss as measured by NVC [50]. Combining PDUS and NFC results by Lescoat et al. has shown strong associations with the primary digital manifestations of SSc, reflecting the severity of vasculopathy. This combined assessment approach helps identify patients with more advanced vascular pathology, offering better predictive capability for the risk of DUs than evaluating either macrovascular or microvascular impairment alone [45].

As already mentioned, the pathophysiology of vascular involvement in SSc includes dysregulation of immune cells from both innate and adaptive immunity, leading to the release of pro-inflammatory and profibrotic enzymes, such as those involved in the Wnt or TGF-β pathways. This dysregulation results in vascular damage and fibrosis. Taking these into account, UAO has been identified as a marker of severe vasculopathy and a predictor of DUs, particularly in patients with limited cutaneous systemic sclerosis (lcSSc) [45].

Bandini et al. demonstrated that abdominal ultrasound and CDUS can non-invasively assess splanchnic vessels, revealing morphological and functional differences in mesenteric arteries in SSc patients compared to healthy controls, suggesting "bowel vasculopathy" [51]. Additionally, renal arteries in SSc patients often show vascular damage without clinical symptoms, indicated by increased intrarenal stiffness but normal renal function. Hughes et al. described an overlap condition of SSc with Antineutrophil cytoplasmic autoantibodies (ANCAs), potentially representing a poor prognostic vascular phenotype [52].

Finally, CT is commonly used as an essential component of the diagnostic assessment of patients with suspected SSc-PAH. It allows for the visualization of associated ILD and excludes significant thromboembolic disease through CT Pulmonary Angiography (CTPA). Other features indicative of pulmonary hypertension (PH) can also be assessed using CTPA. Condliffe et al. proposed a combined index of the ratio of the diameter of the main pulmonary artery (dPA) and the diameter of the Adjacent Aorta (dAA), along with Tricuspid Gradient Measured at Echocardiography (TGECHO). It has been proven to have significant predictive value for mean Pulmonary Arterial Pressure (mPAP) in a diverse group of patients suspected to have PH [53]. However, the combined index has not been implemented widely in clinical practice.

5. Treatment Approaches in Vascular Abnormalities in SSc Patients

5.1. Pharmacological Treatments

Considering the multi-organ involvement, fibrosis, and vasculopathy in SSc, treatment should address these issues if they present [54]. Table 1 presents the current treatment options for SSc patients and their effectiveness for vascular abnormalities and complications [55–59].

In the initial stages of SSc, activation of the endothelium results in the upregulation of vasoactive mediators, such as endothelin 1. ET-1 receptor antagonists are therefore utilized to reverse this deleterious effect [60]. This class includes aniracetam with selective type A receptor action and bosentan and macitentan, which are dual antagonists at both type A and B receptors. In vivo studies in SSc patients demonstrated that aniracetam was associated with decreased pain, disability, and activity and the number of new DUs [33]. On the other hand, in vitro experiments showed reduced expression of mesenchymal markers in microvascular endothelial cells (MVECs) from SSc patients that were preincubated with bosentan or macitentan, pointing towards a potential mechanism to disrupt the EndoMT pathway [21].

Table 1. Treatment modalities for systemic sclerosis and their usefulness for improving vascular involvement.

Groups	Medications	Mechanism of Action	Useful for Vascular Complications of SSc
Vasodilators	Calcium channel blockers (e.g., Nifedipine, Amlodipine)	Relax blood vessels, improve blood flow	Yes, useful for Raynaud's phenomenon and digital ulcers
	Prostacyclin analogs (Prostanoids) (e.g., Iloprost, Epoprostenol, Treprostinil)	Vasodilation, platelet inhibition	Yes, used for severe Raynaud's phenomenon and pulmonary hypertension
	Endothelin receptor antagonists (e.g., Bosentan, Macitentan)	Block endothelin-mediated vasoconstriction	Yes, used for pulmonary arterial hypertension (PAH) and digital ulcers
	Phosphodiesterase Inhibitors (i.e., Sildenafil, Tadalafil)	Enhance nitric-oxide-mediated vasodilation	Yes, primarily for PAH treatment
ACE Inhibitors	Enalapril, Captopril	Inhibit angiotensin-converting enzyme, reduce blood pressure	Yes, useful in scleroderma renal crisis
Immunosuppressants	Mycophenolate mofetil, Cyclophosphamide	Suppress immune response to slow fibrosis progression	Limited, mainly for skin and lung involvement, not directly for vascular issues
Anti-Platelet Agents	Aspirin, Clopidogrel	Prevent blood clot formation	May provide some benefits for digital ulcers
Angiotensin II Receptor Blockers (ARBs)	Losartan, Valsartan	Block angiotensin II, reduce vascular resistance	Useful for controlling hypertension, limited for other vascular complications
Antifibrotic Agents	Nintedanib	Inhibit pathways leading to fibrosis	Primarily for lung fibrosis, limited direct vascular benefits
Anticoagulants	Warfarin	Prevent blood clot formation	Limited, mainly for secondary complications like thrombosis
Statins	Atorvastatin, Simvastatin	Improve endothelial function, reduce cholesterol levels	May have some vascular benefits, but not widely used specifically for SSc
Antifibrotic Immunomodulators	Tocilizumab (IL-6 inhibitor)	Block IL-6-mediated inflammation, slow fibrosis	Limited efficacy in direct vascular complications, useful in lung involvement
B-cell-Depleting Agents	Rituximab	Deplete B-cells, reduce autoantibody production	Limited direct vascular benefit, under investigation for broader effects
T-cell Modulators	Abatacept (CTLA-4 Ig)	Inhibit T-cell activation, reduce immune-mediated tissue damage	Currently, there is limited evidence for vascular benefits, mainly for skin and joint disease
Janus Kinase (JAK) Inhibitors	Tofacitinib, Baricitinib	Inhibit the JAK-STAT pathway, reducing immune signaling	Limited evidence for vascular benefit, mainly used for inflammation and fibrosis
TNF-alpha Inhibitors	Infliximab, Adalimumab	Block TNF-alpha, reducing inflammation	Not typically used for SSc due to lack of efficacy in vascular or fibrotic complications

Table 1. *Cont.*

Groups	Medications	Mechanism of Action	Useful for Vascular Complications of SSc
IL-1 Inhibitors	Anakinra (IL-1 receptor antagonist)	Block IL-1 signaling, reduce inflammation	Not commonly used for SSc vascular issues, limited data on efficacy
Anti-Th17 Agents	Secukinumab (IL-17 inhibitor)	Inhibit IL-17 activity, reduce inflammation	Minimal evidence for impact on vascular complications in SSc
Calcineurin Inhibitors	Tacrolimus, Cyclosporine	Suppress T-cell activation, reduce immune responses	Rarely used for SSc, limited benefit for vascular complications
PDGF receptor-α and -β, FGF receptor-1–3, and VEGFR-1–3 inhibitors	Nintedanib	Block signaling, improves spirometry parameters	Mainly for ILD
Botulinum toxin		Inhibits the release of acetylcholine from presynaptic nerve endings and reduces vascular smooth muscle contraction, thereby improving local circulation	Pain relief and promotes healing of limb ulcers.
Adipose tissue-derived mesenchymal stem cells		Healing of the DU and pain relief in some patients. It improves perioral fibrosis	Promise for treating SSc vascular involvement; healing digital ulcers, and pain relief in some patients. It improves perioral fibrosis

Other therapeutic options for SSc are phosphodiesterase inhibitors, which prevent cGMP hydrolysis by phosphodiesterase-5a and, therefore, prolong the activity of vasodilators, including NO [61]. In clinical practice, PDE-5A inhibitors have been shown to improve the frequency, duration, disability, and discomfort experienced in RP and promote the healing of DUs. Sildenafil has been applied in the treatment of SSc-PAH to improve cardiopulmonary function. According to a recent study, combined therapy of tadalafil plus ambrisentan for SSc-PAH demonstrated superior efficacy than single therapy with either agent [21].

Among the immunomodulator options, mycophenolate mofetil (MMF) inhibits inosine monophosphate dehydrogenase, thus suppressing the synthesis of guanosine nucleotides in lymphocytes and preventing cytokine release that would culminate in EC injury. A secondary effect of MMF is that it interferes with the glycosylation needed for the adhesion of lymphocytes and monocytes to ECs and downregulates the expression of adhesion molecules, hindering leukocyte recall to the vascular endothelium [21].

Cyclophosphamide (CYC) is an alkylating agent that affects the action of Tregs and lowers the levels of IFN-γ and IL-12 secretion. Although CYC is primarily used for SSc-related ILD, it has also exhibited a significant effect on vascular complications. In clinical practice, it demonstrated improved nail fold capillary patterns, increased serum levels of CCN1 and circulating EPCs, and reduced serum levels of endothelial damage markers [21].

Tocilizumab is a monoclonal antibody that interferes with the action of the IL-6 receptor, which has been implicated in the EC activation process and the fibroblast-to-myofibroblast differentiation process [33]. In a case report, the application of tocilizumab showed improvement in DUs, PAH, and ILD [62,63].

Treatments for vascular lesions currently focus on improving vascular endothelial function, reducing ischemia damage to visceral organs, and improving skin symptoms such as perioral sclerosis and fingertip ulcers. These treatments may target immunological or vasoactive substance pathways. It is important to remember, though, that various processes indicate various treatment results. There is a great deal of individual variability in the clinical presentation of SSc. An evidence-based strategy is needed to address the various organ involvement requirements and provide the right medicine combinations [33].

5.2. Specific Treatment Options for SSc-Associated Conditions

5.2.1. Pulmonary Hypertension

Pulmonary hypertension has a devastating effect on the overall morbidity and mortality indices in SSc patients, making its early diagnosis and management a focal point in SSc therapy. The therapeutic options available for the treatment of SSc-PAH comprise four distinct groups of medications: endothelin receptor antagonists (ERAs), phosphodiesterase 5 (PDE5) inhibitors, prostacyclin analogs and receptor agonists, as well as soluble guanylate cyclase (sGC) stimulators [54]. Supportive therapy may also be required, and it involves the management of volume overload with diuretics, antiarrhythmic medications for atrial arrhythmias, and supplementation with oxygen for respiratory failure if indicated.

As Naranjo et al. noted, the suggested approach by the 6th World Symposium on Pulmonary Hypertension includes targeted therapy according to the identified risk of each patient based on a specialized risk stratification algorithm, most commonly the FPHN and REVEAL 2.0 risk systems. Achieving a low-risk level is the principal goal of the therapy, as it has been shown to improve mortality significantly. Monotherapy is generally inadequate, except for some select patients, and, usually, SSc patients with PAH classified as low-to-intermediate risk are offered combination therapy. In the group of patients identified as having high risk, a parenteral prostacyclin analog is added to the combination therapy. Patient response is evaluated initially within 1 to 3 months of therapy onset and, following that, at a 3- to 6-month interval [64].

Endothelin receptor antagonists (ERAs) block the endothelin pathway by interfering with endothelin receptor type A (ETA) and endothelin receptor type B (ETB), conferring a vasodilatory and antiproliferative effect [65]. The results of the BREATHE-1 trial proved bosentan's efficacy—an oral nonselective ETA/B antagonist—by showing ameliorated hemodynamic parameters and 6 min walk distance (6MWD) [65]. Accordingly, ARIES-1/ARIES-2 trials demonstrated that ambrisentan, preferentially targeting ETA, improved the 6MWD, although the effect was noted to be better in Idiopathic PAH (IPAH) patients when compared to SSc-PAH. In SSc patients, ambrisentan was able to slow disease progression and worsening of the clinical condition.

Macitentan, a newer nonselective ETA/B receptor antagonist, was studied in the SERAPHIN trial, where the results were consistent with a significant advantage in mortality and morbidity reduction over placebo. Macitentan has so far demonstrated superior efficacy in IPAH treatment when compared to the other ERAs, and as Bahi et al. reported, despite the lack of a dedicated trial, it is expected to have a similar effect in SSc-PAH [64,65]. A potential pitfall in the use of ERAs remains their toxicological profile, with the potential teratogenic effect limiting their use in pregnant women [54].

Prostacyclin analogs are also employed in SSc management. In SSc-PAH, prostacyclin levels are depleted, resulting in vasoconstriction and smooth muscle cell proliferation in the pulmonary artery and limiting cyclic adenosine monophosphate (cAMP) synthesis [65]. Epoprostenol, treprostinil, and iloprost are prostacyclin analogs, whereas selexipag is an agonist at the prostacyclin receptor. Epoprostenol is administered intravenously because of its short half-life, while intravenous and inhaled forms of iloprost exist. Additionally, treprostinil is manufactured in oral, intravenous, subcutaneous, and inhalational forms. Epoprostenol has demonstrated a beneficial effect on PAH by ameliorating exercise tolerance, hemodynamic function, and overall survival. Its widespread use is limited by its adverse effect profile, including infections, sepsis, and hypotension [64,65].

A randomized trial involving 470 PAH patients (including CTD-PAH) on continuous subcutaneous administration of treprostinil showed an improvement in the 6MWD, dyspnea indices, and hemodynamic parameters, even though the proportion of patients with SSc-PAH was limited [64]. Inhaled treprostinil has also demonstrated a potential advantage for treating patients with combined SSc-PAH and SSc-ILD in a trial involving group 3 PH patients with SSc-ILD [65]. Similarly, intravenous infusion of iloprost improved 6MWD and reduced sPAP, while the inhaled form could have a role in acute PAH crisis management, as suggested by Jin et al. [66]. However, the narrow range of data available on inhaled prostacyclin analogs to treat the subgroup of SSc-specific PAH is quite problematic, and more trials are needed to clarify their effectiveness and potential limitations.

Selexipag is an oral prostacyclin receptor agonist that mediates pulmonary vasodilation. The subgroup analysis of the GRIPHON study in CTD-PAH patients demonstrated a significant reduction in the mortality and morbidity risk (−41%), while delaying disease progression and improving the cardiovascular parameters [66].

The nitric oxide pathway, PDE5 inhibitors, and guanylate cyclase agonists in SSc patients are also studied. In PAH, NO synthesis is downregulated, resulting in reduced cGMP levels. PDE5 inhibitors can mitigate this process, while guanylate cyclase agonists act on the soluble guanylate cyclase and elevate cGMP levels. The result is pulmonary vasodilation and inhibition of the proliferative processes [65].

Phosphodiesterase inhibitors, i.e., sildenafil, improved the 6MWD and the hemodynamic function (mPAP) in SUPER-1/SUPER-2 and PHIRST-1/PHIRST-2 studies both in PAH patients and in the subgroup of SSc-PAH cases. Additionally, PHIRST-1/PHIRST-2 reported a beneficial effect on the quality of life and delayed clinical worsening in the PAH population with similar results in CTD-PAH patients [64]. Tadalafil also showed improvement in the 6MWD, quality of life, and slower clinical worsening with the added effect of a longer-acting agent in IPAH. In SSc-PAH, combination therapy with tadalafil and ambrisentan, currently employed as a first-line option, seems to be especially effective. Although the evidence for using vardenafil in SSc-PAH is lacking, it has also shown similar benefits regarding improved hemodynamics and 6MWD [65].

The guanylate cyclase stimulator, Riociguat, acts on soluble guanylate cyclase (sGC), increasing cGMP levels. The PATENT-1/PATENT-2 trials demonstrated that riociguat has a beneficial effect in CTD-PAH, including in the SSc-PAH subgroup, by increasing the 6MWD and improving the functional class and the hemodynamic parameters.

Additionally, the RIVER study in PAH patients (14% were CTD-PAH patients) associated long-term riociguat therapy with improved RV function and decreased right heart size [65].

Multiple trials have demonstrated (e.g., the AMBITION trial) that initiating combination therapy early in the course of SSc-PAH with ERAs and PDE5 inhibitors significantly improves response and delays disease worsening [65]. In addition, Naranjo et al. illustrated that combination therapy in SSc-PAH patients without prior treatment increased the 6MWD, ameliorating the structure and function of the RV and the associated hemodynamic parameters. The follow-up ATPAHSS-O trial (SSc-PAH) additionally demonstrated improvement in pro-BNP levels.

Furthermore, the GRIPHON and SERAPHIN trials showed a reduction in mortality and morbidity following the addition of selexipag and macitentan to routine therapy, respectively [64]. As SSc-PAH has a particularly complex pathogenesis, future therapeutic approaches will likely include medications targeting different contributing pathways, e.g., a TGF-β signaling targeting agent, an immunomodulator, and a vasodilating agent [65].

Adjunct therapy for SSc includes the following. As SSc patients are predisposed to gastric antral vascular ectasias and ulcerative esophagitis, routine use of anticoagulation is not normally suggested unless specific clinical conditions require it. Additionally, the REVEAL Registry concluded that prolonged use of warfarin confers an unfavorable prognosis in SSc-PAH. Furthermore, although corticosteroids have benefitted survival and hemodynamics in other CTD-PAH patients, the results were not reproducible in SSc-PAH. Similarly, despite the broad usage of calcium channel blockers (CCBs) in RP, current recommendations do not promote their use in SSc-PAH due to their effect on esophageal motility [64].

Supplementation with iron has been suggested as a means to relieve hypoxic stress in PAH. However, the clinical trial of intravenous iron demonstrated no improvement in the hemodynamic parameters and functional class by week 12. Conversely, the episodes of dyspnea were reduced, and a better quality of life was reported, most notably in iron-deficient patients with recurrent gastrointestinal bleeding and SSc-PAH [65].

5.2.2. Raynaud's Phenomenon

The dihydropyridine group of CCBs, with nifedipine being the prototype, is considered the first-line option in the treatment of RP. This is further supported by the results of a 2017 meta-analysis that evaluated the use of CCB in the treatment of primary and secondary RP. It was concluded that nifedipine, compared to placebo, reduced the frequency of the attacks in secondary RP by −4.19 and their severity, and the response was dose-dependent [67].

PDE5 inhibitors are classically regarded as second-line treatment in mild RP and as a second or third option (in combination therapy with prostacyclins) for severe RP. In 2013, a meta-analysis evaluated the effectiveness of sildenafil, tadalafil, and vardenafil by analyzing six RCT studies (244 patients, 92% of whom had SSc-related RP). The data from the meta-analysis demonstrated that sildenafil and tadalafil successfully lowered the frequency (−0.49), severity (−0.46 based on Raynaud condition score), and daily duration of the attacks (−14.62 min) [54].

In 2018, a randomized, n-of-1, double-blind trial conducted by Roustit et al. compared on-demand single doses of sildenafil prior to or during exposure to attack triggers versus placebo in patients with primary and secondary RP. The results demonstrated that, although there was a 90% probability that sildenafil was more effective compared to placebo, due to the high heterogeneity and relatively small effect size, on-demand PDE5 inhibitors were not, in fact, superior [68].

Current approaches suggest the use of prostacyclin analogs as rescue medication in cases of severe, refractory RP. The effectiveness of oral prostacyclin analogs, as well as selexipag, has not been demonstrated in secondary RP and, so far, only intravenous iloprost has yielded satisfactory therapeutic outcomes for SSc-related RP.

Alprostadil, a synthetic form of prostaglandin E1, has failed to show consistent benefit, with conflicting data arising from two trials. Ancillary treatments, such as topical application of nitrates (e.g., nitroglycerin and glyceryl trinitrate), demonstrated a beneficial effect (in a meta-analysis involving ~200 patients with secondary RP), with improved clinical status and hemodynamic function. Limitations include debilitating headaches and a contraindicated combination with a PDE5 inhibitor [54].

Aspirin, targeting platelet activation, might have a role in treating RP, and atorvastatin might be able to delay vascular injury. Pentoxifylline and fluoxetine might also benefit some patients, but the decision should be based on individual protocols. An advantageous effect in the severity and frequency of RP episodes was, indeed, demonstrated by a small, randomized trial comparing fluoxetine to nifedipine. Conversely, subset analysis of the RISE-SSc RCT showed no improvement in RP when comparing riociguat to placebo. Angiotensin II receptor type 1 blockers are regarded as a rescue option for treating mild RP in the case of nifedipine failure. However, their effectiveness is considered low [67].

5.2.3. Scleroderma Renal Crisis

Scleroderma renal crisis is associated with significant morbidity and comprises one out of the four main causes of death in SSc patients. As such, timely diagnosis and management are paramount [69]. Current guidelines on the management of SSc-associated renal crisis involve hospitalization and initiation of therapy with ACEIs; commonly, a short-acting agent is used (e.g., captopril). The goal is to achieve a 24 h reduction in systolic blood pressure by 20 mm Hg and to reach and maintain a blood pressure (BP) of 120/70 mm Hg by day 3 without hypotension. When the goal BP is met, the dose can be stabilized with a long-acting ACEI [70]. If BP remains uncontrolled with maximum acceptable doses of ACEI, adding a dihydropyridine calcium channel blocker may be useful. Due to their potential for stimulating the RAAS, diuretics should not be used unless volume control is necessary. ACEIs, due to their vasodilatory effect on the efferent arteriole, can decrease renal function to the point where dialysis is unavoidable.

Therapy should continue while on dialysis, as per the guidelines, since almost half of the patients have been shown to partially recover within 3 to 18 months. ACEIs may mask the diagnosis of scleroderma renal crisis when used prior to an established acute crisis by maintaining a normal BP, leading to delayed diagnosis and increased risk of adverse outcomes, including death [70]. As the levels of circulating endothelin-1 have been reported to be elevated in SSc, ERAs can have a beneficial effect in managing acute SSc renal crisis.

Additionally, prostacyclins can have a role in rapidly lowering BP and improving renal blood flow. The recovery of renal function following a scleroderma renal crisis may take up to 2 years. Therefore, renal transplantation should not be considered before this time has passed [69,70].

5.2.4. Other Vascular Complications in Scleroderma

A multidisciplinary approach in the care of wounds (i.e., DUs) is indicated, especially on the occasion of large ulcers and strategies for wound care, e.g., the TIME algorithm (Tissue, Infection, Moisture, Edge) could have a beneficial effect [67]. Pain management and wound debridement should be employed as needed. As the risk of secondary infection is significant (up to two out of three patients), dressings incubated with iodine or silver nitrate can be used. Based on the local resistance patterns, empirical antibiotic therapy is another option when severe infection occurs.

Pharmacological treatment includes using a first-line CCB, followed by the addition of PDE5 inhibitors. Third-line treatment involves the utilization of prostacyclins, whereas bosentan and sympathectomy can both be considered prophylactically [67].

5.3. Non-Pharmacological Treatments for SSc

Therapeutic patient education should be pursued whenever applicable. It involves functionally re-educating the patient to avoid or modify certain habits to prevent and/or reduce disease exacerbation via lifestyle modification. General provisions include cold protection with gloves (incl. heated gloves), thermal clothing and space heaters, microtrauma protection, smoking cessation, and avoidance of vasoconstrictor drugs [70].

In the fight against exertional dyspnea, respiratory rehabilitation has shown significant advantages. Physical therapy and rehabilitation can be utilized symptomatically to increase regional blood flow and teach the patients to mobilize exercises for heat generation. Other techniques have also been suggested, including biofeedback, laser treatment, and acupuncture, but results have not been adequately satisfactory [54].

In summary, recent advancements have introduced novel agents and treatment strategies for addressing micro- and macrovascular abnormalities in SSc. These emerging therapies include endothelial progenitor cell therapy, antifibrotic drugs, and biologics targeting specific pathways implicated in vascular damage. Ongoing clinical trials are crucial for evaluating the safety and efficacy of these innovative treatments. Additionally, combination therapies and personalized medicine approaches are being explored to enhance therapeutic outcomes. Future research should focus on identifying biomarkers for early detection and monitoring response to treatment, ultimately aiming to improve the quality of life for patients with SSc [47]. However, despite recent advancements in our understanding of the underlying disrupted molecular pathways in SSc, there is still a great unmet medical need, as there is currently no treatment that addresses the fibrosis component of the illness. Novel studies reveal some inflammatory pathways that can be addressed by repurposing medications [71,72].

6. Conclusions

The management of micro- and macrovascular abnormalities in SSc remains a significant challenge due to the complex pathophysiology of the disease. Current therapeutic options, including pharmacological agents and biologics, have shown varying degrees of efficacy in mitigating vascular damage and improving patient outcomes. Emerging therapies, such as endothelial progenitor cell therapy and novel antifibrotic drugs, offer promising new avenues for treatment. Additionally, personalized medicine and combination therapies also potentially optimize treatment strategies. However, despite recent advancements in understanding the disrupted molecular pathways in SSc, a significant unmet medical need remains, as no treatment currently effectively targets the fibrotic component of the disease. Further research is needed to identify reliable biomarkers for early detection and accurately monitor therapeutic responses. By continuing to explore and develop targeted therapies, there is hope for significantly improving the quality of life and prognosis for patients with this complex autoimmune disease.

Author Contributions: Conceptualization, K.B., R.S. and T.V.; methodology, I.E.K.; software, E.S.; validation, P.S., K.B. and T.V.; formal analysis, K.B.; investigation, I.E.K.; resources, E.S.; data curation, P.S.; writing—original draft preparation, K.B., I.E.K., E.S. and P.S.; writing—review and editing, R.S. and T.V.; visualization, K.B.; supervision, R.S.; project administration, T.V.; funding acquisition, T.V. All authors have read and agreed to the published version of the manuscript.

Funding: This study is financed by the European Union-NextGenerationEU, through the National Recovery and Resilience Plan of the Republic of Bulgaria, project No BG-RRP-2.004-0008.

Acknowledgments: Parts of the figure were drawn by using pictures from Servier Medical Art. Servier Medical Art by Servier is licensed under a Creative Commons BY 4.0 (https://creativecommons.org/licenses/by/4.0/ (accessed on 10 September 2024)).

Conflicts of Interest: The authors declare no conflicts of interest.

References

1. Denton, C.P.; Khonn, D. Systemic Sclerosis. *Lancet* **2017**, *390*, 1685–1699. [CrossRef] [PubMed]
2. Van den Hoogen, F.; Khanna, D.; Fransen, J.; Johnson, S.R.; Baron, M.; Tyndall, A.; Matucci-Cerinic, M.; Naden, R.P.; Medsger, T.A., Jr.; Carreira, P.E.; et al. 2013 classification criteria for systemic sclerosis: An American college of rheumatology/European league against rheumatism collaborative initiative. *Ann. Rheum. Dis.* **2013**, *72*, 1747–1755. [CrossRef] [PubMed]
3. Araujo, F.C.; Camargo, C.; Kayser, C. Validationof the ACR/EULAR classification criteria for systemic sclerosis in patients with early scleroderma. *Rheumatol. Int.* **2017**, *37*, 1825–1833. [CrossRef] [PubMed]
4. Rubio-Rivas, M.; Royo, C.; Simeon, C.P.; Corbella, X.; Fanollosa PLa, V. Epidemiology of systemic sclerosis: A systemic review of population-based studies. *Clin. Epidemiol.* **2020**, *12*, 257–267.
5. Pattanaik, D.; Brown, M.; Pastlethuaite, B.C.; Postkethuaite, A.E. Pathogenesis of systemic sclerosis. *Front. Immunol.* **2015**, *6*, 272. [CrossRef] [PubMed]
6. Tsou, P.S.; Varga, J.; O'Reilly, S. Advances in epigenetics in systemic sclerosis: Molecular mechanisms and therapeutic potential. *Nat. Rev. Rheumatol.* **2021**, *17*, 596–607. [CrossRef]
7. Raschi, E.; Privitera, D.; Bodio, C.; Lonati, P.A.; Borghi, M.O.; Ingegnoli, F.; Meroni, P.L.; Chighizola, C.B. Scleroderma-specific autoantibodies embedded in immune complexes mediate endothelial damage: An early event in the pathogenesis of systemic sclerosis. *Arthritis Res. Ther.* **2020**, *22*, 265. [CrossRef]
8. Dib, H.; Tamby, M.C.; Bussone, G.; Regent, A.; Berezné, A.; Lafine, C.; Broussard, C.; Simonneau, G.; Guillevin, L.; Witko-Sarsat, V.; et al. Targets of anti-endothelial cell antibodies in pulmonary hypertension and scleroderma. *Eur. Respir. J.* **2012**, *39*, 1405–1414. [CrossRef]
9. Cutolo, M.; Soldano, S.; Smith, V. Pathophysiology of systemic sclerosis: Current understanding and new insights. *Expert. Rev. Clin. Immunol.* **2019**, *15*, 753–764. [CrossRef] [PubMed]
10. Bellando-Randone, S.; Della-Torre, E.; Balanescu, A. The role of interleukin-17 in the pathogenesis of systemic sclerosis: Pro-fibrotic or antifibrotic? *J. Scleroderma Relat. Disord.* **2021**, *6*, 227–235. [CrossRef] [PubMed] [PubMed Central]
11. Kurzinski, K.; Torok, K.S. Cytokine profiles in localized scleroderma and relationship to clinical features. *Cytokine* **2011**, *55*, 157–164. [CrossRef] [PubMed] [PubMed Central]
12. Ko, J.; Noviani, M.; Chellamuthu, V.R.; Albani, S.; Low, A.H.L. The Pathogenesis of Systemic Sclerosis: The Origin of Fibrosis and Interlink with Vasculopathy and Autoimmunity. *Int. J. Mol. Sci.* **2023**, *24*, 14287. [CrossRef] [PubMed] [PubMed Central]
13. Brown, M.; O'Reilly, S. The immunopathogenesis of fibrosis in systemic sclerosis. *Clin. Exp. Immunol.* **2019**, *195*, 310–321. [CrossRef] [PubMed] [PubMed Central]
14. Bălănescu, P.; Bălănescu, E.; Bălănescu, A. IL-17 and Th17 cells in systemic sclerosis: A comprehensive review. *Rom. J. Intern. Med.* **2017**, *55*, 198–204. [CrossRef] [PubMed]

15. Lei, L.; Zhao, C.; Qin, F.; He, Z.Y.; Wang, X.; Zhong, X.N. Th17 cells and IL-17 promote the skin and lung inflammation and fibrosis process in a bleomycin-induced murine model of systemic sclerosis. *Clin. Exp. Rheumatol.* **2016**, *34* (Suppl. S100), 14–22. [PubMed]
16. O'Reilly, S.; Ciechomska, M.; Cant, R.; van Laar, J.M. Interleukin 6 (IL 6) trans signaling drives a STAT3 dependent pathway that leads to hyperactive transforming growth factor-β (TGF-β) signaling promoting SMAD3 activation and fibrosis via Gremlin protein. *J. Biol. Chem.* **2014**, *289*, 9952–9960. [CrossRef] [PubMed] [PubMed Central]
17. Denton, C.P.; Ong, V.H.; Xu, S.; Chen-Harris, H.; Modrusan, Z.; Lafyatis, R.; Khanna, D.; Jahreis, A.; Siegel, J.; Sornasse, T. Therapeutic interleukin-6 blockade reverses transforming growth factor-beta pathway activation in dermal fibroblasts: Insights from the faSScinate clinical trial in systemic sclerosis. *Ann. Rheum. Dis.* **2018**, *77*, 1362–1371. [CrossRef] [PubMed] [PubMed Central]
18. Odell, I.D.; Agrawal, K.; Sefik, E.; Odell, A.V.; Caves, E.; Kirkiles-Smith, N.C.; Horsley, V.; Hinchcliff, M.; Pober, J.S.; Kluger, Y.; et al. IL-6 trans-signaling in a humanized mouse model of scleroderma. *Proc. Natl. Acad. Sci. USA* **2023**, *120*, e2306965120. [CrossRef]
19. Steadman, T.; O'Reilly, S. Elevated interleukin-11 in systemic sclerosis and role in disease pathogenesis. *J. Dermatol.* **2023**, *50*, 1255–1261. [CrossRef] [PubMed]
20. Ye, W.; Wang, Q.; Zhao, L.; Wang, C.; Zhang, D.; Zhou, M.; Chen, F.; Wang, W.; Zhu, Z.; Guo, W.; et al. Blockade of IL-11 Trans-Signaling or JAK2/STAT3 Signaling Ameliorates the Profibrotic Effect of IL-11. *Immunol. Investig.* **2023**, *52*, 703–716. [CrossRef] [PubMed]
21. Zanin-Silva, D.C.; Santana-Gonçalves, M.; Kawashima-Vasconcelos, M.Y.; Oliveira, M.C. Management of Endothelial Dysfunction in Systemic Sclerosis: Current and Developing Strategies. *Front. Med.* **2021**, *8*, 788250. [CrossRef] [PubMed] [PubMed Central]
22. Muruganandam, M.; Ariza-Hutchinson, A.; Patel, R.A.; Sibbitt, W.L., Jr. Biomarkers in the Pathogenesis, Diagnosis, and Treatment of Systemic Sclerosis. *J. Inflamm. Res.* **2023**, *16*, 4633–4660. [CrossRef] [PubMed]
23. Ramadhiani, R.; Ikeda, K.; Hirata, K.I.; Emoto, N. Endothelial Cell Senescence Exacerbates Pulmonary Fibrosis Potentially Through Accelerated Endothelial to Mesenchymal Transition. *Kobe J. Med. Sci.* **2021**, *67*, E84–E91. [PubMed]
24. Tsou, P.S.; Shi, B.; Varga, J. Role of cellular senescence in the pathogenesis of systemic sclerosis. *Curr. Opin. Rheumatol.* **2022**, *34*, 343–350. [CrossRef]
25. Chiu, Y.H.; Spierings, J.; van Laar, J.M.; de Vries-Bouwstra, J.K.; van Dijk, M.; Goldschmeding, R. Association of endothelial to mesenchymal transition and cellular senescence with fibrosis in skin biopsies of systemic sclerosis patients: A cross-sectional study. *Clin. Exp. Rheumatol.* **2023**, *41*, 1612–1617. [CrossRef]
26. Brindle, N.P.; Saharinen, P.; Alitalo, K. Signaling and functions of angiopoietin-1 in vascular protection. *Circ. Res.* **2006**, *98*, 1014–1023. [CrossRef]
27. Di Maggio, G.; Confalonieri, P.; Salton, F.; Trotta, L.; Ruggero, L.; Kodric, M.; Geri, P.; Hughes, M.; Bellan, M.; Gilio, M.; et al. Biomarkers in Systemic Sclerosis: An Overview. *Curr. Issues Mol. Biol.* **2023**, *45*, 7775–7802. [CrossRef] [PubMed] [PubMed Central]
28. Prajjwal, P.; Marsool, M.D.M.; Yadav, V.; Kanagala, R.S.D.; Reddy, Y.B.; John, J.; Lam, J.R.; Karra, N.; Amiri, B.; Islam, M.U.; et al. Neurological, cardiac, musculoskeletal, and renal manifestations of scleroderma along with insights into its genetics, pathophysiology, diagnostic, and therapeutic updates. *Health Sci. Rep.* **2024**, *7*, e2072. [CrossRef] [PubMed] [PubMed Central]
29. López-Isac, E.; Acosta-Herrera, M.; Kerick, M.; Assassi, S.; Satpathy, A.T.; Granja, J.; Mumbach, M.R.; Beretta, L.; Simeón, C.P.; Carreira, P.; et al. GWAS for systemic sclerosis identifies multiple risk loci and highlights fibrotic and vasculopathy pathways. *Nat. Commun.* **2019**, *10*, 4955. [CrossRef]
30. Ishikawa, Y.; Tanaka, N.; Asano, Y.; Kodera, M.; Shirai, Y.; Akahoshi, M.; Hasegawa, M.; Matsushita, T.; Saito, K.; Motegi, S.-I.; et al. GWAS for systemic sclerosis identifies six novel susceptibility loci including one in the Fcγ receptor region. *Nat. Commun.* **2024**, *15*, 319. [CrossRef]
31. Ota, Y.; Kuwana, M. Updates on genetics in systemic sclerosis. *Inflamm. Regen.* **2021**, *41*, 17. [CrossRef]
32. Shumnalieva, R.; Kachakova, D.; Kaneva, R.; Kolarov, Z.; Monov, S. Serum miR-21 and miR-29a expression in systemic sclerosis patients. *Clin. Exp. Rheumatol.* **2023**, *41*, 1688–1694. [CrossRef] [PubMed]
33. Ren, H.E.; Liu, L.; Xiao, Y.; Shi, Y.; Zeng, Z.; Ding, Y.; Zou, P.; Xiao, R. Further insight into systemic sclerosis from the vasculopathy perspective. *Biomed. Pharmacother.* **2023**, *166*, 115282. [CrossRef] [PubMed]
34. Del Galdo, F.; Sotgia, F.; de Almeida, C.J.; Jasmin, J.; Musick, M.; Lisanti, M.P.; Jiménez, S.A. Decreased expression of caveolin 1 in patients with systemic sclerosis: Crucial role in the pathogenesis of tissue fibrosis. *Arthritis Rheum.* **2008**, *58*, 2854–2865. [CrossRef] [PubMed]
35. Saygin, D.; Highland, K.; Tonelli, A. Microvascular involvement in Systemic Sclerosis and Systemic Lupus Erythematosus. *Microcirculation* **2019**, *26*, e12440. [CrossRef]
36. Trojanowska, M. Cellular and molecular aspects of vascular dysfunction in systemic sclerosis. *Nat. Rev. Rheumatol.* **2010**, *6*, 453–460. [CrossRef]
37. Mathon, L.; Berezne, A.; Kahaleh, B.; Guillevin, L.; Humbort, M. Endothelial cells and microparticles in systemic sclerosis. *Autoimmun. Rev.* **2009**, *8*, 595–599.
38. Herrick, A.L. The pathogenesis, diagnosis and treatment of Raynaud phenomenon. *Nat. Rev. Rheumatol.* **2012**, *8*, 469–479. [CrossRef]

39. Cutolo, M.; Pizzorni, C.; Silli, A. Capillaroscopy. *Best Pract. Res. Clin. Rheumatol.* **2008**, *22*, 1093–1108. [CrossRef]
40. Roustit, M.; Gracowski, J.L. Assessment of endothelial and neurovascular function in human skin microcirculation. *Trends Pharmacol. Sci.* **2013**, *33*, 373–383. [CrossRef]
41. D'Alessandro, R.; Garcia Gonzalez, E.; Falsetti, P.; Conticini, E.; d'Alessandro, M.; Selvi, E.; Bellisai, F.; Berlengiero, V.; Vallifuoco, G.; Pata, A.P.; et al. Peripheral Macrovascular Involvement in Systemic Sclerosis: A Cohort Study by Color and Spectral Doppler Ultrasonography. *Life* **2023**, *13*, 487. [CrossRef] [PubMed] [PubMed Central]
42. Colaci, M.; Zanoli, L.; Lo Gullo, A.; Sambataro, D.; Sambataro, G.; Aprile, M.L.; Castellino, P.; Malatino, L. The Impaired Elasticity of Large Arteries in Systemic Sclerosis Patients. *J. Clin. Med.* **2022**, *11*, 3256. [CrossRef] [PubMed] [PubMed Central]
43. Bertolino, J.; Scafi, M.; Benyamine, A.; Aissi, K.; Boufi, M.; Schleinitz, N.; Sarlon, G.; Rossi, P.; Granel, B. Atteintes macrovasculaires de la sclérodermie: État de la question en 2019 [Systemic sclerosis and macrovascular involvement: Status of the issue in 2019]. *J. Med. Vasc.* **2019**, *44*, 400–421. (In French) [CrossRef] [PubMed]
44. Matucci-Cerinic, M.; Kahaleh, B.; Wigley, F.M. Review: Evidence that systemic sclerosis is a vascular disease. *Arthritis Rheum.* **2013**, *65*, 1953–1962. [CrossRef] [PubMed]
45. Lescoat, A.; Coiffier, G.; de Carlan, M.; Droitcourt, C.; Ballerie, A.; Cazalets, C.; Perdriger, A.; Jégo, P. Combination of Capillaroscopic and Ultrasonographic Evaluations in Systemic Sclerosis: Results of a Cross-Sectional Study. *Arthritis Care Res.* **2018**, *70*, 938–943. [CrossRef] [PubMed]
46. Haque, A.; Kiely, D.G.; Kovacs, G.; Thompson, A.A.R.; Condliffe, R. Pulmonary hypertension phenotypes in patients with systemic sclerosis. *Eur. Respir. Rev.* **2021**, *30*, 210053. [CrossRef] [PubMed] [PubMed Central]
47. Lechartier, B.; Humbert, M. Pulmonary arterial hypertension in systemic sclerosis. *Presse Med.* **2021**, *50*, 104062. [CrossRef] [PubMed]
48. Coghlan, J.G.; Denton, C.P.; Grünig, E.; Bonderman, D.; Distler, O.; Khanna, D.; Müller-Ladner, U.; Pope, J.E.; Vonk, M.C.; Doelberg, M.; et al. DETECT study group. Evidence-based detection of pulmonary arterial hypertension in systemic sclerosis: The DETECT study. *Ann. Rheum. Dis.* **2014**, *73*, 1340–1349. [CrossRef] [PubMed] [PubMed Central]
49. Pattanaik, D.; Brown, M.; Postlethwaite, A.E. Vascular involvement in systemic sclerosis (scleroderma). *J. Inflamm. Res.* **2011**, *4*, 105–125. [CrossRef] [PubMed] [PubMed Central]
50. Schioppo, T.; Orenti, A.; Boracchi, P.; De Lucia, O.; Murgo, A.; Ingegnoli, F. Evidence of macro- and micro-angiopathy in scleroderma: An integrated approach combining 22-MHz power Doppler ultrasonography and video-capillaroscopy. *Microvasc. Res.* **2019**, *122*, 125–130. [CrossRef] [PubMed]
51. Bandini, G.; Cometi, L.; Accogli, E.; Domanico, A.; Tofani, L.; Bruni, C.; Bellando-Randone, S.; Lepri, G.; Orlandi, M.; Guiducci, S.; et al. Ultrasound evaluation of bowel vasculopathy in systemic sclerosis. *Eur. J. Intern. Med.* **2022**, *100*, 62–68. [CrossRef] [PubMed]
52. Hughes, M.; Kahaleh, B.; Denton, C.P.; Mason, J.C.; Matucci-Cerinic, M. ANCA in systemic sclerosis, when vasculitis overlaps with vasculopathy: A devastating combination of pathologies. *Rheumatology* **2021**, *60*, 5509–5516. [CrossRef] [PubMed]
53. Condliffe, R.; Radon, M.; Hurdman, J.; Davies, C.; Hill, C.; Akil, M.; Guarasci, F.; Rajaram, S.; Swift, A.J.; Wragg, Z.; et al. CT pulmonary angiography combined with echocardiography in suspected systemic sclerosis-associated pulmonary arterial hypertension. *Rheumatology* **2011**, *50*, 1480–1486. [CrossRef] [PubMed]
54. Pope, J.E.; Denton, C.P.; Johnson, S.R.; Fernandez-Codina, A.; Hudson, M.; Nevskaya, T. State-of-the-art evidence in the treatment of systemic sclerosis. *Nat. Rev. Rheumatol.* **2023**, *19*, 212–226. [CrossRef] [PubMed]
55. Chung, L.; Spino, C.; McLain, R.; Johnson, S.R.; Denton, C.P.; Molitor, J.A.; Steen, V.D.; Lafyatis, R.; Simms, R.W.; Kafaja, S.; et al. Safety and efficacy of abatacept in early diffuse cutaneous systemic sclerosis (ASSET): Open-label extension of a phase 2, double-blind randomised trial. *Lancet Rheumatol.* **2020**, *2*, e743–e753. [CrossRef]
56. Zamanian, R.T.; Badesch, D.; Chung, L.; Domsic, R.T.; Medsger, T.; Pinckney, A.; Keyes-Elstein, L.; D'Aveta, C.; Spychala, M.; White, R.J.; et al. Safety and Efficacy of B-Cell Depletion with Rituximab for the Treatment of Systemic Sclerosis-associated Pulmonary Arterial Hypertension: A Multicenter, Double-Blind, Randomized, Placebo-controlled Trial. *Am. J. Respir. Crit. Care Med.* **2021**, *204*, 209–221. [CrossRef]
57. Moriana, C.; Moulinet, T.; Jaussaud, R.; Decker, P. JAK inhibitors and systemic sclerosis: A systematic review of the literature. *Autoimmun. Rev.* **2022**, *21*, 103168. [CrossRef]
58. Strunz, P.P.; Labinsky, H.; Nagler, L.K.; Portegys, J.; Froehlich, M.; Gernert, M.; Schmalzing, M. Case Report: Effectiveness of secukinumab in systemic sclerosis with early skin progress after autologous hematopoietic stem cell transplantation and end-stage kidney disease. *Front. Immunol.* **2023**, *14*, 1294496. [CrossRef] [PubMed] [PubMed Central]
59. Hofmann, N.N.; Ambühl, R.A.; Jordan, S.; Distler, O. Calcineurin inhibitors in systemic sclerosis—A systematic literature review. *Ther. Adv. Musculoskelet. Dis.* **2022**, *14*, 1759720X221092374. [CrossRef] [PubMed] [PubMed Central]
60. Volkmann, E.R.; Andréasson, K.; Smith, V. Systemic sclerosis. *Lancet* **2023**, *401*, 304–318. [CrossRef] [PubMed] [PubMed Central]
61. LiverTox: Clinical and Research Information on Drug-Induced Liver Injury [Internet]. Bethesda (MD): National Institute of Diabetes and Digestive and Kidney Diseases; 2012-. Phosphodiesterase Type 5 (PDE5) Inhibitors. Available online: https://www.ncbi.nlm.nih.gov/books/NBK548192/ (accessed on 2 August 2024).
62. Kudsi, M.; Khalayli, N.; Tarcha, R.; Al-Darwish, L. Tocilizumab in systemic sclerosis treatment: A case report. *Ann. Med. Surg.* **2023**, *85*, 4586–4588. [CrossRef] [PubMed] [PubMed Central]

63. Fernández-Lázaro, D.; Iglesias-Lázaro, M.; Garrosa, E.; Rodríguez-García, S.; Jerves Donoso, D.; Gutiérrez-Abejón, E.; Jorge-Finnigan, C. Impact of Innovative Treatment Using Biological Drugs for the Modulation of Diffuse Cutaneous Systemic Sclerosis: A Systematic Review. *Medicina* **2023**, *59*, 247. [CrossRef] [PubMed] [PubMed Central]
64. Naranjo, M.; Hassoun, P.M. Systemic Sclerosis-Associated Pulmonary Hypertension: Spectrum and Impact. *Diagnostics* **2021**, *11*, 911. [CrossRef] [PubMed] [PubMed Central]
65. Bahi, M.; Li, C.; Wang, G.; Korman, B.D. Systemic Sclerosis-Associated Pulmonary Arterial Hypertension: From Bedside to Bench and Back Again. *Int. J. Mol. Sci.* **2024**, *25*, 4728. [CrossRef] [PubMed]
66. Jin, Q.; Chen, D.; Zhang, X.; Zhang, F.; Zhong, D.; Lin, D.; Guan, L.; Pan, W.; Zhou, D.; Ge, J. Medical Management of Pulmonary Arterial Hypertension: Current Approaches and Investigational Drugs. *Pharmaceutics* **2023**, *15*, 1579. [CrossRef]
67. Fernández-Codina, A.; Cañas-Ruano, E.; Pope, J.E. Management of Raynaud's phenomenon in systemic sclerosis-a practical approach. *J. Scleroderma Relat. Disord.* **2019**, *4*, 102–110. [CrossRef] [PubMed] [PubMed Central]
68. Roustit, M.; Giai, J.; Gaget, O.; Khouri, C.; Mouhib, M.; Lotito, A.; Blaise, S.; Seinturier, C.; Subtil, F.; Paris, A.; et al. On-Demand Sildenafil as a Treatment for Raynaud Phenomenon: A Series of n-of-1 Trials. *Ann. Intern. Med.* **2018**, *169*, 694–703. [CrossRef] [PubMed]
69. Nagaraja, V. Management of scleroderma renal crisis. *Curr. Opin. Rheumatol.* **2019**, *31*, 223–230. [CrossRef] [PubMed]
70. Hachulla, E.; Agard, C.; Allanore, Y.; Avouac, J.; Bader-Meunier, B.; Belot, A.; Berezne, A.; Bouthors, A.S.; Condette-Wojtasik, G.; Constans, J.; et al. French recommendations for the management of systemic sclerosis. *Orphanet J. Rare Dis.* **2021**, *16* (Suppl. S2), 322. [CrossRef] [PubMed] [PubMed Central]
71. Zhu, J.L.; Black, S.M.; Chen, H.W.; Jacobe, H.T. Emerging treatments for scleroderma/systemic sclerosis. *Fac. Rev.* **2021**, *10*, 43. [CrossRef]
72. O'Reilly, S. Emerging therapeutic targets in systemic sclerosis. *J. Mol. Med.* **2024**, *102*, 465–478. [CrossRef] [PubMed]

sclerosis

Review

Insights and Future Perspectives in Calcinosis Cutis Associated with Systemic Sclerosis

Luna Lazar [1], Mette Mogensen [2,3], Mikael Ploug Boesen [4] and Anne Braae Olesen [1,*]

1 Department of Dermatology, Aarhus University Hospital, 8200 Aarhus, Denmark
2 Department of Dermatology, Bispebjerg Hospital, Copenhagen University Hospitals, 2400 Copenhagen, Denmark
3 Department of Clinical Medicine, University of Copenhagen, 2400 Copenhagen, Denmark
4 Department of Radiology, Bispebjerg Hospital, Copenhagen University Hospitals, 2400 Copenhagen, Denmark; mikael.ploug.boesen@regionh.dk
* Correspondence: anne.braae@rm.dk

Abstract: Introduction: Calcinosis cutis (CC), the pathological deposition of calcium salts in the skin, is a frequent and challenging complication of systemic sclerosis (SSc). Despite its high prevalence, the underlying pathophysiology remains poorly understood, complicating treatment strategies. Material and Methods: This narrative review synthesizes the literature on CC in the context of SSc. The current understanding and treatment of CC in SSc is reviewed, focusing on the role of hypoxia in its pathogenesis and the therapeutic potential of sodium thiosulfate (STS). Results and Discussion: Research indicates a potential link between hypoxia and the development of CC in SSc, shedding light on novel pathogenic mechanisms. Additionally, promising results from treatments such as STS spurs interest in conducting larger, randomized controlled trials to validate these findings.

Keywords: dystrophic calcifications; calcinosis cutis; systemic sclerosis; scleroderma; treatment; hypoxia; chronic inflammation; sodium thiosulfate

1. Introduction

Systemic sclerosis (SSc) is a multisystem autoimmune disease characterized by widespread vasculopathy, fibrosis, and immune dysregulation [1]. Calcinosis cutis (CC), the deposition of insoluble calcium salts in the skin and subcutaneous tissues, is a common yet understudied manifestation of SSc and other autoimmune diseases [2]. These deposits can lead to significant morbidity, including pain, ulcerations, and recurrent infections, severely impacting the quality of life of affected individuals. CC typically presents as firm, palpable nodules or plaques that may be localized or widespread [3]. These deposits are often found in areas of the body subjected to repetitive trauma or pressure, such as the fingers, elbows, knees, and buttocks. The physical burden of calcinosis cutis is profound, causing chronic pain, restricted joint mobility, and recurrent infections due to ulcerations overlying the calcium deposits [4,5]. The psychosocial impact is also significant, as visible lesions can lead to stigmatization and emotional distress [6]. Despite the high prevalence and substantial burden of calcinosis cutis in SSc, the underlying pathophysiology remains poorly understood, complicating efforts to develop effective therapy and preventive measures of CC [7]. Various factors have been implicated in development of CC, including chronic inflammation, immune dysregulation, and vascular abnormalities. However, emerging research suggests that hypoxia, a common feature in SSc due to persistent vascular insufficiency, may play a crucial role in the pathogenesis of this condition [8]. Figure 1. Calcinosis cutis lesions.

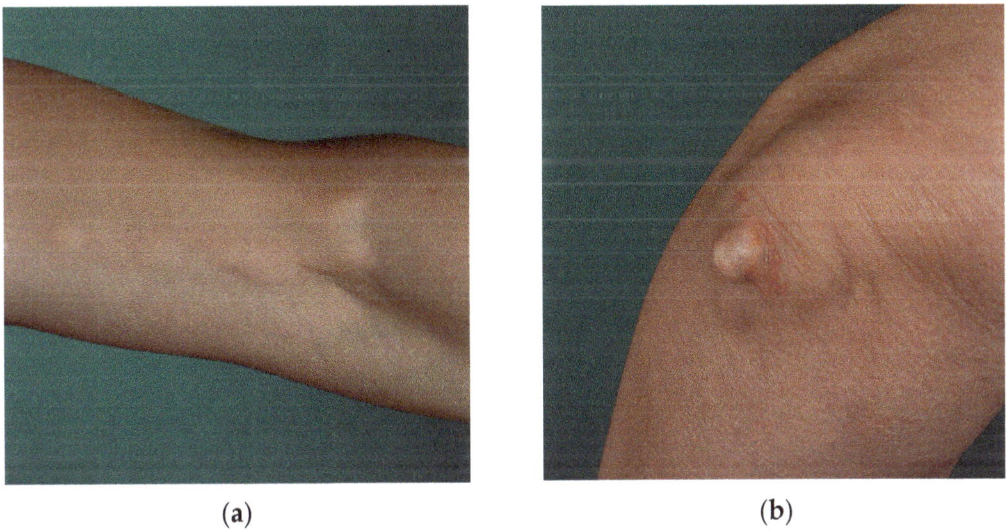

Figure 1. Multiple calcinosis cutis (CC) lesions in two female SSc patients: (**a**) linear CC lesions on the upper arm; (**b**) nodular CC lesion on the elbow with ulcerations. Photos shown with permission from patients.

Hypoxia, reduced oxygen availability in tissues, is a significant pathological feature in SSc [8–10]. The microvascular damage characteristic of SSc leads to chronic hypoxia, resulting from the occlusion and destruction of small blood vessels. This impaired tissue perfusion and oxygen delivery creates a persistent low-oxygen environment. Cells respond to hypoxia through various adaptive mechanisms, often mediated by hypoxia-inducible factors (HIFs). HIFs are transcription factors that activate the expression of genes involved in angiogenesis, metabolism, and cell survival under low oxygen conditions [9,11,12]. In SSc, the chronic activation of these pathways may contribute to pathological processes such as CC [9]. Understanding the role of hypoxia in SSc and its impact on CC provides a framework for exploring targeted therapies.

In the following, we aim to provide a comprehensive overview of the current understanding of CC in SSc, focusing on the potential role of hypoxia in its pathogenesis and the emerging therapeutic potential of sodium thiosulfate (STS). We will discuss the evidence supporting the hypoxia hypothesis, including findings from nailfold capillaroscopy, and explore the mechanisms of action and clinical evidence for STS and other treatment options. Additionally, we highlight the need for larger, well-designed clinical trials to validate these findings and establish evidence-based treatment guidelines for CC in SSc. By advancing our understanding and treatment of this challenging condition, our vision is to improve outcomes and quality of life for patients with SSc.

2. Materials and Methods

This narrative review synthesizes the current literature on CC in the context of SSc. To conduct a comprehensive analysis, we performed a systematic search of three major databases: PubMed, Embase, and Web of Science. The search encompassed studies published from 1980 to the present and focused on capturing all relevant research, reviews, and case reports related to CC in SSc. We used a combination of keywords and Medical Subject Headings (MeSH) to ensure an inclusive search strategy. The primary search terms included "Systemic Sclerosis" and "Calcinosis Cutis", along with related terms such as "Scleroderma, Systemic", "Dystrophic Calcification", "Skin Calcification", and "Autoimmune Disease". The search was conducted across all fields, including titles, abstracts, and full texts to identify a broad range of literature addressing the clinical manifestations, pathophysiology, diagnostic approaches, and treatment options for CC in SSc. The search results were carefully reviewed to select peer-reviewed studies, reviews, and case reports that provided insights into the relationship between CC and SSc. We included articles that offered detailed discussions on pathogenesis, clinical features, diagnostic tools, therapeutic interventions, and prognostic factors specific to CC in SSc. Studies unrelated to CC in SSc, or those focusing on other conditions, were excluded from the review. From the selected articles, we extracted relevant information, paying particular attention to the role of immune and vascular dysfunction in the development of CC. We also examined emerging therapeutic approaches and potential correlations between CC localization, disease duration, and exacerbations. The extracted data were synthesized to provide a detailed overview, highlighting established knowledge as well as gaps for future research.

3. Results

3.1. Pathophysiology: The Hypoxia Hypothesis

The exact mechanisms leading to CC in SSc remain elusive. However, recent studies suggest that hypoxia, a hallmark of SSc due to chronic vascular insufficiency, may play a crucial role [4,5,7,13]. Under hypoxic conditions, HIFs stabilize and activate the transcription of various genes involved in angiogenesis, metabolism, and cell survival [12]. In SSc, chronic hypoxia and the resultant upregulation of HIFs could promote the expression of pro-osteogenic factors such as vascular endothelial growth factor (VEGF) [11,14]. These factors might induce the differentiation of fibroblasts and vascular smooth muscle cells into osteoblast-like cells, potentially leading to the deposition of calcium in the skin and subcutaneous tissues, characteristic of CC. However, the direct role of HIFs in this specific context needs further investigation to confirm their contribution to CC in SSc.

Nailfold capillaroscopy (NFC) is a non-invasive imaging technique that allows for the direct observation of the microcirculation in the nailfold area [15,16]. It is particularly useful in SSc for assessing microvascular changes and has been instrumental in linking vascular abnormalities to the development of CC. Studies have shown that certain NFC patterns, particularly severe capillary loss and extensive avascular areas, are significantly associated with the presence of CC in SSc patients [17–19]. The reduced capillary density and avascular areas observed in NFC reflect a state of chronic tissue hypoxia. The presence of giant capillaries and microhemorrhages indicates ongoing attempts at vascular repair and remodeling. These findings support the hypothesis that chronic hypoxia due to microvascular damage plays a critical role in the pathogenesis of CC.

In addition to hypoxia, chronic inflammation and immune dysregulation are central to the pathogenesis of SSc. Cytokines such as interleukin-6 and tumor necrosis factor-alpha are elevated in SSc and have been implicated in promoting CC [20–22]. These pro-inflammatory cytokines can enhance the osteogenic differentiation of mesenchymal cells and stimulate the production of extracellular matrix components that facilitate calcification.

CC, while present in both SSc and dermatomyositis (DM), likely arises from different pathological mechanisms in each disease. In SSc, the hypoxia hypothesis suggests that chronic low oxygen conditions due to microvascular damage lead to calcium deposition in tissues. In contrast, CC in DM may involve distinct pathophysiological processes not primarily driven by tissue hypoxia. DM is an inflammatory myopathy characterized by muscle weakness and skin manifestations occurring also in a juvenile form [23]. The development of CC in DM is thought to be linked more closely to chronic inflammation and immune complex deposition rather than to ischemia and hypoxia. Inflammatory cytokines and immune complexes may contribute to CC by damaging tissues and creating a local environment conducive to calcium salt precipitation. In DM, the release of calcium from damaged muscle cell mitochondria is a significant contributor [8]. Studies report a decrease in CC when patients are treated with anti-inflammatory treatments [24–26].

3.2. Diagnosis and Characteristics

CC is diagnosed based on clinical examination supported by imaging techniques. While guidelines are sparse, the imaging gold standard is radiography, and other types of imaging such as ultrasound, computed tomography and magnetic resonance could provide extended information such as involvement of underlying structures. Larger studies comparing diagnostic accuracy are lacking. Diagnosis is occasionally confirmed through biopsy to identify calcium deposits in the skin or underlying tissues [27–31]. Figure 2. Calcinosis cutis imaging.

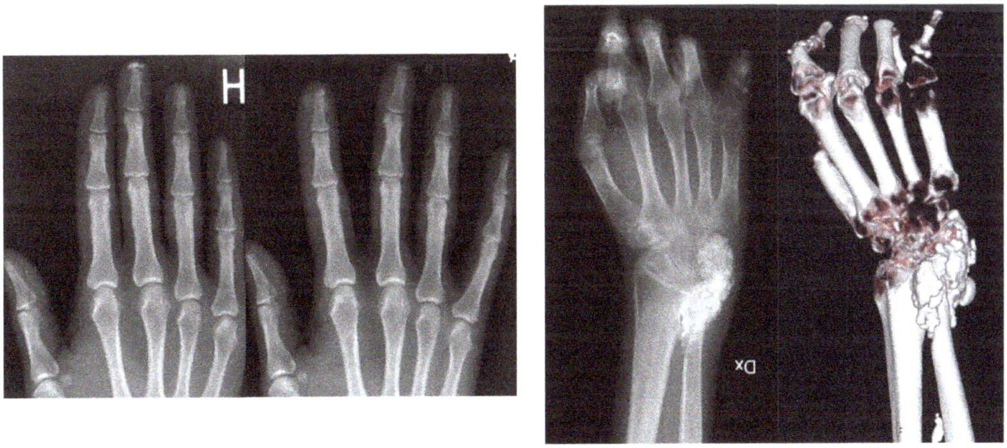

(**a**) (**b**)

Figure 2. (**a**) Radiographic and computed tomography (CT) image of the same hand and wrist in a 48-year-old female Ssc patient. Conventional radiography showing multilobulated calcifications in the distal radioulnar joint and ulnar side of the wrist, measuring 3 × 5 × 2 cm. To the right, a CT 3D multiplanar visualization with bone algorithm. (**b**) Radiographic image of the hand of a 65-year-old female SSc patient showing calcinosis observed in the distal parts of the first, third, and fourth fingers of the right hand. On the right side, a new radiography examination four years later shows new calcinosis formation at the distal part of the second finger, with some deposits measuring up to 4 mm. Furthermore, reduced density of calcinosis at the distal end of the third finger.

Calcinosis is present in several autoimmune connective tissue diseases. Certain patient profiles are more predisposed to developing CC, particularly those with SSc and DM. In SSc, CC is more frequently seen in patients with limited cutaneous involvement, and the presence of anti-centromere antibodies has been strongly associated with its development [32]. Anti-PM/Scl, an autoantibody present in SSc, DM, and more common in patients with overlap syndromes have been found to be associated with calcinosis consistently [33,34].

Regarding clinical manifestations, CC is often observed in patients with long-standing Raynaud's phenomenon, digital ulcers, and sclerodactyly [35,36]. The calcifications in DM are generally more extensive and can be associated with muscle weakness and skin rashes, distinguishing them from the more limited CC in SSc [37]. CC occurs more frequently in SSc patients with longer disease duration [36]. CC severity is not predicted by the severity of the underlying autoimmune connective tissue disease [3]. CC in SSc predominantly follow patterns of trauma and ischemia affecting the hands, fingers, elbows, and knees. In contrast, DM-related CC typically involves the trunk and extremities. The primary mineral component of these deposits also differs. Hydroxyapatite is predominant in SSc, while carbonate apatite is more common in DM [38,39].

3.3. Promising Treatments

CC in SSc presents a significant clinical challenge due to its complex pathogenesis and limited treatment options. Current therapeutic strategies aim to reduce symptoms, prevent complications, and decrease the burden of calcium deposits. Recent excellent systematic reviews provide an organized and comprehensive overview of the various treatments and their level of evidence [40,41]. This section reviews the various treatments for CC, their known or expected mechanism of action, and focuses on STS, the risk profile, and different administration methods.

3.3.1. Potential Preventive Actions

Vasodilation plays a key role in reducing tissue hypoxia. By improving blood flow to affected areas, vasodilators can help alleviate the ischemic conditions that promote calcium deposition. This therapeutic approach aims to enhance oxygen delivery to tissues, potentially mitigating the factors that enhance calcification. Calcium channel blockers, such as nifedipine or diltiazem, are among the most frequently used treatments for CC in SSc [41]. These medications are believed to inhibit the influx of calcium ions into cells, potentially reducing calcium deposition in tissues. The effectiveness of calcium channel blockers is variable; while some patients report a reduction in the size and number of calcium deposits, others do not experience any significant benefits [42]. Common side effects include hypotension, dizziness, and gastrointestinal disturbances [3,41]. Phosphodiesterase type 5 (PDE5) inhibitors, such as sildenafil, have also been explored as a potential treatment for CC in SSc. These medications work by promoting vasodilation and improving blood flow, similar to calcium channel blockers, but through a different mechanism—by increasing the levels of cyclic guanosine monophosphate (cGMP) in blood vessels [43]. PDE5 inhibitors may help reduce tissue hypoxia, thereby decreasing the conditions that favor calcium deposition. While their use in treating CC is less common, they have shown early promise in improving vascular function [36,44].

For patients prone to CC, minimizing trauma to the skin and soft tissues is crucial in preventing the development or worsening of calcium deposits. The gentle handling of the skin, avoiding repetitive pressure or friction, and protecting vulnerable areas from injury can reduce the risk of trauma-induced calcification. Educating patients about these preventive measures is essential. Using cushioned supports or specialized protective gear in daily activities may further help mitigate the impact on areas prone to CC, thereby minimizing the formation of new calcified lesions or the aggravation of existing ones [4].

3.3.2. Mechanical Destruction/Removal of CC

Surgical Interventions

The surgical removal of calcinosis deposits can provide symptomatic relief, especially in cases where the deposits are causing significant pain, recurrent infections, or ulcerations [3,45]. However, surgery is often considered a last resort due to the risks associated with the procedure, including infection/delayed healing, nerve damage, scarring, and, in particular, the potential recurrence of CC in the same anatomical location. Surgical interventions range from minimally invasive techniques to more extensive excisions, depending on the size and location of the deposits [40,46].

Lithotripsy

Extracorporeal shock wave lithotripsy (ESWL) is a non-invasive medical procedure used for treating CC, generating high-energy shock waves onto the targeted CC lesions. These shock waves are delivered to the skin surface using a device that is placed over the affected area. Previous results demonstrated some effect on CC lesion size and a great effect on pain reduction [47–50].

3.3.3. Chemical Destruction/Removal of CC

Sodium Thiosulfate

STS, traditionally used intravenous to treat calciphylaxis in chronic kidney disease, has emerged as a promising therapeutic option for CC in SSc. STS is a water-soluble salt and reducing agent that reacts with oxidizing agents and has been used to treat CC since 2005. Preliminary studies and case reports have demonstrated significant reductions in calcium deposits and associated symptoms following treatment with STS [40,41,51–58]. Although the exact mechanism of action is unknown, STS is believed to work primarily by forming soluble complexes with calcium, facilitating the dissolution and excretion of calcium deposits [2]. Additionally, its antioxidant properties help reduce oxidative stress, which may mitigate inflammation and vascular damage contributing to CC. Furthermore, STS may improve vascular function and tissue oxygenation, counteracting the hypoxic environment that promotes calcification [59].

Administration of Sodium Thiosulfate

STS can be administered in various ways, including intravenous, topical, and intralesional methods. The topical application of STS may be beneficial for localized calcinosis deposits, providing direct treatment to affected areas with potentially fewer systemic side effects [40,58,60–63]. Intralesional injections involve directly administering the drug upon the calcium deposits, which may be effective for treating isolated, symptomatic lesions. The administration of intralesional STS for treating CC in SSc involves a regimen designed to gradually soften and reduce calcium deposits. Our approach recommends multiple treatments, administered at 1–2-week intervals, with a total of 4–8 sessions depending on the severity and extent of the CC lesions. Dosage increases during the sessions as more room is gradually allowed ranging from 0.05 mL to 10 mL using a preferred concentration of 150 mg/mL [51,56]. This repeated administration is necessary as the calcinosis deposits gradually soften over the course of the treatment, transitioning from a rock-hard consistency to a more toothpaste-like texture. Some studies have reported using a single administration of STS [51] and some very low concentrations (0.1 mg/mL), but the outcomes have generally been less effective compared to the repeated treatment regimen [40].

While STS is an inexpensive treatment, a significant challenge in using STS is its availability as a magistral (compounded) preparation. The compounded nature of the drug means that its availability can vary widely between different countries and even within regions. This variability in access can hinder the consistent application of this treatment modality, making it less reliable for patients who may benefit from it. Moreover, STS is officially registered only as an intravenous medication in most countries, presenting additional challenges. When used intravenously, STS acts systemically, which has a different risk profile compared to topical or intralesional administration. Systemic treatment is generally more extensive and should typically be reserved for cases with widespread calcinosis, such as when a SSc patient has 100 or more lesions. The systemic approach can be more appropriate in such severe cases due to the extensive nature of the disease, but it also requires careful monitoring for potential systemic side effects and complications. Studies report mixed effectiveness of intravenous STS in SSc patients [41].

Risk Profile of Sodium Thiosulfate

Topical and intralesional STS treatments are generally associated with only mild side effects and are considered safe. Infection occurred in 9% (5/53) of patients after intralesional STS administration [51,53,56], which was managed with antibiotics [53]. Injection-associated pain was reported in more than 11% of patients receiving intralesional STS and was transient in all cases [56]. Blistering is rare and tends to occur with higher STS concentrations. We observed blistering of the skin 4–7 days after switching from injection with STS 150 mg/mL to injection with 250 mg/mL [56]. Skin irritation, inflammation, or redness occurred and resolved without intervention [51]. One study noted skin discoloration, but the prevalence was not reported [40]. Allergic reactions to STS are a rare, potential risk. No published results document this adverse reaction. Similarly, skin necrosis is a potential risk, but no published results have shown this adverse reaction.

Sodium Thiosulfate in the Context of Hypoxia

If the hypoxia hypothesis is correct, STS could address CC through several mechanisms. The calcium-chelating properties of STS may dissolve and soften calcified deposits, making them easier to resorb. Additionally, its antioxidant effects could reduce oxidative stress caused by hypoxia, interrupting the cycle of tissue damage and calcium buildup [8].

The response to STS treatment appears to differ slightly between SSc and DM, likely due to the distinct pathophysiological mechanisms in each disease [41]. In SSc, where vascular dysfunction and hypoxia play a significant role in calcinosis formation, the ability of STS to improve tissue oxygenation and reduce oxidative stress may explain its more pronounced effectiveness. In contrast, calcinosis in DM is often linked to chronic inflammation and immune dysregulation rather than hypoxia, and lesions decrease in response to anti-inflammatory treatments, which differs from SSc [24–26]. Figure 3. Calcinosis cutis treatment.

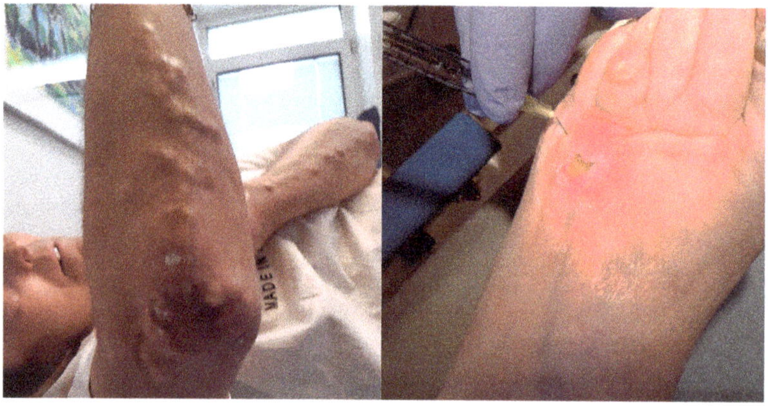

(a) (b)

Figure 3. Calcinosis cutis lesions in relation to treatment: (**a**) extensive, widespread lesions on both forearms with inflammation, making treatment difficult; (**b**) intralesional sodium thiosulfate treatment being performed on a severely ulcerated lesion on the foot. Photos shown with permission from patients.

3.3.4. Other Treatments

Bisphosphonates, including alendronate and pamidronate, work by inhibiting osteoclast-mediated bone resorption, which may help reduce calcification in soft tissues, but is mainly used for osteoporosis treatment. The clinical evidence for their effectiveness in treating CC is mixed. Side effects associated with bisphosphonates include gastrointestinal issues, osteonecrosis of the jaw, and hypocalcemia [41,64]. Warfarin, an anticoagulant, has been used in some cases based on the hypothesis that it can inhibit calcium deposition by preventing the formation of insoluble calcium salts. However, the evidence supporting the use of warfarin for CC is limited, and it is not widely recommended due to the risk of bleeding complications [41,65]. Colchicine, an anti-inflammatory agent, has been used to treat CC, particularly when inflammation is a prominent feature. Anecdotal evidence suggests that colchicine may provide some benefit in reducing inflammation and pain associated with CC. However, gastrointestinal upset and neutropenia are potential side effects [3,41].

4. Discussion

CC in SSc remains a medically challenging condition with limited effective treatment options. Conventional therapies, including calcium channel blockers, bisphosphonates, warfarin, colchicine, and surgical interventions, have shown variable effectiveness, and are often associated with significant side effects. STS is as a promising treatment, with early evidence suggesting it may effectively reduce calcium deposits and alleviate symptoms in patients who already have developed CC. However, a limitation of STS treatment is that, even when effective in reducing existing CC in some patients, it does not prevent the formation of new lesions.

The hypoxia hypothesis provides a compelling explanation for the efficacy of STS in treating CC. Hypoxia, or reduced oxygen availability, is a significant factor in the pathogenesis of SSc. It promotes the formation of reactive oxygen species, leading to oxidative stress, inflammation, and subsequent tissue damage. These conditions favor the deposition of calcium in the skin and soft tissues. STS appears to counteract these processes through several mechanisms. Its calcium-chelating properties increase the solubility of calcium salts, facilitating the dissolution and excretion of calcified deposits. This action can transform hard deposits into a softer consistency, aiding in their resorption over time. Additionally, STS may reduce oxidative stress and protect tissues from further damage. By improving vascular function and tissue oxygenation, STS possibly mitigates the ischemic conditions that favor calcinosis, promoting a healthier tissue environment less prone to calcification. Furthermore, its potential anti-inflammatory effects may disrupt the cycle of tissue damage and calcification, reducing the inflammatory environment that supports calcium deposition. These multifaceted actions make STS a promising therapeutic option for managing CCs in SSc, addressing multiple pathways implicated in the formation and persistence of CC.

CC in SSc shares similarities with calcinosis observed in other autoimmune diseases, but distinct differences exist in terms of localization, disease progression, and treatment options. Treatment options for CC in SSc are largely focused on addressing the underlying vascular damage and hypoxia, with calcium channel blockers, STS, and surgical removal being commonly explored [41]. In DM, however, treatment often revolves around controlling inflammation and muscle involvement, with immunosuppressive agents like corticosteroids or methotrexate playing a more central role [66]. While surgical interventions may be considered in both diseases, they may be more challenging in SSc due to the fibrosis and poorer wound healing associated with the disease [44].

Comparatively, CC in overlap syndromes, such as patients with features of both SSc and DM, can present a hybrid pattern of CC, with more extensive skin and soft tissue involvement, often complicating treatment and leading to variable outcomes [3]. This highlights the need for personalized treatment strategies tailored to the specific autoimmune profile and disease presentation.

Future Research Directions

Future research should aim to confirm the efficacy and safety of STS in treating CC through larger, randomized controlled trials. These studies should explore optimal dosing regimens, long-term outcomes, and potential side effects. Understanding the long-term safety profile of STS is crucial for ensuring sustained patient safety and treatment efficacy. Additionally, further investigations are needed to elucidate the precise mechanisms by which STS exerts its therapeutic effects. Understanding how STS interacts with the biochemical pathways involved in calcinosis formation will help optimize its use and potentially lead to the development of more efficient treatments. Furthermore, future research must further explore the underlying pathophysiology to better understand the different types of CC.

The accurate diagnosis and assessment of CC are essential for effective treatment. Diagnostic challenges include differentiating CC from other skin and soft tissue conditions and determining the extent and activity of calcified deposits. Advanced imaging techniques, such as high-resolution ultrasound, CT scans, and MRI, can significantly improve diagnostic accuracy and monitor treatment response [27–31]. Future research should focus on standardizing imaging protocols and establishing reliable biomarkers to assess disease activity and treatment efficacy.

Conducting placebo-controlled studies with STS presents significant challenges. One major issue is the burning pain associated with STS injections, which results from its tissue toxicity. This pain can make it difficult to blind patients and physicians to the treatment being administered, potentially introducing bias into the study results. Effective blinding is critical in clinical trials to ensure that the outcomes are not influenced by participant and physician expectations. Therefore, meticulously planned study designs or alternative methods to manage pain and maintain blinding are necessary to ensure the reliability of clinical trial data. Further research should also explore combination therapies that may enhance the efficacy of STS or target additional pathways involved in CC formation. Through comprehensive studies, international cooperation, and continued innovation, we hope to provide more effective and safer treatment options for patients suffering from this rare debilitating condition.

Author Contributions: Conceptualization, L.L., M.M. and A.B.O.; methodology, L.L., M.M. and A.B.O.; validation, L.L., M.M., M.P.B. and A.B.O.; formal analysis, L.L., M.M. and A.B.O.; investigation, L.L., M.M. and A.B.O.; resources, L.L., M.M., M.P.B. and A.B.O.; data curation, L.L., M.M. and A.B.O.; writing—original draft preparation, L.L., M.M. and A.B.O.; writing—review and editing, L.L., M.M., M.P.B. and A.B.O.; visualization, L.L., M.M., M.P.B. and A.B.O.; supervision, M.M., M.P.B. and A.B.O.; project administration, L.L.; funding acquisition, L.L., M.M., M.P.B. and A.B.O. All authors have read and agreed to the published version of the manuscript.

Funding: Our ongoing clinical CC research project was funded by an unrestricted grant from LEO Foundation, Denmark, 2023, EU clinical trial no.: 2023-510255-34-00.

Institutional Review Board Statement: Not applicable.

Data Availability Statement: No new data were created or analyzed in this study. Data sharing is not applicable to this article. Further inquiries can be directed to the corresponding author.

Conflicts of Interest: The authors declare no conflicts of interest. All grants received are unrestricted. The funders had no role in the design of the study; in the collection, analyses, or interpretation of data; in the writing of the manuscript; or in the decision to publish the results.

References

1. Cutolo, M.; Sulli, A.; Pizzorni, C.; Paolino, S.; Smith, V. Systemic sclerosis: Markers and targeted treatments. *Acta Reumatol. Port.* **2016**, *41*, 18–25. [PubMed]
2. Davuluri, S.; Lood, C.; Chung, L. Calcinosis in systemic sclerosis. *Curr. Opin. Rheumatol.* **2022**, *34*, 319–327. [CrossRef] [PubMed]
3. Balin, S.J.; Wetter, D.A.; Andersen, L.K.; Davis, M.D. Calcinosis cutis occurring in association with autoimmune connective tissue disease: The Mayo Clinic experience with 78 patients, 1996–2009. *Arch. Dermatol.* **2012**, *148*, 455–462. [CrossRef]
4. Valenzuela, A.; Song, P.; Chung, L. Calcinosis in scleroderma. *Curr. Opin. Rheumatol.* **2018**, *30*, 554–561. [CrossRef]
5. Valenzuela, A.; Chung, L. Calcinosis: Pathophysiology and management. *Curr. Opin. Rheumatol.* **2015**, *27*, 542–548. [CrossRef]
6. Hughes, M.; Herrick, A.L. Diagnosis and management of systemic sclerosis-related calcinosis. *Expert Rev. Clin. Immunol.* **2023**, *19*, 45–54. [CrossRef]
7. Burgess, K.A.; Herrick, A.L.; Watson, R.E.B. Systemic sclerosis skin is a primed microenvironment for soft tissue calcification-a hypothesis. *Rheumatology* **2021**, *60*, 2517–2527. [CrossRef] [PubMed]
8. Valenzuela, A.; Chung, L. Subcutaneous calcinosis: Is it different between systemic sclerosis and dermatomyositis? *J. Scleroderma Relat. Disord.* **2022**, *7*, 7–23. [CrossRef]
9. Beyer, C.; Schett, G.; Gay, S.; Distler, O.; Distler, J.H. Hypoxia. Hypoxia in the pathogenesis of systemic sclerosis. *Arthritis Res. Ther.* **2009**, *11*, 220. [CrossRef]
10. Siao-Pin, S.; Damian, L.O.; Muntean, L.M.; Rednic, S. Acroosteolysis in systemic sclerosis: An insight into hypoxia-related pathogenesis. *Exp. Ther. Med.* **2016**, *12*, 3459–3463. [CrossRef]
11. Maciejewska, M.; Sikora, M.; Stec, A.; Zaremba, M.; Maciejewski, C.; Pawlik, K.; Rudnicka, L. Hypoxia-Inducible Factor-1alpha (HIF-1alpha) as a Biomarker for Changes in Microcirculation in Individuals with Systemic Sclerosis. *Dermatol. Ther.* **2023**, *13*, 1549–1560. [CrossRef] [PubMed]

12. Copur, S.; Ucku, D.; Cozzolino, M.; Kanbay, M. Hypoxia-inducible factor signaling in vascular calcification in chronic kidney disease patients. *J. Nephrol.* **2022**, *35*, 2205–2213. [CrossRef]
13. Marjanovic, E.; Moore, T.L.; Manning, J.B.; Dinsdale, G.; Wilkinson, S.; Dickinson, M.R.; Herrick, A.L.; Murray, A.K. Systemic sclerosis-related digital calcinosis; a pilot study of cutaneous oxygenation and perfusion. *Rheumatology* **2020**, *59*, 3573–3575. [CrossRef] [PubMed]
14. Davies, C.A.; Jeziorska, M.; Freemont, A.J.; Herrick, A.L. The differential expression of VEGF, VEGFR-2, and GLUT-1 proteins in disease subtypes of systemic sclerosis. *Hum. Pathol.* **2006**, *37*, 190–197. [CrossRef]
15. Smith, V.; Ickinger, C.; Hysa, E.; Snow, M.; Frech, T.; Sulli, A.; Cutolo, M. Nailfold capillaroscopy. *Best Pract. Res. Clin. Rheumatol.* **2023**, *37*, 101849. [CrossRef]
16. Lazar, L.T.; Guldberg-Moller, J.; Lazar, B.T.; Mogensen, M. Nailfold capillaroscopy as diagnostic test in patients with psoriasis and psoriatic arthritis: A systematic review. *Microvasc. Res.* **2023**, *147*, 104476. [CrossRef]
17. Valentini, G.; Vettori, S.; Cuomo, G.; Iudici, M.; D'Abrosca, V.; Capocotta, D.; Del Genio, G.; Santoriello, C.; Cozzolino, D. Early systemic sclerosis: Short-term disease evolution and factors predicting the development of new manifestations of organ involvement. *Arthritis Res. Ther.* **2012**, *14*, R188. [CrossRef]
18. Samoes, B.; Guimaraes da Fonseca, D.; Beirao, T.; Costa, F.; Vieira, R.; Terroso, G.; Ferreira, R.M.; Nicolau, R.; Saraiva, A.; Salvador, M.J.; et al. Assessment of calcinosis in Portuguese patients with systemic sclerosis—A multicenter study. *Clin. Rheumatol.* **2023**, *42*, 2125–2134. [CrossRef] [PubMed]
19. Morardet, L.; Avouac, J.; Sammour, M.; Baron, M.; Kahan, A.; Feydy, A.; Allanore, Y. Late Nailfold Videocapillaroscopy Pattern Associated with Hand Calcinosis and Acro-Osteolysis in Systemic Sclerosis. *Arthritis Care Res.* **2016**, *68*, 366–373. [CrossRef]
20. Ibrahim-Achi, Z.; de Vera-Gonzalez, A.; Gonzalez-Delgado, A.; Lopez-Mejias, R.; Gonzalez-Gay, M.A.; Ferraz-Amaro, I. Interleukin-6 serum levels are associated with disease features and cardiovascular risk in patients with systemic sclerosis. *Clin. Exp. Rheumatol.* **2023**, *42*, 1564–1570. [CrossRef]
21. Kosalka-Wegiel, J.; Licholai, S.; Pacholczak-Madej, R.; Dziedzina, S.; Milewski, M.; Kuszmiersz, P.; Korona, A.; Gasior, J.; Matyja-Bednarczyk, A.; Kwiatkowska, H.; et al. Serum IL-17 and TNFalpha as prognostic biomarkers in systemic sclerosis patients: A prospective study. *Rheumatol. Int.* **2024**, *44*, 119–128. [CrossRef]
22. Masri, M.F.B.; Ng, S.A.; Chin, C.W.; Low, A.H. Biomarkers in the evaluation of cardiac involvement in systemic sclerosis. *Rheumatol. Immunol. Res.* **2024**, *5*, 99–106. [CrossRef]
23. Pandya, R.; Kleitsch, J.; Lim, D.; Werth, V.P. Clinical characteristics and symptom progression of dermatomyositis subtypes: A retrospective analysis of a prospective database. *J. Am. Acad. Dermatol.* **2024**, *91*, 31–36. [CrossRef]
24. Rodriguez-Lozano, A.L.; Mata-Aguilera, X.; Rivas-Larrauri, F.; Bustamante-Ogando, J.C.; Gutierrez-Hernandez, A.; Bojalil-Cabildo, A.; Scheffler-Mendoza, S.; Yamazaki-Nakashimada, M. Subcutaneous immunoglobulin for the treatment of calcinosis associated with juvenile dermatomyositis. *Int. J. Rheum. Dis.* **2024**, *27*, e15239. [CrossRef]
25. Shobha, V.; Kodali, R.; Amin, S.N.; Srivastava, P.; Sharma, B.; Goel, R.; Ganapati, A.; Dhote, S.; Janardana, R.; Rajasekhar, L.; et al. Effectiveness of generic tofacitinib in idiopathic inflammatory myositis (IIM)-a retrospective analysis from Indian Myositis Registry (MyoIN). *Clin. Rheumatol.* **2024**, *43*, 2245–2252. [CrossRef]
26. Shiari, R.; Khalili, M.; Zeinali, V.; Shashaani, N.; Samami, M.; Moghaddamemami, F.H. Local injection of infliximab into calcinosis lesions in patients with juvenile dermatomyositis (JDM): A clinical trial. *Pediatr. Rheumatol. Online J.* **2024**, *22*, 2. [CrossRef]
27. Rowe, S.P.; Fritz, J.; Fishman, E.K. Soft Tissue Calcinosis Universalis Visualized with Novel 3-D Computed Tomography Cinematic Rendering. *J. Rheumatol.* **2019**, *46*, 539–540. [CrossRef]
28. Atzeni, I.M.; Hogervorst, E.M.; Stel, A.J.; de Leeuw, K.; Bijl, M.; Bos, R.; Westra, J.; van Goor, H.; Bolling, M.C.; Slart, R.; et al. [(18)F]Sodium Fluoride PET has the potential to identify active formation of calcinosis cutis in limited cutaneous systemic sclerosis. *Semin. Arthritis Rheum.* **2022**, *55*, 152027. [CrossRef]
29. Cosedis Enevoldsen, F.; Therkildsen, J.; Klose-Jensen, R.; Lynggaard Elkjaer, A.; Uggerby Naeser, E.; Klicman, R.F.; Thorup Aaen, K.; Sondergaard, K.H.; Hauge, E.M. High-resolution peripheral quantitative computed tomography for the assessment of acro-osteolysis and calcinosis in patients with systemic sclerosis. *Jt. Bone Spine* **2024**, *91*, 105699. [CrossRef]
30. Fairchild, R.; Chung, M.; Sharpless, L.; Li, S.; Chung, L. Ultrasound Detection of Calcinosis and Association with Ulnar Artery Occlusion in Patients with Systemic Sclerosis. *Arthritis Care Res.* **2021**, *73*, 1332–1337. [CrossRef]
31. Hughes, M.; Hodgson, R.; Harris, J.; Porter, N.; Jackson, S.; Kirwadi, A.; Manning, J.; Peytrignet, S.; Herrick, A.L. Imaging calcinosis in patients with systemic sclerosis by radiography, computerised tomography and magnetic resonance imaging. *Semin. Arthritis Rheum.* **2019**, *49*, 279–282. [CrossRef]
32. Sakata, K.; Kaneko, Y.; Yasuoka, H.; Takeuchi, T. Association of radiographic findings in hand X-ray with clinical features and autoantibodies in patients with systemic sclerosis. *Clin. Rheumatol.* **2020**, *39*, 113–118. [CrossRef]
33. Lazzaroni, M.-G.; Marasco, E.; Campochiaro, C.; DeVries-Bouwstra, J.; Gonzalez-Perez, M.-I.; Rojas-Serrano, J.; Hachulla, E.; Zanatta, E.; Barsotti, S.; Furini, F.; et al. The clinical phenotype of systemic sclerosis patients with anti-PM/Scl antibodies: Results from the EUSTAR cohort. *Rheumatology* **2021**, *60*, 5028–5041. [CrossRef]
34. Cavazzana, I.; Vojinovic, T.; Airo, P.; Fredi, M.; Ceribelli, A.; Pedretti, E.; Lazzaroni, M.G.; Garrafa, E.; Franceschini, F. Systemic Sclerosis-Specific Antibodies: Novel and Classical Biomarkers. *Clin. Rev. Allergy Immunol.* **2023**, *64*, 412–430. [CrossRef]

35. Morrisroe, K.; Stevens, W.; Sahhar, J.; Ngian, G.-S.; Ferdowsi, N.; Hill, C.L.; Roddy, J.; Walker, J.; Proudman, S.; Nikpour, M. Digital ulcers in systemic sclerosis: Their epidemiology, clinical characteristics, and associated clinical and economic burden. *Arthritis Res. Ther.* **2019**, *21*, 299. [CrossRef]
36. Valenzuela, A.; Baron, M.; Herrick, A.L.; Proudman, S.; Stevens, W.; Rodriguez-Reyna, T.S.; Vacca, A.; Medsger, T.A.; Hinchcliff, M.; Hsu, V.; et al. Calcinosis is associated with digital ulcers and osteoporosis in patients with systemic sclerosis: A Scleroderma Clinical Trials Consortium study. *Semin. Arthritis Rheum.* **2016**, *46*, 344–349. [CrossRef]
37. Chung, M.P.; Richardson, C.; Kirakossian, D.; Orandi, A.B.; Saketkoo, L.A.; Rider, L.G.; Schiffenbauer, A.; von Mühlen, C.A.; Chung, L. Calcinosis Biomarkers in Adult and Juvenile Dermatomyositis. *Autoimmun. Rev.* **2020**, *19*, 102533. [CrossRef]
38. Lee, P.; Green, L.; Marzec, B.; Meldrum, F.; Del Galdo, F.; Alcacer-Pitarch, B. Dystrophic calcinosis: Structural and morphological composition, and evaluation of ethylenediaminetetraacetic acid ('EDTA') for potential local treatment. *Arthritis Res. Ther.* **2024**, *26*, 102. [CrossRef]
39. Eidelman, N.; Boyde, A.; Bushby, A.J.; Howell, P.G.; Sun, J.; Newbury, D.E.; Miller, F.W.; Robey, P.G.; Rider, L.G. Microstructure and mineral composition of dystrophic calcification associated with the idiopathic inflammatory myopathies. *Arthritis Res. Ther.* **2009**, *11*, R159. [CrossRef]
40. Nowaczyk, J.; Zawistowski, M.; Fiedor, P. Local, non-systemic, and minimally invasive therapies for calcinosis cutis: A systematic review. *Arch. Dermatol. Res.* **2022**, *314*, 515–525. [CrossRef]
41. Traineau, H.; Aggarwal, R.; Monfort, J.B.; Senet, P.; Oddis, C.V.; Chizzolini, C.; Barbaud, A.; Francès, C.; Arnaud, L.; Chasset, F. Treatment of calcinosis cutis in systemic sclerosis and dermatomyositis: A review of the literature. *J. Am. Acad. Dermatol.* **2020**, *82*, 317–325. [CrossRef] [PubMed]
42. Vayssairat, M.; Hidouche, D.; Abdoucheli-Baudot, N.; Gaitz, J.P. Clinical significance of subcutaneous calcinosis in patients with systemic sclerosis. Does diltiazem induce its regression? *Ann. Rheum. Dis.* **1998**, *57*, 252–254. [CrossRef]
43. Seftel, A.D. Phosphodiesterase type 5 inhibitor differentiation based on selectivity, pharmacokinetic, and efficacy profiles. *Clin. Cardiol.* **2004**, *27*, I14–I19. [CrossRef]
44. Valenzuela, A.; Chung, L. Management of Calcinosis Associated with Systemic Sclerosis. *Curr. Treat. Options Rheumatol.* **2016**, *2*, 85–96. [CrossRef]
45. Bender, T.; Burt, M. A case report and review of calcinosis cutis. *J. Surg. Case Rep.* **2024**, *2024*, rjae068. [CrossRef]
46. Merlino, G.; Germano, S.; Carlucci, S. Surgical management of digital calcinosis in CREST syndrome. *Aesthetic Plast. Surg.* **2013**, *37*, 1214–1219. [CrossRef]
47. Sultan-Bichat, N.; Menard, J.; Perceau, G.; Staerman, F.; Bernard, P.; Reguiaï, Z. Treatment of calcinosis cutis by extracorporeal shock-wave lithotripsy. *J. Am. Acad. Dermatol.* **2012**, *66*, 424–429. [CrossRef]
48. Beatty, P.; Killion, L.; Power, R.; Roche, M. Dystrophic calcinosis cutis successfully treated with extracorporeal shockwave lithotripsy. *Clin. Exp. Dermatol.* **2021**, *46*, 1656–1658. [CrossRef]
49. Delgado-Márquez, A.M.; Carmona, M.; Vanaclocha, F.; Postigo, C. Effectiveness of extracorporeal shock wave lithotripsy to treat dystrophic calcinosis cutis ulcers. *Actas Dermosifiliogr.* **2015**, *106*, 140–143. [CrossRef]
50. Chan, A.Y.; Li, E. Electric shock wave lithotripsy (ESWL) as a pain control measure in dermatomyositis with calcinosis cutis-old method, new discovery. *Clin. Rheumatol.* **2005**, *24*, 172–173. [CrossRef]
51. Baumgartner-Nielsen, J.; Olesen, A.B. Treatment of Skin Calcifications with Intra-lesional Injection of Sodium Thiosulphate: A Case Series. *Acta Derm. Venereol.* **2016**, *96*, 257–258. [CrossRef]
52. Darrieurtort-Laffite, C.; Bertrand-Vasseur, A.; Garraud, T.; Planche, L.; Le Goff, B. Tolerance and effect of sodium thiosulfate in calcific tendinitis of the rotator cuff. *Clin. Rheumatol.* **2020**, *39*, 561–569. [CrossRef]
53. Goossens, J.; Courbebaisse, M.; Caudron, E.; Bahans, C.; Vacquerie, V.; Melchior, J.; Salle, P.V.; Moesch, C.; Daudon, M.; Frocht, V.; et al. Efficacy of intralesional sodium thiosulfate injections for disabling tumoral calcinosis: Two cases. *Semin. Arthritis Rheum.* **2017**, *47*, 451–455. [CrossRef]
54. Granja, B.V.; De Matos, P.R.; Azevedo, F.; Baudrier, T.; Mota, A. Intralesional sodium thiosulfate for the treatment of calciphylaxis: A case report and review of the literature. *Int. J. Dermatol.* **2024**, *63*, 132–134. [CrossRef]
55. Lopez-Sundh, A.E.; Quintana-Sancho, A.; Duran-Vian, C.; Reguero-DelCura, L.; Corrales-Martinez, A.F.; Gomez-Fernandez, C.; Gonzalez-Lopez, M.A. Clinical and ultrasound response to intralesional sodium thiosulfate for the treatment of calcinosis cutis in the setting of systemic sclerosis. A case-based review. *Clin. Rheumatol.* **2021**, *40*, 2985–2989. [CrossRef]
56. Olesen, A.B.; Fage, S. Dysthrophic calcification in Systemic Sclerosis—Intralesional Injections of Sodium Thiosulfate may have significant Positive Effects on your patients. *Med. Res. Arch.* **2020**, *8*, 8. [CrossRef]
57. Paula, E.; Denys, P.; Anama, D.P.; Maria, D.; Carolina, V.; Ana, T.; Luis, M.; Guido, M.C. Intralesional Sodium Thiosulfate as Adjuvant Therapy in Severe Calciphylaxis. *J. Drugs Dermatol.* **2023**, *22*, e28–e30. [CrossRef]
58. Ricardo, J.W.; Sun, H.Y.; Gorji, M.; Sebaratnam, D.F. Topical sodium thiosulfate as treatment of calcinosis cutis: Case series and systematic review. *J. Am. Acad. Dermatol.* **2022**, *87*, 443–444. [CrossRef]
59. Cicone, J.S.; Petronis, J.B.; Embert, C.D.; Spector, D.A. Successful treatment of calciphylaxis with intravenous sodium thiosulfate. *Am. J. Kidney Dis.* **2004**, *43*, 1104–1108. [CrossRef]
60. Del Barrio-Diaz, P.; Moll-Manzur, C.; Alvarez-Veliz, S.; Vera-Kellet, C. Topical sodium metabisulfite for the treatment of calcinosis cutis: A promising new therapy. *Br. J. Dermatol.* **2016**, *175*, 608–611. [CrossRef]

61. Gauffenic, A.; Ratsimbazafy, V.; Ostertag, A.; Linglart, A.; Bourrat, E.; Leroy, C.; Liote, F.; Latourte, A.; Richette, P.; Ea, H.K.; et al. Effectiveness of topical sodium thiosulfate for ectopic calcifications and ossifications. Results of the CATSS-O study. *Semin. Arthritis Rheum.* **2023**, *63*, 152306. [CrossRef] [PubMed]
62. von Hodenberg, C.; Neufeld, M.; Wohlrab, J.; Meyer, D.; Ehrchen, J.; Sunderkotter, C. Topical sodium thiosulfate: A reliable treatment for digital calcinosis cutis—A case series with six patients. *J. Dtsch. Dermatol. Ges.* **2020**, *18*, 1181–1183. [CrossRef]
63. Wolf, E.K.; Smidt, A.C.; Laumann, A.E. Topical sodium thiosulfate therapy for leg ulcers with dystrophic calcification. *Arch. Dermatol.* **2008**, *144*, 1560–1562. [CrossRef]
64. Rauch, L.; Hein, R.; Biedermann, T.; Eyerich, K.; Lauffer, F. Bisphosphonates for the Treatment of Calcinosis Cutis-A Retrospective Single-Center Study. *Biomedicines* **2021**, *9*, 1698. [CrossRef]
65. Lassoued, K.; Saiag, P.; Anglade, M.C.; Roujeau, J.C.; Touraine, R.L. Failure of warfarin in treatment of calcinosis universalis. *Am. J. Med.* **1988**, *84*, 795–796. [CrossRef]
66. Gutierrez, A., Jr.; Wetter, D.A. Calcinosis cutis in autoimmune connective tissue diseases. *Dermatol. Ther.* **2012**, *25*, 195–206. [CrossRef]

sclerosis

MDPI

Review

A Narrative Review of Therapeutic Options in Systemic Sclerosis Associated Interstitial Lung Disease

Robert Harrington *, Patricia Harkins and Richard Conway

Department of Rheumatology, St. James's Hospital, D08 NHY Dublin, Ireland; pharkins@stjames.ie (P.H.); riconway@stjames.ie (R.C.)
* Correspondence: rharrington@stjames.ie

Abstract: Background: Interstitial lung disease (ILD) has replaced scleroderma renal crisis as the leading cause of mortality in systemic sclerosis (SSc), with a 10-year mortality of 40%. There have been well-powered randomised control trials (RCTs) demonstrating the effect of cyclophosphamide (CYC), mycophenolic acid (MMF), nintedanib and tocilizumab (TCZ) in SSc-ILD but a paucity of sufficiently powered studies investigating other agents in the disease. **Methods:** This is a narrative review which examines the existing evidence for immunosuppressive treatments, transplant and adjunctive therapies in SSc-ILD by reviewing the key landmark trials in the last two decades. **Results:** MMF for 2 years is as effective as oral CYC for 1 year. Rituximab (RTX) is non-inferior to CYC. TCZ appears to have a beneficial effective regardless of the extent of lung involvement. **Conclusions:** There is now a strong evidence base supporting the use of MMF as the first line option in SSc-ILD. RTX, CYC and TCZ are viable therapeutic options if there is ILD progression on MMF. Anti-fibrotic and pulmonary arterial (PAH) treatments likely add long-term synergistic benefits. There remains a role for lung transplantation in select patients.

Keywords: systemic sclerosis; scleroderma; interstitial lung disease; rituximab; cyclophosphamide; tocilizumab; mycophenolic acid

1. Introduction

SSc is an autoimmune connective tissue disease characterised by microvascular damage and progressive fibrosis of the skin and internal organs, including the heart, lungs, kidneys and the gastrointestinal tract [1–3]. Pulmonary fibrosis has replaced scleroderma renal crisis (SRC) as the leading cause of mortality in SSc, with a reported prevalence of up to 30% and a 10-year mortality of 40% [4]. A review of 9260 SSc patients from the European Trials and Research Group (EUSTAR)database revealed a prevalence of SSc-ILD of 50.2% [5]. Post-mortem studies suggest an even higher frequency of pulmonary involvement, with fibrosis reported in greater than 75% of cases [6].

While the aetiology and pathogenesis are not fully understood, the main risk factors for the progression of SSc-ILD are the diffuse cutaneous SSc (dcSSc) phenotype, the anti-Scl-70 antibody (anti-topoisomerase 1), male gender, African heritage, cardiac involvement and raised acute phase reactants [7,8]. Recent evidence from the EUSTAR cohort now clearly shows that ILD can appear at any time after SSc diagnosis, with stable incidence at any point during disease course, independent of disease duration [9]. This underscores the importance of continued interval screening for new-onset ILD in SSc.

The predominant pattern of ILD reported on high-resolution computed tomography (HRCT) in SSc is non-specific interstitial pneumonia (NSIP). It is observed in up to 75% of SSc-ILD cases and it is characterised by irregular ground-glass attenuation, traction bronchiectasis and sparing of the subpleural regions [10–12]. The consensus opinion is that NSIP in SSc-ILD represents inflammation rather than established fibrosis. Established fibrosis typically produces a usual interstitial pneumonia (UIP) pattern on HRCT. Therefore, this suggests a degree of potential reversibility with timely immunosuppressive treatment in SSc-ILD.

The use of corticosteroids (CS) in SSc still remains controversial as there is an association with higher doses of CS and scleroderma renal crisis (SRC). To avoid this, and the sequelae of long-term CS, there is a real need to identify and stratify the best immunosuppressive agents for SSc-ILD. There have been well-powered RCTs demonstrating the effect of CYC, MMF, nintedanib and TCZ in SSc ILD, but a paucity of sufficiently powered studies investigating other agents in the disease. This article will review the key landmark RCTs that have directed the treatment of SSc-ILD along with the American Thoracic Society (ATS), American College of Rheumatology (ACR) and the European League Against Rheumatism (EULAR) guidelines for SSc-ILD.

2. Landmark Trials

Prior to the landmark RCTs demonstrating the efficacy of CYC and MMF in SSc-ILD, smaller cohort studies demonstrated that cyclosporine A (CYA) could be used to treat SSc. CYA was originally isolated from the fungus Tolypocladium inflatum in the 1970s and was introduced to solid organ transplant medicine and bone marrow transplantation in the 1980s [13]. An early Italian cohort study from 2001 of nine patients demonstrated that low-dose CyA treatment at 2.5 mg/kg/day was well tolerated without any significant negative effect on blood pressure and renal function [14]. There was a progressive improvement in lung score in seven patients with abnormal baseline pulmonary function prior to treatment. This improvement persisted beyond 3 years. Since this time, larger trials and RCTs have added greatly to the evidence base, which informs our choice of treatment options used today in clinical practice. The key landmark trials are highlighted in Table 1. The first of these is the large scleroderma lung study 1 (SLS), which investigated the role of CYC in the treatment of SSc-ILD.

Table 1. Landmark trials relating to SSc-ILD.

Overview of Landmark Trials in SSc-ILD					
Trial	**Year**	***n***	**Treatment**	**Comparator**	**Result**
SLS 1	2006	158	CYC (oral)	Placebo	Significant but modest beneficial effect on lung function Effect maintained through 24 months
SLS 2	2016	126	MMF	CYC (oral)	MMF for 2 years was as effective as oral CYC for 1 year MMF is safer and better tolerated with a lower toxicity profile
SENSCIS	2019	576	Nintedanib	Placebo	At 1-year the nintedanib group lost 52 mls from baseline FVC compared to 93 mls for the placebo group
FOCUSSCED	2020	210	TCZ (SC)	Placebo	TCZ appears to have a beneficial effect regardless of the extent of lung involvement
RECITAL (SSc-ILD Subgroup)	2023	37	RTX	CYC	RTX is non-inferior to CYC

2.1. Scleroderma Lung Study 1 (SLS1)

SLS1 was a 2-year double-blind, randomised, placebo-controlled trial funded by the National Institute of Health, which examined the effects of oral cyclophosphamide on pulmonary function in patients with SSc-ILD [15]. The trial enrolled 158 patients across 13 centres. It included those with mild to moderate ILD and evidence of active disease, such as active alveolitis on bronchoalveolar lavage (BAL) or ground-glass opacities (GGOs), on HRCT. All patients included were deemed to have at least moderate dyspnoea.

The patients were randomised to either 12 months of CYC or 12 months of placebo followed by a 12-month observation period off treatment. Oral CYC was dosed at ≤ 2 mg per kg body weight. In total, 145 of 158 completed 6 months of treatment and were included in the analysis. The mean absolute difference in forced vital capacity (FVC) % predicted between the groups was 2.53% in favour of CYC ($p < 0.03$). This difference in FVC was maintained at 24 months. There was no significant difference between the two groups in diffusion capacity for carbon monoxide (DLCO).

Interestingly, while this difference may seem small, there were also treatment-related differences in dyspnoea scores and quality of life scores. The mean focal score, as per the transitional dyspnoea index, showed a clinically significant improvement (i.e., >1 unit) of $+1.4 \pm 0.23$ units in the CYC group compared with a clinically significant deterioration (i.e., >1 unit) of -1.5 ± 0.43 units in the placebo group. The CYC group also scored more favourably on the health assessment questionnaire (HAQ) disability score at the 12-month mark.

At oral CYC dosing ≤ 2 mg per kg body weight, the difference in adverse events between the two groups was perhaps lower than expected. The CYC group only experienced significantly more leukopenia and neutropenia than placebo. While the rate of haematuria was numerically higher in the CYC group, surprisingly, this difference was not statistically significant. Of course, a 2-year trial cannot account for the long-term effects of CYC. A particular concern is the established association between CYC treatment and bladder cancer. This is problematic when there are no clear guidelines as to how to best screen or monitor these patients for bladder cancer development years after initial treatment [16].

In summary, at the time of publication, given there was no reasonable alternative with a solid evidence base, the risk–benefit profile was in favour of CYC treatment in SSc-ILD patients. CYC demonstrated a favourable effect on lung volumes (i.e., FVC) but not gas transfer (i.e., DLCO). CYC did have a real, measurable effect on dyspnoea and quality of life scores. After the publication of SLS1 in 2006, CYC became the standard of care in SSc-ILD.

2.2. *Scleroderma Lung Study 2 (SLS2)*

SLS2 was a 2-year double-blind, parallel-group, RCT comparing MMF with oral CYC in 126 SSc-ILD patients [17]. Prior to SLS2, uncontrolled studies had shown that MMF had the potential to be an effective alternative to CYC, particularly given the demonstrated favourable safety profile in solid organ transplants [18]. SLS2 was designed to investigate the comparative efficacy and safety of MMF, administered for 2 years versus oral CYC, given for 1 year and followed thereafter by placebo for a further year.

The trial was performed in 14 US centres from 2009 to 2015. All patients enrolled had FVC values $\geq$45% and <80% predicted, exertional dyspnoea $\geq$ grade 2 on the Mahler Baseline Dyspnoea Index (BDI) and GGOs on HRCT. Notably, MMF was titrated up to 1.5 g BD in the treatment arm and oral CYC was titrated to a target dose of around 2 mg/kg/day, which was in line with SLS1.

It was hypothesised that a 2-year course of MMF would be safer, better tolerated and produce longer-lasting improvements than CYC. At 24 months, the mean values of FVC % predicted were similar in both groups: 2.17 vs. 2.86 ($p = 0.24$). While MMF compared favourably to CYC in terms of DLCO % predicted at 6 and 18 months, the 12 and 24-month results did not differ. Both CYC and MMF showed significant improvements in dyspnoea and disability, as per the health assessment questionnaire disability index (HAQ-DI). There was a 6-fold increased risk of leukopenia with CYC treatment compared to MMF, but there were no other differences in reported adverse events. The CYC group were 1.7 times more likely to discontinue treatment compared with the MMF group.

The bottom line was that 65% of those in the CYC arm and 72% of those in the MMF arm had either stable or improving pulmonary function based on measured FVC predicted values [17]. Ultimately, while there was no difference in all-cause mortality, MMF would become the first-line treatment in SSc-ILD given its better tolerance and more favourable safety profile.

2.3. SENSCIS

The Nintedanib for Systemic-Sclerosis-Associated Interstitial Lung Disease (SENSCIS) trial was a randomised, double-blind, placebo controlled trial encompassing results from 32 countries. SENSCIS investigated the efficacy and safety of nintedanib in a cohort of 576 SSc-ILD patients [19]. Over half (51.9%) of the patients enrolled had dcSSc but all had HRCT evidence of ≥10% fibrosis of the lungs along with FVCs of at least 40% predicted and DLCOs of 30 to 89% predicted.

SENSCIS recruited all patients from November 2015 through October 2017. A key point to highlight here is that less than half (48.4%) of those enrolled were receiving MMF at baseline. SLS2, which showed the efficacy and favourable safety profile of MMF in SSc-ILD was published in 2016. The 48.4% figure on MMF at baseline is, therefore, perhaps still lower than one would expect, given the results from SLS2.

The treatment arm received nintedanib at 150 mg orally twice per day and the control arm received oral placebo tablets. The primary end point was the annual rate of FVC decline. The nintedanib group experienced an annual rate of FVC decline of −52.4 millilitres (mls) compared with −93.3 mls in the placebo group. The preserved 40.9 mls in the first year is a significant difference ($p = 0.04$).

A subgroup analysis showed that in patients receiving both MMF and nintedanib, the adjusted mean annual rate of decline in FVC was −40.2 mls versus −66.5 mls in those receiving MMF and placebo [20]. In those not receiving MMF, the annual rate of decline in FVC was −63.9 mls with nintedanib and −119.3 mls with placebo. These results suggest a synergistic effect of combining MMF and nintedanib on FVC.

However, SENSCIS failed to show a beneficial effect of nintedanib on patient-reported outcomes such as the Functional Assessment of Chronic Illness Therapy Dyspnoea Questionnaire (FACIT-Dyspnoea) and quality of life scores (HAQ-DI). Moreover, the tolerability of nintedanib from a gastrointestinal (GI) perspective proved problematic during SENSCIS, with diarrhoea experienced by 75.7% of the nintedanib group [19]. Even with anti-diarrhoeal agents, real-world experience suggests that at least a third of patients experience significant GI upset, so much so that continuing the medication can become problematic. Lastly, SENSCIS only demonstrated the effect of nintedanib in the first year of treatment and at the time of publication in 2019, it was unclear whether the effect would be cumulative over multiple years of treatment or not.

2.4. FOCUSSCED

The Tocilizumab in Systemic Sclerosis (FOCUSSCED) trial was a phase 3 placebo-controlled RCT investigating the effect of TCZ in patients with SSc and progressive skin disease [21]. In total, 210 patients were recruited from November 2015 to February 2017. Of these, 136 (65%) had ILD, and the majority with known fibrosis (77%) had pulmonary involvement with >10% of the volume of the lung fields affected on HRCT. However, the mean baseline FVC predicted was 80.3% in the TCZ group and 83.9% in the placebo group, which is only reflective of mild lung involvement. Similarly, the mean baseline DLCO was 74.4% in the TCZ group and 76.8% in the placebo group.

Patients were randomised to receive TCZ at 162 mg subcutaneous injection weekly or weekly placebo subcutaneous injection. PFTs and HRCT were performed at baseline and repeated at week 48. Among those with ILD at baseline, the least squares mean (LSM) change from baseline to week 48 in FVC was +0.07 in the TCZ group compared with −6.40 in the placebo group ($p < 0.0001$). This effect was also independent of the degree of fibrosis at the pre-treatment baseline. Therefore, TCZ appears to have a beneficial effect on SSc-ILD regardless of the extent of lung involvement prior to commencing treatment. However, this should be tempered by the fact that the patients enrolled in FOCUSSCED had milder baseline ILD than in SLS1, SLS2 and SENSCIS. To illustrate this point, the SENSCIS cohort had a mean baseline FVC of 72% along with 35 to 37% baseline lung fibrosis on HRCT, whereas FOCUSSCED had a mean baseline FVC of 82% along with 2 to 17% baseline lung fibrosis on HRCT [19].

Lastly, there were no differences between TCZ and placebo for patient or physician-reported outcomes at 48 weeks. Importantly, this includes the HAQ-DI and the Saint George's Respiratory Questionnaire. Even if TCZ seems to have a numerically beneficial effect on ILD, this does not translate to improvement in quality-of-life metrics in this cohort of SSc patients with early baseline ILD.

2.5. RECITAL

The Rituximab versus Intravenous Cyclophosphamide in Patients with Connective Tissue Disease-associated Interstitial Lung Disease (RECITAL) trial was a phase 2b randomised, double-blind, multicentre UK-based trial that aimed to assess whether or not RTX is superior to CYC in severe or progressive connective tissue disease-associated ILD (CTD-ILD). This included three broad groups: idiopathic inflammatory myopathies (IIM), mixed connective tissue disease (MCTD) and SSc. This was unusual as the RECITAL trial published the end results as a composite of the three diseases showing the effect of RTX in CTD-ILD.

SSc accounted for 38% of the trial recruits (37/97). The subgroup analysis of SSc-ILD patients was presented at the American College of Rheumatology (ACR) Congress in Philadelphia in November 2022. It reported a 24-week change from baseline FVC of −26.0 mls (95% CI −186.8, 134.6) in the RTX group versus −3.3 mls (95% CI −154.8, 148.2) in the CYC group.

These results did not support their hypothesis that RTX is superior to CYC in this patient group. However, RECITAL does support the idea that RTX is non-inferior to CYC. Given SLS2 showed that CYC and MMF are similar in terms of efficacy, this does support the idea of RTX as a second-line agent in SSc-ILD along with CYC [18,22].

3. Guidelines

3.1. American Thoracic Society

The updated American Thoracic Society (ATS) guidelines from 2023 make a strong recommendation for the use of MMF in SSc-ILD but only a conditional recommendation for the use of CYC in the treatment of SSc-ILD [23]. Similarly, RTX, TCZ, nintedanib, as well as the combination of MMF and nintedanib, were all given only conditional recommendations. Pirfenidone was met with the consensus opinion that further research is required to increase the evidence base before any recommendation can be made.

3.2. American College of Rheumatology

The new ACR guidelines from 2023 recommend MMF as the preferred first-line treatment. Alternatively, TCZ and RTX may be used as a first-line treatment [24]. Additional options thereafter include CYC and azathioprine (AZA). ACR also makes a conditional recommendation for the use of nintedanib in SSc-ILD. Importantly, there is a strong recommendation against the use of glucocorticoids as a first-line treatment. Lastly, there is a conditional recommendation for referral to an experienced centre for autologous haematopoietic stem cell transplant (AHSCT) if ILD is progressing on first-line treatment.

3.3. European League against Rheumatism

The updated European League Against Rheumatism (EULAR) guidelines place MMF, RTX and CYC in the same group as a first-line treatment [25]. TCZ is categorised as a second-line treatment. Nintedanib is also strongly recommended. While HSCT is included in the first-line group for reserve patients, there is no mention yet of chimeric antigen receptor T cell (CAR-T) treatment as it is still a nascent medical technology.

The treatment recommendations for SSc-ILD from above guidelines are compared in Table 2.

Table 2. Comparison of SSc-ILD treatment guidelines.

Comparison of SSc-ILD Treatment Guidelines					
Guideline	**1st Line**	**2nd Line**	**Anti-Fibrotics**	**HSCT**	**CAR-T**
ATS [23]	MMF	CYC RTX TCZ	Nintedanib (Conditional)	N/A	N/A
ACR & CHEST [24]	MMF TCZ RTX	CYC AZA	Nintedanib (Conditional)	Consider if progressing despite 1st line	N/A
EULAR [25]	RTX MMF CYC	TCZ	Nintedanib (May use in conjunction with 1st line immunosuppression)	Consider in severe cases	N/A

4. Screening and Treatment Paradigm

A recent modified Delphi consensus from a panel of expert pulmonologists and rheumatologists in the field recommends ILD screening in all systemic sclerosis patients [26]. Initial screening should include a history of respiratory symptoms, chest auscultation for crackles, HRCT Thorax and PFTs. Routine screening for pulmonary hypertension should be part of the process when dyspnoea is not explained by the progression of ILD.

Often, treatment criteria will focus on a combination of PFT results and HRCT evidence of ILD. The same expert panel suggest the commencement of treatment if FVC < 80% with any degree of ILD or symptoms, or there is >20% total lung involvement on HRCT, or there is >10% lung involvement on HRCT with abnormal PFTs. They also recommended initiating treatment in high-risk patients with early diffuse cutaneous disease and any evidence of mild ILD.

The ACR systemic autoimmune rheumatic disease (SARD) ILD guidelines offer practical advice regarding the frequency of monitoring for progression in SSc-ILD [23]. PFT testing with spirometry, lung volumes and diffusion capacity should be performed every 3–6 months for the first year and then less frequently once stable. Ambulatory desaturation testing can be performed every 3–12 months, and interval HRCT should be guided by PFT trend. CXR, 6 min walk test and bronchoscopy are generally not helpful and are conditionally recommended against in this guideline, except in a few exceptional circumstances, where they provide additional diagnostic utility.

We present our preferred treatment hierarchy in Figure 1. MMF is our preferred first-line agent, given the lower relative toxicity when compared with CYC. MMF is also an oral therapy that can be very beneficial and convenient for the patient. Nintedanib may also be offered in conjunction with MMF if tolerated from a gastrointestinal perspective. We will discuss lung transplant, HSCT and the potential of CAR-T cells in a separate section as rescue treatments.

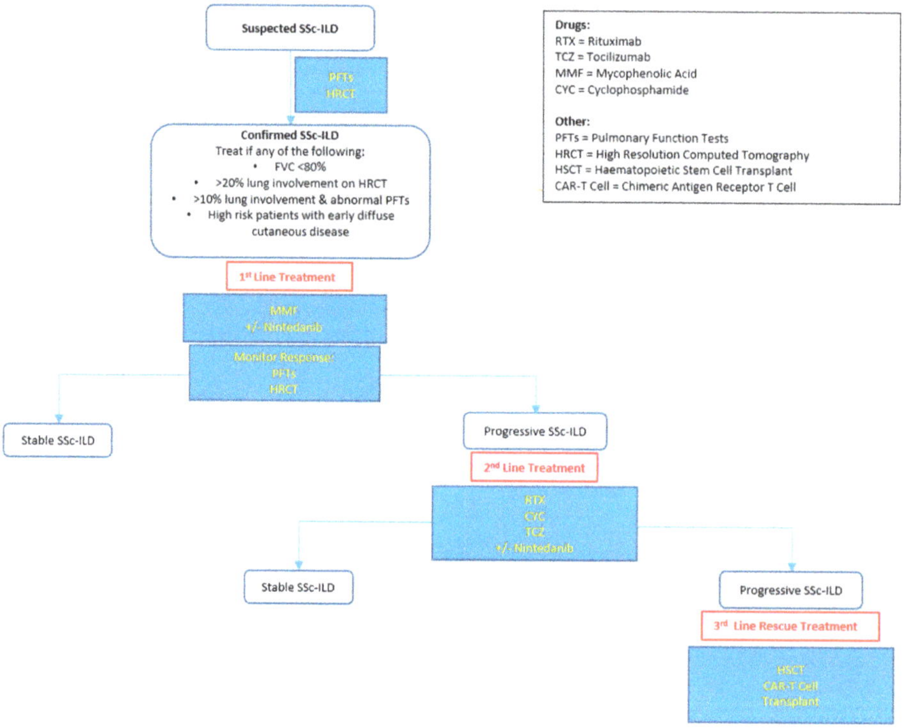

Figure 1. Proposed SSc-ILD treatment hierarchy.

5. Transplant

5.1. Lung Transplant

Historically, SSc-ILD patients were deemed to be poor candidates given the systemic nature of the disease and the concerns of high extra pulmonary morbidity and mortality [27]. While the immunosuppressive treatment paradigm has come a long way, there remains the grave concern of graft failure and death from bronchiolitis obliterans (BO). This fear is compounded by studies suggesting a link between gastro-oesophageal reflux (GORD) and BO; it is well established that gastrointestinal dysmotility and GORD are often features of SSc, hence the concern [28].

Data from the International Society for Heart and Lung Transplantation (ISHLT) from 2019 reported that only 0.9% of all lung transplants were for connective tissue disease (CTD)-related ILD and lower still for SSc-ILD specifically [29]. Despite this, the recent evidence base suggests that SSc-ILD patients have similar short- and long-term survival with lung transplant when compared to patients with other forms of pulmonary fibrosis. A retrospective cohort study from the University of Pittsburgh Medical Centre (UPMC) compared the post-transplant outcomes of 72 SSc-ILD patients with 311 patients with other forms of interstitial lung disease. Interestingly, they found the 1-year survival of 81% for SSc compared well with the 79% 1-year survival rate in the other causes of the ILD group. Similarly, the 5-year survival rate was favourable for the SSc-ILD patient compared to other causes of ILD: 66% vs. 58% [30]. A second retrospective cohort study from the University of California Los Angeles (UCLA) group again showed reassuring survival data. The group of SSc-ILD patients was smaller at 35, but they demonstrated 1-, 3- and 5-year survival rates post-transplant of 94%, 77% and 70%, respectively. These results were comparable to those seen in patients with other forms of ILD. Notably, 60% of the SSc-ILD patients in this cohort had severe oesophageal dysmotility. This perhaps suggests that previous fears of GORD-related BO and graft failure were overestimated [31].

The 2021 ISHLT consensus document proposed that lung transplant is now a viable option for a select group of patients with CTD, including those with advanced SSc-ILD [29]. The combined 2023 ACR and American College of Chest Physicians (CHEST) guideline for the treatment of SARD-ILD makes a conditional recommendation for referral for lung transplant after failure of all immunosuppressive treatments and consideration of suitability for HSCT [23]. Interestingly, the 2017 EULAR recommendations for the treatment of systemic sclerosis, which are due to be updated, do not mention lung transplant at all, although it does acknowledge HSCT as a viable option [32]. The 2019 European Respiratory Society (ERS) evidence-based consensus recommendations for the identification and management of interstitial lung disease in systemic sclerosis do acknowledge the role of lung transplant in these patients [33]. After the progression of ILD despite MMF or CYC treatment, these patients may then be considered candidates for either rituximab, lung transplant or HSCT.

5.2. HSCT

Hematopoietic stell cell transplant (HSCT) has been used in severe refractory autoimmune diseases for the past quarter of a century. While the introduction of biologic therapies in recent times has reduced the role of HSCT, there remain a few diseases where HSCT may still be used. SSc-ILD is one of those rare diseases where HSCT features in the treatment guidelines.

There are three RCTs demonstrating the clear benefits of HSCT in progressive diffuse SSc. This are shown in Table 3. While not all patients in these trials have ILD, the impact of treatment on lung disease is reported as a secondary outcome. All three trials demonstrated a beneficial effect on FVC with HSCT treatment compared to the comparator groups of CYC monotherapy. Notably, at least in the context of these short RCTs, there does not appear to be the same beneficial effect on DLCO.

Table 3. Overview of HSCT RCTs in SSc.

Study	n	Baseline ILD on HRCT	Baseline FVC	Trial End FVC
ASSIST [34]	HSCT n = 10 CYC n = 9	HSCT 70% CYC 89%	Median FVC %pred. HSCT 62% CYC 67%	Median Change at 1 yr HSCT +20% CYC −9%
ASTIS [35]	HSCT n = 79 CYC n = 77	HSCT 87% CYC 80%	Mean FVC %pred. HSCT 82% CYC 81%	Mean Change at 2 yrs HSCT +6.3% CYC −2.8%
SCOT [36]	HSCT n = 36 CYC n = 39	HSCT 100% CYC 95%	Mean FVC %pred. HSCT 74% CYC 74%	Change at 54 Months HSCT 13/36 improved (↑FVC >10%) HSCT 4/36 decline (↓FVC ≥10%) CYC 8/39 improved (↑FVC >10%) CYC 8/39 decline (↓FVC ≥10%)

The ASSIST study (American Scleroderma Stem Cell versus Immune Suppression Trial) defined an increase of greater than 10% in FVC at 12 months as a significant improvement. Overall, 80% of the HSCT treatment group (n = 8) met this threshold, whereas the CYC group (n = 9) showed a mean decrease in FVC [34].

The ASTIS trial (Autologous Stem Cell Transplantation International Scleroderma) demonstrated a mean increase in FVC of +6.3% at 2 years in the HSCT group (n = 79) compared with a mean decrease of −2.8% in the CYC control group (n = 77) (p = 0.004) [35].

The SCOT trial (Scleroderma: Cyclophosphamide Or Transplantation) randomised 36 patients to the HSCT arm and 39 to the CYC arm [36]. It defined a significant improvement in FVC at the trial end of 54 months to be an increase of greater than 10%. It also defined a significant decline in FVC at the trial end to be a decrease of $\geq$10%. Overall, 13/36 HSCT patients experienced a significant improvement, and only 4/36 HSCT patients experienced a significant decline in FVC. This compares favourably to the CYC group, where 8/39 patients experienced a significant improvement, and 7/39 experienced a significant decline.

While many large observational studies exist, they tell us little about the efficacy of HSCT compared to first-line treatments and, as a result, are less insightful. Both the combined guidelines from ACR and CHEST and the guidelines from EULAR recommend HSCT for the treatment of SSc-ILD patients. The ACR and CHEST guidelines recommend HSCT if ILD is progressing despite the trial of first-line treatments, MMF, TCZ and RTX [24]. The EULAR recommendations make a more general recommendation to consider HSCT in severe cases of SSc-ILD. However, the EULAR peer review report for their guidelines has deemed the quality of the scientific evidence for HSCT in SSc-ILD to be grade A or excellent [32]. Notably, the ATS guidelines for SSc-ILD do not make any reference to HSCT as a treatment option [33].

6. CAR-T Cells

Autologous chimeric antigen receptor (CAR)-T cell therapy is a nascent treatment beginning to gain traction in the treatment of autoimmune rheumatic diseases. While it has been hailed as a transformative medical technology in the world of haematology, it is showing early promise in the treatment of systemic lupus erythematosus (SLE), idiopathic inflammatory myopathies (IIM) and now also SSc.

The group pioneering this technology in Europe is the Friedrich-Alexander University Hospital Erlangen-Nürnberg group. The early results with their first seven patients were presented at EULAR's 2024 Congress in Vienna in June, and their results were published in their scientific abstract for the conference [37]. This small group included seven diffuse systemic sclerosis patients ranging in age from 23 to 60. Overall, six out of seven were positive for anti-Scl70 and one was positive for RNA polymerase 3. Notably, all had interstitial lung disease, three had cardiac involvement and one had renal involvement. Prior treatments included MMF, MTX, RTX and cyclophosphamide. Interestingly, CAR-T cell treatment did not completely deplete circulating autoantibodies in all patients. Nevertheless, serial PFTs showed reassuring stability in both FVC and DLCO up to 400 days post initial CAR-T treatment. One patient also had positron emission tomography (PET) performed at baseline prior to treatment and then again at 3 months after treatment. The 3-month follow-up PET showed markedly reduced uptake throughout the lung fields. It should be noted that all seven patients have not received any form of immunosuppressive maintenance treatment since their initial CAR-T cell infusions.

These are very promising results in a small cohort of severe refractory SSc patients. To see the efficacy of CAR-T cell therapy pitted against the current standard of care in an RCT of treatment naïve SSc-ILD patients would be fascinating. The logistics and granting of ethics for such a trial may prove difficult to obtain for the time being. The question of whether CAR-T and HSCT are competitive or complementary is not so easy to answer at present. It is too early yet to truly appreciate the potential toxicity, morbidity and mortality with CAR-T cell therapy compared to HSCT. SSc-ILD patients may very well be one of those niche cohorts that could benefit in the future from this promising medical technology.

7. Adjunctive Therapies and Other Considerations

7.1. Pulmonary Hypertension

Pulmonary arterial hypertension (PAH) affects approximately 30% of SSc-ILD patients [38]. A meta-analysis of 22 studies reported survival rates of 81% for 1 year, 64% for 2 years and 52% for 3 years in SSc-ILD patients with PAH [39]. There are currently four major categories of medication for PAH and they are shown in Table 4. These are prostacyclin analogues, phosphodiesterase inhibitors (PDE5i), endothelin receptor antagonists (ERAs) and guanylate cyclase stimulators.

Table 4. PAH therapeutics in SSc-ILD.

PAH Therapeutics in SSc-ILD	
Prostacyclin Analogues	Epoprostenol Treprostinil Iloprost
Phosphodiesterase Inhibitors	Sildenafil Tadalafil
Endothelin Receptor Antagonists	Bosentan Ambrisentan Macitentan
Guanylate Cyclase Stimulators	Riociguat

Combination therapy is now routine in clinical practice in idiopathic pulmonary arterial hypertension (IPAH). The evidence base is growing for the use of combination therapy in SSc-PAH. The AMBITION trial, which included a small cohort of CTD patients, demonstrated that a combination of ambrisentan and tadalafil improved haemodynamics, 6 min walk test (6MWT) distance and reduced the risk of clinical deterioration when compared to monotherapy [40]. A small prospective, open-label trial of 24 patients with SSc-PAH without prior PAH treatment demonstrated improvements in haemodynamics, 6MWT distance and right ventricle (RV) structure and function with combination treatment with ambrisentan and tadalafil [41]. The follow-up ATPAHSS-O trial, which again solely focused on SSc-PAH patients, showed improvements in RV and left ventricle (LV) function on cardiac MRI along with 6MWT distance, pro-BNP and haemodynamics with ambrisentan and tadalafil combination treatment [42].

While the current EULAR SSc guidelines give PDE5i, ERAs and prostanoids a strong level A recommendation, the eagerly awaited updated EULAR SSc guidelines are set to give riociguat a level B recommendation for PAH treatment [25]. The role of both anticoagulation and corticosteroids in SSc-PAH remains contentious, and neither are commonly used in clinical practice.

7.2. Oxygen

There is no specific guidance for SSc-ILD patients and supplemental oxygen. In clinical practice, oxygen is provided to those patients with severe hypoxaemia at rest, as is the case with all forms of ILD. While there is no evidence to suggest supplemental oxygen provides a survival benefit in SSc-ILD, there is evidence showing that ambulatory oxygen does improve quality of life and reduce dyspnoea. AmbOX was a prospective, open-label, mixed-method, crossover randomised controlled clinical trial carried out at three centres across the United Kingdom [43]. Approximately 10% of the patients enrolled in this trial had CTD. This trial used the King's Brief Interstitial Lung Disease questionnaire (K-BILD). It demonstrated that ambulatory oxygen seemed to be associated with improved health-related quality of life measures in patients with ILD, including CTD-ILD. While we do not have similar robust trials solely in SSc-ILD, we assume for now that these results are translatable and applicable to SSc-ILD patients.

7.3. Pulmonary Rehabilitation

Many SSc-ILD patients are referred for pulmonary rehabilitation but there is a paucity of evidence to suggest that this improves quality of life. There are, however, a few small single-centre trials that demonstrate an improvement in aerobic capacity with moderate-intensity exercise. These studies were performed in SSc patients rather than specifically SSc-ILD patients [44,45].

7.4. GORD Treatment

In addition to immunosuppressive therapies, the management of GORD in SSc-ILD patients is paramount. The oesophageal involvement, reflux and gastric dysmotility seen in dc-SSc all increase the risk of aspiration pneumonitis, which can cause ILD progression [46,47]. Apart from the conservative measures of smaller meals, eating dinner well before lying supine to sleep at night and raising the head of the bed, the use of proton pump inhibitors (PPI) and pro-motility agents may be beneficial.

7.5. Pneumocystis Jirovecii Pneumonia Prophylaxis

The risk of pneumocystis jirovecii pneumonia (PJP) should be carefully considered in SSc-ILD patients on strong or combination immunosuppression or high-dose corticosteroids. The mortality rate with PJP in patients with rheumatic diseases is 39.6%, and this may be even higher in SSc-ILD patients. There is a risk of medication-related adverse events with PJP prophylaxis, regardless of whether co-trimoxazole, dapsone or atovaquone is prescribed. In general, the number needed to harm (NNH) with first-line PJP prophylaxis, co-trimoxazole, is 131. Fortunately, the number needed to treat (NNT) in SSc to prevent one case of PJP is 36 [48]. This shows a favourable risk–benefit ratio that supports the prescribing of PJP prophylaxis in SSc-ILD patients with strong immunosuppression.

7.6. Vaccination

Seasonal influenza vaccines and SARS-CoV-2 vaccines are strongly recommended for SSc-ILD patients. It is also prudent for SSc-ILD patients to strongly consider receiving the pneumococcal polysaccharide (Pneumovax 23) vaccine, which protects against the 23 serotypes of streptococcus pneumoniae. A booster shot is not required for 5 years after initial vaccination. The Centre for Disease Control (CDC) recommend respiratory syncytial virus (RSV) vaccination for all adults 75 years of age and older and adults with certain risk factors between the ages of 60 and 75 [49]. Given the morbidity and mortality associated with RSV in patients with ILD, SSc-ILD patients should again strongly consider the RSV vaccine.

A comprehensive review article from Italy goes further, identifying SSc-ILD patients as a frail immunocompromised cohort who are overlooked by the current vaccination literature and guidelines [50]. It makes a strong recommendation for vaccination in SSc-ILD patients against the six following pathogens: SARS-CoV-2, influenza, streptococcus pneumoniae, neisseria meningitidis, haemophilus influenzae and diphtheria–tetanus–pertussis.

7.7. Symptomatic Dyspnoea Management

There are no specific high-quality trials examining the effect of low-dose opioids or benzodiazepines (BDZs) on dyspnoea in SSc-ILD patients. Again, it is assumed that evidence from trials in other forms of ILD demonstrating a beneficial effect on dyspnoea is applicable to SSc-ILD patients. In one longitudinal study in fibrosing ILD patients on long-term oxygen, both opioids and low-dose BDZs appear to be safe [51].

8. Conclusions

There is a strong evidence base now for the use of MMF as a first-line treatment in SSc-ILD. RTX, CYC and TCZ are advised if there is ILD progression on MMF. Antifibrotic treatment with nintedanib likely adds synergistic long-term benefits and may be used if tolerated from a GI perspective. SSc-ILD patients may still be considered for lung transplant despite concerns regarding GORD, BO and graft failure. Careful assessment and consideration for PPIs and pro-kinetics should be made on a case-by-case basis to minimise GORD and the risk of aspiration. There is also a favourable risk–benefit ratio that supports the prescribing of PJP prophylaxis in patients on strong immunosuppression.

CAR-T cell therapy is a promising medical technology that may replace HSCT in the coming decades for select SSc-ILD cases. PAH is common in SSc-ILD patients, and while current guidelines give a strong recommendation for PDE5i, ERAs and prostanoids, it is likely that future guidelines will recommend combination therapy if tolerated.

Seasonal influenza and SARS-CoV-2 vaccines are strongly recommended. Consideration should be given for both the pneumococcal polysaccharide vaccine and the RSV vaccine. In addition to long-term oxygen or ambulatory oxygen, low-dose opioids and low-dose BDZs may be appropriate to reduce dyspnoea and improve quality of life.

Author Contributions: Conceptualisation, R.C. and R.H.; methodology, R.H. and P.H.; writing—original draft preparation, R.H. and P.H.; writing—review and editing, R.C.; supervision, R.C. All authors have read and agreed to the published version of the manuscript.

Funding: This research received no external funding.

Conflicts of Interest: The authors declare no conflicts of interest.

References

1. Denton, C.P.; Khanna, D. Systemic sclerosis. *Lancet* **2017**, *390*, 1685–1699. [CrossRef]
2. Gabrielli, A.; Avvedimento, E.V.; Krieg, T. Scleroderma. *N. Engl. J. Med.* **2009**, *360*, 1989–2003. [CrossRef] [PubMed]
3. Varga, J.; Abraham, D. Systemic sclerosis: A prototypic multisystem fibrotic disorder. *J. Clin. Investig.* **2007**, *117*, 557–567. [CrossRef] [PubMed]
4. Perelas, A.; Silver, R.M.; Arrossi, A.V.; Highland, K.B. Systemic sclerosis-associated interstitial lung disease. *Lancet Respir. Med.* **2020**, *8*, 304–320. [CrossRef] [PubMed]
5. Lescoat, A.; Huscher, D.; Schoof, N.; Airò, P.; de Vries-Bouwstra, J.; Riemekasten, G.; Hachulla, E.; Doria, A.; Rosato, E.; Hunzelmann, N.; et al. Systemic sclerosis-associated interstitial lung disease in the EUSTAR database: Analysis by region. *Rheumatology* **2023**, *62*, 2178–2188; Erratum in *Rheumatology* **2023**, *62*, 3219–3220. https://doi.org/10.1093/rheumatology/kead247. [CrossRef] [PubMed]
6. D'Angelo, W.A.; Fries, J.F.; Masi, A.T.; Shulman, L.E. Pathologic observations in systemic sclerosis (scleroderma): A study of fifty-eight autopsy cases and fifty-eight matched controls. *Am. J. Med.* **1969**, *46*, 428–440. [CrossRef] [PubMed]
7. McNearney, T.A.; Reveille, J.D.; Fischbach, M.; Friedman, A.W.; Lisse, J.R.; Goel, N.; Tan, F.K.; Zhou, X.; Ahn, C.; Feghali-Bostwick, C.A.; et al. Pulmonary involvement in systemic sclerosis: Associations with genetic, serologic, sociodemographic, and behavioral factors. *Arthritis Rheum.* **2007**, *57*, 318–326. [CrossRef]
8. Khanna, D.; Tashkin, D.P.; Denton, C.P.; Renzoni, E.A.; Desai, S.R.; Varga, J. Etiology, risk factors, and biomarkers in systemic sclerosis with interstitial lung disease. *Am. J. Respir. Crit. Care Med.* **2020**, *201*, 650–660. [CrossRef]
9. Bruni, C.; Petelytska, L.; Velauthapillai, A.; Tofani, L.; Hachulla, E.; Müller-Ladner, U.; Siegert, E.; Allanore, Y.; Riemekasten, G.; Bergmann, C.; et al. OP0019 Incidence and Risk Factors for New Onset Interstitial Lung Disease in Systemic Sclerosis: Insights from an Analysis of the Eustar Cohort. *Ann. Rheum. Dis.* **2024**, *83*, 66–68.
10. Fujita, J.; Yoshinouchi, T.; Ohtsuki, Y.; Tokuda, M.; Yang, Y.; Yamadori, I.; Bandoh, S.; Ishida, T.; Takahara, J.; Ueda, R. Non-specific interstitial pneumonia as pulmonary involvement of systemic sclerosis. *Ann. Rheum. Dis.* **2001**, *60*, 281–283. [CrossRef]
11. Bouros, D.; Wells, A.U.; Nicholson, A.G.; Colby, T.V.; Polychronopoulos, V.; Pantelidis, P.; Haslam, P.L.; Vassilakis, D.A.; Black, C.M.; du Bois, R.M. Histopathologic subsets of fibrosing alveolitis in patients with systemic sclerosis and their relationship to outcome. *Am. J. Respir. Crit. Care Med.* **2002**, *165*, 1581–1586. [CrossRef] [PubMed]
12. Travis, W.D.; Costabel, U.; Hansell, D.M.; King, T.E., Jr.; Lynch, D.A.; Nicholson, A.G.; Ryerson, C.J.; Ryu, J.H.; Selman, M.; Wells, A.U.; et al. An official American Thoracic Society/European Respiratory Society statement: Update of the international multidisciplinary classification of the idiopathic interstitial pneumonias. *Am. J. Respir. Crit. Care Med.* **2013**, *188*, 733–748. [CrossRef] [PubMed]
13. Watts, R.; Clunie, G.; Hall, F.; Marshall, T. *Rheumatology*; Oxford University Press: Oxford, UK, 2009; p. 558, ISBN 978-0-19-922999-4.
14. Filaci, G.; Cutolo, M.; Basso, M.; Murdaca, G.; Derchi, L.; Gianrossi, R.; Ropolo, F.; Zentilin, P.; Sulli, A.; Puppo, F.; et al. Long-term treatment of patients affected by systemic sclerosis with cyclosporin A. *Rheumatology* **2001**, *40*, 1431–1432. [CrossRef] [PubMed]
15. Tashkin, D.P.; Elashoff, R.; Clements, P.J.; Goldin, J.; Roth, M.D.; Furst, D.E.; Arriola, E.; Silver, R.; Strange, C.; Bolster, M.; et al. Scleroderma Lung Study Research Group. Cyclophosphamide versus placebo in scleroderma lung disease. *N. Engl. J. Med.* **2006**, *354*, 2655–2666. [CrossRef] [PubMed]
16. Talar-Williams, C.; Hijazi, Y.M.; Walther, M.M.; Linehan, W.M.; Hallahan, C.W.; Lubensky, I.; Kerr, G.S.; Hoffman, G.S.; Fauci, A.S.; Sneller, M.C. Cyclophosphamide-induced cystitis and bladder cancer in patients with Wegener granulomatosis. *Ann. Intern. Med.* **1996**, *124*, 477–484. [CrossRef] [PubMed]
17. Tashkin, D.P.; Roth, M.D.; Clements, P.J.; Furst, D.E.; Khanna, D.; Kleerup, E.C.; Goldin, J.; Arriola, E.; Volkmann, E.R.; Kafaja, S.; et al. Sclerodema Lung Study II Investigators. Mycophenolate mofetil versus oral cyclophosphamide in scleroderma-related interstitial lung disease (SLS II): A randomised controlled, double-blind, parallel group trial. *Lancet Respir. Med.* **2016**, *4*, 708–719. [CrossRef] [PubMed] [PubMed Central]

18. Staatz, C.E.; Tett, S.E. Pharmacology and toxicology of mycophenolate in organ transplant recipients: An update. *Arch. Toxicol.* **2014**, *88*, 1351–1589. [CrossRef] [PubMed]
19. Distler, O.; Highland, K.B.; Gahlemann, M.; Azuma, A.; Fischer, A.; Mayes, M.D.; Raghu, G.; Sauter, W.; Girard, M.; Alves, M.; et al. Nintedanib for Systemic Sclerosis-Associated Interstitial Lung Disease. *N. Engl. J. Med.* **2019**, *380*, 2518–2528. [CrossRef] [PubMed]
20. Highland, K.B.; Distler, O.; Kuwana, M.; Allanore, Y.; Assassi, S.; Azuma, A.; Bourdin, A.; Denton, C.P.; Distler, J.H.W.; Hoffmann-Vold, A.M.; et al. Efficacy and safety of nintedanib in patients with systemic sclerosis-associated interstitial lung disease treated with mycophenolate: A subgroup analysis of the SENSCIS trial. *Lancet Respir. Med.* **2021**, *9*, 96–106. [CrossRef] [PubMed]
21. Roofeh, D.; Lin, C.J.F.; Goldin, J.; Kim, G.H.; Furst, D.E.; Denton, C.P.; Huang, S.; Khanna, D.; focuSSced Investigators. Tocilizumab Prevents Progression of Early Systemic Sclerosis-Associated Interstitial Lung Disease. *Arthritis Rheumatol.* **2021**, *73*, 1301–1310. [CrossRef] [PubMed] [PubMed Central]
22. Maher, T.; Tudor, V.; Saunders, P.; Gibbons, M.; Fletcher, S.; Parfrey, H.; Denton, C.; Hoyles, R.; Renzoni, E.; Kokosi, M.; et al. Rituximab versus Cyclophosphamide for the Treatment of Connective Tissue Disease Associated Interstitial Lung Disease (RECITAL): A Sub-group Analysis of a Multi-centre Randomised Controlled Trial [abstract]. *Arthritis Rheumatol.* **2022**, *74* (Suppl. S9), A4779. Available online: https://acrabstracts.org/abstract/rituximab-versus-cyclophosphamide-for-the-treatment-of-connective-tissue-disease-associated-interstitial-lung-disease-recital-a-sub-group-analysis-of-a-multi-centre-randomised-controlled-trial/ (accessed on 6 March 2024).
23. Raghu, G.; Montesi, S.B.; Silver, R.M.; Hossain, T.; Macrea, M.; Herman, D.; Barnes, H.; Adegunsoye, A.; Azuma, A.; Chung, L.; et al. Treatment of Systemic Sclerosis-associated Interstitial Lung Disease: Evidence-based Recommendations. An. Official American Thoracic Society Clinical Practice Guideline. *Am. J. Respir. Crit. Care Med.* **2024**, *209*, 137–152. [CrossRef] [PubMed] [PubMed Central]
24. Interstitial Lung Disease Guideline. ACR. 2023. Available online: https://rheumatology.org/interstitial-lung-disease-guideline (accessed on 6 June 2024).
25. Del Galdo, F.; Lescoat, A.; Conaghan, P.G.; Ananyeva, L.P.; Balbir-Gurman, A.; Bertoldo, E.; Boyadzhieva, V.; Castellví, I.; Colic, J.; Denton, C.P.; et al. OP0234 2023 Update of Eular Recommendations for the Treatment of Systemic Sclerosis. In Proceedings of the Annals of the Rheumatic Diseases (ARD). EULAR 2023 European Congress of Rheumatology, Milan, Italy, 31 May–3 June 2023; BMJ Publishing Group: London, UK, 2023; pp. 154–155.
26. Rahaghi, F.F.; Hsu, V.M.; Kaner, R.J.; Mayes, M.D.; Rosas, I.O.; Saggar, R.; Steen, V.D.; Strek, M.E.; Bernstein, E.J.; Bhatt, N.; et al. Expert consensus on the management of systemic sclerosis-associated interstitial lung disease. *Respir. Res.* **2023**, *24*, 6. [CrossRef] [PubMed] [PubMed Central]
27. De Cruz, S.; Ross, D. Lung transplantation in patients with scleroderma. *Curr. Opin. Rheumatol.* **2013**, *25*, 714–718. [CrossRef] [PubMed]
28. Meyer, K.C.; Raghu, G.; Verleden, G.M.; Corris, P.A.; Aurora, P.; Wilson, K.C.; Brozek, J.; Glanville, A.R.; Committee IAEBTF. An international ISHLT/ATS/ERS clinical practice guideline: Diagnosis and management of bronchiolitis obliterans syndrome. *Eur. Respir. J.* **2014**, *44*, 1479–1503. [CrossRef]
29. Crespo, M.M.; Lease, E.D.; Sole, A.; Sandorfi, N.; Snyder, L.D.; Berry, G.J.; Le Pavec, J.; Venado, A.E.; Cifrian, J.M.; Goldberg, H.; et al. ISHLT consensus document on lung transplantation in patients with connective tissue disease: Part I: Epidemiology, assessment of extrapulmonary conditions, candidate evaluation, selection criteria, and pathology statements. *J. Heart Lung Transplant.* **2021**, *40*, 1251–1266. [CrossRef] [PubMed]
30. Crespo, M.M.; Bermudez, C.A.; Dew, M.A.; Johnson, B.A.; George, M.P.; Bhama, J.; Morrell, M.; D'cUnha, J.; Shigemura, N.; Richards, T.J.; et al. Lung Transplant in Patients with Scleroderma Compared with Pulmonary Fibrosis. Short- and Long-Term Outcomes. *Ann. Am. Thorac. Soc.* **2016**, *13*, 784–792. [CrossRef] [PubMed]
31. Miele, C.H.; Schwab, K.; Saggar, R.; Duffy, E.; Elashoff, D.; Tseng, C.-H.; Weigt, S.; Charan, D.; Abtin, F.; Johannes, J.; et al. Lung Transplant Outcomes in Systemic Sclerosis with Significant Esophageal Dysfunction. A Comprehensive Single-Center Experience. *Ann. Am. Thorac. Soc.* **2016**, *13*, 793–802. [CrossRef] [PubMed] [PubMed Central]
32. Kowal-Bielecka, O.; Fransen, J.; Avouac, J.; Becker, M.; Kulak, A.; Allanore, Y.; Distler, O.; Clements, P.; Cutolo, M.; Czirjak, L.; et al. Update of EULAR recommendations for the treatment of systemic sclerosis. *Ann. Rheum. Dis.* **2017**, *76*, 1327–1339. [CrossRef]
33. Hoffmann-Vold, A.-M.; Maher, T.M.; Philpot, E.E.; Ashrafzadeh, A.; Distler, O.; Kreuter, M. Evidence-based consensus recommendations for the identification and management of interstitial lung disease in systemic sclerosis. *Eur. Respir. J.* **2019**, *54* (Suppl. S63), PA5195. [CrossRef]
34. Burt, R.K.; Shah, S.J.; Dill, K.; Grant, T.; Gheorghiade, M.; Schroeder, J.; Craig, R.; Hirano, I.; Marshall, K.; Ruderman, E.; et al. Autologous non-myeloablative haemopoietic stem-cell transplantation compared with pulse cyclophosphamide once per month for systemic sclerosis (ASSIST): An open-label, randomised phase 2 trial. *Lancet* **2011**, *378*, 498–506. [CrossRef] [PubMed]
35. Van Laar, J.M.; Farge, D.; Sont, J.K.; Naraghi, K.; Marjanovic, Z.; Larghero, J.; Schuerwegh, A.J.; Marijt, E.W.; Vonk, M.C.; Schattenberg, A.V. Autologous hematopoietic stem cell transplantation vs intravenous pulse cyclophosphamide in diffuse cutaneous systemic sclerosis: A randomized clinical trial. *JAMA* **2014**, *311*, 2490–2498. [CrossRef]
36. Sullivan, K.M.; Goldmuntz, E.A.; Keyes-Elstein, L. Autologous stem-cell transplantation for severe scleroderma. *N. Engl. J. Med.* **2018**, *378*, 1066–1067. [CrossRef] [PubMed]

37. Auth, J.; Müller, F.; Taubmann, J.; Völkl, S.; Fakhouri, S.C.; Bucci, L.; Aigner, M.; Atzinger, A.; Bayerl, N.; Wirsching, A. OP0320 Efficacy of CD19-targeting CAR T cell treatment in patients with diffuse systemic sclerosis (dSSc)—An open label, single-center pilot study. *Ann. Rheum. Dis.* **2024**, *83*, 204–205.
38. PHAROS Investigators; Hinchcliff, M.; Fischer, A.; Schiopu, E.; Steen, V.D.; Alkassab, F.; Bolster, M.B.; Chung, L.; Csuka, M.E.; Derk, C.T.; et al. Pulmonary Hypertension Assessment and Recognition of Outcomes in Scleroderma (PHAROS): Baseline Characteristics and Description of Study Population. *J. Rheumatol.* **2011**, *38*, 2172–2179. [CrossRef] [PubMed]
39. Lefèvre, G.; Dauchet, L.; Hachulla, E.; Montani, D.; Sobanski, V.; Lambert, M.; Hatron, P.-Y.; Humbert, M.; Launay, D. Survival and Prognostic Factors in Systemic Sclerosis-Associated Pulmonary Hypertension: A Systematic Review and Meta-Analysis. *Arthritis Rheum.* **2013**, *65*, 2412–2423. [CrossRef] [PubMed]
40. Galie, N.; Barbera, J.A.; Frost, A.E.; Ghofrani, H.A.; Hoeper, M.M.; McLaughlin, V.V.; Peacock, A.J.; Simonneau, G.; Vachiery, J.L.; Grunig, E.; et al. Initial Use of Ambrisentan plus Tadalafil in Pulmonary Arterial Hypertension. *N. Engl. J. Med.* **2015**, *373*, 834–844. [CrossRef]
41. Hassoun, P.M.; Zamanian, R.T.; Damico, R.; Lechtzin, N.; Khair, R.; Kolb, T.M.; Tedford, R.J.; Hulme, O.L.; Housten, T.; Pisanello, C.; et al. Ambrisentan and Tadalafil Up-front Combination Therapy in Scleroderma-associated Pulmonary Arterial Hypertension. *Am. J. Respir. Crit. Care Med.* **2015**, *192*, 1102–1110. [CrossRef]
42. Sato, T.; Ambale-Venkatesh, B.; Lima, J.A.; Zimmerman, S.L.; Tedford, R.J.; Fujii, T.; Hulme, O.L.; Pullins, E.H.; Corona-Villalobos, C.P.; Zamanian, R.T.; et al. The impact of ambrisentan and tadalafil upfront combination therapy on cardiac function in scleroderma associated pulmonary arterial hypertension patients: Cardiac magnetic resonance feature tracking study. *Pulm. Circ.* **2018**, *8*, 8307. [CrossRef] [PubMed]
43. Visca, D.; Mori, L.; Tsipouri, V.; Fleming, S.; Firouzi, A.; Bonini, M.; Pavitt, M.J.; Alfieri, V.; Canu, S.; Bonifazi, M.; et al. Effect of ambulatory oxygen on quality of life for patients with fibrotic lung disease (AmbOx): A prospective, open-label, mixed-method, crossover randomised controlled trial. *Lancet Respir. Med.* **2018**, *6*, 759–770. [CrossRef] [PubMed]
44. Oliveira, N.C.; dos Santos Sabbag, L.M.; de Sa Pinto, A.L.; Borges, C.L.; Lima, F.R. Aerobic exercise is safe and effective in systemic sclerosis. *Int. J. Sports Med.* **2009**, *30*, 728–732. [CrossRef] [PubMed]
45. Pinto, A.L.; Oliveira, N.C.; Gualano, B.; Christmann, R.B.; Painelli, V.S.; Artioli, G.G.; Prado, D.M.; Lima, F.R. Efficacy and safety of concurrent training in systemic sclerosis. *J. Strength. Cond. Res.* **2011**, *25*, 1423–1428. [CrossRef] [PubMed]
46. Zhang, X.J.; Bonner, A.; Hudson, M.; The Canadian Scleroderma Research Group; Baron, M.; Pope, J.; Markland, J.; Docherty, P.; Fritzler, M.; Jones, N.; et al. Association of gastroesophageal factors and worsening of forced vital capacity in systemic sclerosis. *J. Rheumatol.* **2013**, *40*, 850–858. [CrossRef]
47. Savarino, E.; Ghio, M.; Marabotto, E.; Zentilin, P.; Sammito, G.; Cittadini, G.; Sconfienza, L.; Murolo, C.; Gemignani, L.; Indiveri, F.; et al. Possible connection between gastroesophageal reflux and interstitial pulmonary fibrosis in patients with systemic sclerosis. *Recenti Prog. Med.* **2009**, *100*, 512–516. [PubMed]
48. Chan, S.C.W.; Chung, H.Y.; Lau, C.S.; Li, P.H. Epidemiology, mortality and effectiveness of prophylaxis for Pneumocystis jiroveci pneumonia among rheumatic patients: A territory-wide study. *Ann. Clin. Microbiol. Antimicrob.* **2021**, *20*, 78. [CrossRef] [PubMed]
49. CDC. Healthcare Providers: RSV Vaccination for Adults 60 Years of Age and Over | CDC. 2023. Available online: https://www.cdc.gov/vaccines/vpd/rsv/hcp/older-adults.html (accessed on 6 June 2024).
50. Murdaca, G.; Noberasco, G.; Olobardi, D.; Lunardi, C.; Maule, M.; Delfino, L.; Triggiani, M.; Cardamone, C.; Benfaremo, D.; Moroncini, G.; et al. Current Take on Systemic Sclerosis Patients' Vaccination Recommendations. *Vaccines* **2021**, *9*, 1426. [CrossRef] [PubMed] [PubMed Central]
51. Bajwah, S.; Davies, J.M.; Tanash, H.; Currow, D.C.; Oluyase, A.O.; Ekstrom, M. Safety of benzodiazepines and opioids in interstitial lung disease: A national prospective study. *Eur. Respir. J.* **2018**, *52*, 6. [CrossRef]

sclerosis

MDPI

Review

Lung Involvement in Systemic Sclerosis—From Pathogenesis to Prediction

Issa El Kaouri [1], Konstantina Bakopoulou [1], Ivan Padjen [2], Velik Lazarov [3], Paraskevas Panagiotis Sdralis [1], Tsvetelina Velikova [4] and Russka Shumnalieva [1,4,5,*]

[1] Faculty of Medicine, Medical University of Sofia, Boulevard "Akademik Ivan Evstratiev Geshov" 15, 1431 Sofia, Bulgaria; 104166@students.mu-sofia.bg (I.E.K.); 104170@students.mu-sofia.bg (K.B.); 104169@students.mu-sofia.bg (P.P.S.)

[2] Division of Clinical Immunology and Rheumatology, Department of Internal Medicine, University Hospital Centre Zagreb, School of Medicine, University of Zagreb, Kispaticeva 12, 10000 Zagreb, Croatia; ivan_padjen@yahoo.ca

[3] Second Specialised Hospital for Obstetrics and Gynaecology "Sheynovo", ul. Sheinovo 19, 1504 Sofia, Bulgaria; dr.v.lazarov@gmail.com

[4] Medical Faculty, Sofia University, St. Kliment Ohridski, 1 Kozyak Str., 1407 Sofia, Bulgaria; tsvelikova@medfac.mu-sofia.bg

[5] Department of Rheumatology, Clinic of Rheumatology, University Hospital St Ivan Rilski, Urvich Str. 13, 1612 Sofia, Bulgaria

* Correspondence: rshumnalieva@yahoo.com

Abstract: Systemic sclerosis (SSc) is a rare, multifactorial autoimmune disease characterized by widespread vascular damage and fibrosis. Pulmonary involvement is a significant manifestation of SSc, contributing to considerable morbidity and mortality. Therefore, identifying reliable biomarkers is of the utmost importance. This review explores emerging biomarkers to enhance diagnostic accuracy, prognostic assessment, and disease monitoring in SSc lung involvement. We discuss recent findings in immunological biomarkers, inflammatory indicators, and other parameters that can function as potential diagnostic and prognostic tools. A comprehensive understanding of these biomarkers could result in earlier and more accurate detection of pulmonary complications in SSc, aiding in timely intervention. Furthermore, we explore the advances in disease monitoring through innovative biomarkers, focusing on their roles in disease activity and treatment response. Integrating these novel biomarkers into current clinical practice and therapeutic protocols through clinical trials can revolutionize the management of SSc-related lung disease, ultimately improving patient outcomes and quality of life.

Keywords: systemic sclerosis; SSc; scleroderma; pulmonary sclerosis; fibrosis; interstitial lung disease; pulmonary arterial hypertension; PAH

1. Introduction

Systemic sclerosis (SSc) is an autoimmune disease of the connective tissue, affecting multiple systems and organs, generalized by increased fibrosis and vascular changes. It is characterized by functional and structural abnormalities of small blood vessels, skin and internal organ fibrosis, and autoantibody production [1].

It has the highest mortality rate among rheumatic diseases, even though survival rates have improved, particularly for those with diffuse cutaneous SSc (dcSSc). For individuals living with SSc, there is considerable uncertainty regarding their prognosis and the possibility of developing serious or life-altering symptoms. It is a rare disease, classified as an orphan disease, indicating a substantial need for medical attention [1].

Being an infrequent condition, with an annual incidence of 10–50 new cases per million people, SSc has a prevalence of 40–340 individuals per million, and there are differences in occurrence across various regions. Pulmonary involvement in SSc includes mainly the development of pulmonary vascular diseases such as pulmonary artery hypertension (PAH), pulmonary venoocclusive disease (PVOD), interstitial lung disease (ILD), and increased susceptibility to lung neoplasms [2].

Interstitial changes are discoverable in up to 80% of SSc patients via high-resolution CT scans of the chest and in up to 90% of patients upon autopsy [2]. However, only about 30–40% will develop ILD that has clinical significance, which carries a 10-year mortality rate as high as 40%. While ILD becomes more common as SSc progresses, it typically manifests within the first five years following the initial non-Raynaud's symptoms. It is unlikely to appear more than 15 years postdiagnosis. The early appearance of SSc-ILD, especially within the first three years of diagnosis, is increasingly observed and may indicate a more severe disease progression [3]. Demographic factors linked to the development of ILD in SSc patients include sex (being male), African American ethnicity, and diffuse skin involvement. It is also more prevalent among those with nail fold capillary irregularities, digital ulcers, a longer duration of disease, and PAH identified through echocardiogram screening. A genetic predisposition to SSc-ILD has been established, with most risk associated with variations in the HLA region and genes involved in innate immunity, as well as B-cell and T-cell activation and signal transduction [3].

This current paper aims to review the available literature on the pathogenesis of lung involvement in SSc and potential diagnostic and therapeutic options. For this purpose, we performed a comprehensive search across multiple databases, including PubMed, Scopus, and Web of Science. The search period covered articles published from January 1950 to July 2024 to ensure the inclusion of recent and relevant studies. Boolean operators and keywords used in the search included the following: ("Systemic Sclerosis" OR "Scleroderma") AND ("Lung Involvement" OR "Pulmonary Manifestations" OR "Interstitial Lung Disease") AND ("Pathogenesis" OR "Mechanism" OR "Etiology") AND ("Prediction" OR "Prognosis" OR "Biomarkers"). The search aimed to identify original research articles, review papers, and clinical studies. The abstracts and titles were initially screened to exclude irrelevant studies, followed by a full-text review to ensure the inclusion of high-quality papers that directly addressed the topic. In total, 312 papers were retrieved, with 70 meeting the inclusion criteria for this review (Figure 1).

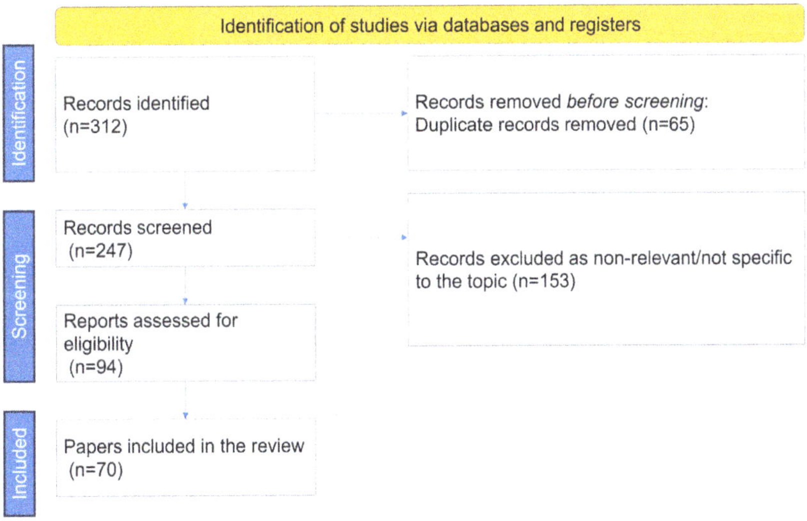

Figure 1. Identification, screening, and selection of papers to include.

2. Pathogenesis of Lung Involvement in SSc

2.1. Interstitial Lung Involvement

In SSc-ILD, the disruption of lung architecture and accumulation of a collagen-rich ECM results from interactions among epithelial, endothelial, and interstitial cells and components of the innate and adaptive immune systems, as Khanna et al. have shown [4].

ILD is commonly implicated with SSc, characterized by the gradual development of fibrosis and scarring of the lung parenchyma. Thickening of the alveolar walls, fibroblast proliferation, accumulation of ECM proteins and fibrosis within the alveolar and interstitial spaces are all pathological hallmarks of SSc-ILD. Histologically, this manifests as usual interstitial pneumonia (UIP) or nonspecific interstitial pneumonia (NSIP), with NSIP being more common in SSc. The lung architecture is disrupted, affecting gas exchange and leading to hypoxia and, therefore, to pulmonary hypertension (PH), thus significantly impacting morbidity and mortality rates [5]. Honeycombing and traction bronchiectasis may develop as fibrosis progresses [6]. The early detection of ILD in SSc is crucial as it allows for interventions that aim to slow down or stop disease progression [7].

ILD-associated PH in SSc is a special entity in the lung involvement in SSc [8,9]. In SSc, PH could also develop as a consequence of hypoxia and/or lung diseases, mostly ILD (group 3 PH). It affects up to 31% of patients with clinically significant SSc-ILD and is related to increased mortality rates compared with SSc-ILD patients without PH [10,11]. The mechanism behind ILD-PH in SSc includes a shared pathophysiology concerning parenchymal and vascular remodeling, with endothelial injury and vascular dysfunction interacting with endothelial dysfunction, oxidative stress, altered immune pathways, perivascular fibrosis, or a genetic predisposition [12,13].

2.2. Mechanisms of Fibrosis in SSc

This pathological process begins with repetitive endothelial and epithelial cell injuries, which activate immune responses, recruit fibroblasts, and lead to their differentiation into myofibroblasts. These myofibroblasts accumulate ECM and contribute to fibrosis. Epithelial cells may undergo apoptosis or epithelial–mesenchymal transition (EMT), leading to further ECM production and resistance to apoptosis, which perpetuates fibrosis [4].

Denton et al. concluded that TGF-β plays a crucial role in fibrosis by promoting ECM accumulation and regulating immune responses. Injured cells secrete TGF-β, which recruits immune cells like macrophages that release more TGF-β, enhancing fibrotic processes [14]. Other cytokines, such as IL-4 and IL-13, produced by type 2 helper T cells and increased thrombin levels contribute to fibroblast proliferation and differentiation [15,16].

Moreover, according to Bhattacharyya et al., the Wnt/β-catenin pathway plays a role in fibroblast activation and tissue remodeling in lung fibrosis [17]. Moving forward, macrophages, essential for lung immunity, are also involved in fibrosis through M1 and M2 polarization. As presented by Khanna et al., M2 macrophages, characterized by markers like CD163 and CD204, accumulate in SSc patients and release fibrotic mediators such as chemokine (C-C motif) ligand 18 (CCL18). Altered macrophage–endothelial interactions can worsen fibrosis and vasculopathy [4]. According to Lafyatis, B lymphocytes also contribute to fibrosis by producing pro-inflammatory cytokines like IL-6, which promote fibrotic pathways and myofibroblast activation [15]. Finally, according to Murguganandam et al., elevated levels of biomarkers such as Krebs von den Lungen 6 (KL-6), surfactant protein D (SP-D), and CCL19 are associated with active SSc-ILD and its progression [18].

2.3. Vascular Abnormalities in SSc: Pathophysiology of Pulmonary Hypertension, Endothelial Cell Dysfunction, and Vascular Remodeling

As we stated above, the pathophysiology of lung involvement in SSc includes PAH, PVOD, and ILD, with marked susceptibility to lung neoplasms [19]. Changes in vasculature or lung interstitium could lead to the development of PH defined as a mean pulmonary arterial hypertension over 25 mm Hg. According to the updated classification of PH by the World Health Organization (WHO), PH is classified into five groups. SSc is most often associated with group 1, pulmonary arterial hypertension (PAH); group 3, PH due to chronic lung diseases and/or hypoxia; and less commonly, group 2, PH due to left heart disease [10].

In SSc, PH could present as an isolated disease manifestation, as PAH (SSc-associated PAH or SSc-PAH), or in combination with ILD (PH-ILD) with the latter subtypes of PH having different prognosis in patients with SSc. Thus, in this review we will focus on PAH and ILD as the main and most serious pulmonary manifestations in SSc.

PAH is one of the primary outcomes of vascular disorders in SSc, along with PVOD [19]. The pathophysiology of SSc-PAH involves a complex interaction of vascular injury, fibrosis, and immune dysregulation [20]. Patients diagnosed with SSc exhibit the highest occurrence of PH group 1 among individuals with collagen vascular diseases. Patients with SSc-PAH also demonstrate a tendency for additional organ involvement, especially in the form of renal dysfunction and intrinsic heart disease, which may lead to end-stage organ failure [19]. This is evidenced by Mulkoju et al. stating that PAH is associated with increased early mortality and is the most prevalent cause of disease-related mortality in specific subtypes of SSc [21].

Various risk factors have been implicated with the development of PAH, including Raynaud's phenomenon, chronic disease, telangiectasia, menopause, older age, reduced diffusion capacity for carbon monoxide (DLco < 50%), DLco/alveolar volume < 70%, and an elevation in right ventricular systolic pressure > 2 mmHg/year [22]. Hemodynamic impairment in these patients is less severe than idiopathic PAH (IPAH). Still, they often exhibit more profound right ventricular dysfunction and higher N-terminal brain natriuretic peptide (NT-pro BNP) levels, indicating severe disease progression [4].

Endothelial cell (EC) dysfunction is pivotal, triggered by factors such as reactive oxygen species, cytokines, and autoantibodies. More specifically, this dysfunction leads to endothelial-to-mesenchymal transition (EndoMT), where ECs transform into myofibroblasts, contributing to ECM overproduction and vascular remodeling [18]. Furthermore, according to Bhattacharyya et al. [17], activated endothelial cells secrete endothelin-1, nitric oxide, and adhesion molecules, which result in vasoconstriction, tissue ischemia, and inflammation. Imbalanced cytokines including endothelial growth factor (VEGF), matrix metalloproteinase (MMP)-9, endothelin-1 (ET-1) and angiostatic factors [pentraxin 3 (PTX3), MMP-12, endostatin, angiostatin, semaphorin 3E (Sema3E), and Slit2], and impaired recruitment of endothelial progenitor cells (EPCs) inhibit proper angiogenesis, aggravating vascular destruction [17]. Doskaliuk et al. emphasize that endothelial cells decrease the presence of endothelial junctional proteins like occludin and vascular endothelial cadherin. Consequently, EndoMT cells lose their ability to act as a barrier, leading to increased plasma leakage and promoting vascular remodeling in PAH [23].

2.4. *Immunological and Inflammatory Processes: Autoantibodies, Immune System Dysregulation, Cytokines, and Inflammatory Mediators*

Autoantibodies are highly important to the pathogenesis of SSc, significantly influencing the development and progression of lung fibrosis and other organ complications [1]. The antibodies, such as antinuclear antibodies (ANAs), anti-centromere antibodies (ACAs), and anti-topoisomerase I (anti-Scl-70) antibodies, are indeed significant in diagnosing and monitoring SSc [22]. However, the correlation between these antibody levels and disease activity, particularly lung involvement, varies [24]. ANAs are found in SSc patients and are associated with various clinical manifestations.

While these antibodies are valuable in identifying subsets of SSc patients and predicting disease patterns, their levels do not always directly correlate with disease activity or severity. For example, anti-Scl-70 antibodies are associated with dcSSc and an increased risk of ILD, yet their presence or titer may not reflect the current activity or progression of ILD [22]. According to Muruganandam et al., the presence of anti-Scl-70 antibodies is mainly associated with a higher risk of developing ILD, affecting up to 85% of SSc patients, and is a leading cause of SSc-related mortality [20]. These autoantibodies contribute to fibrosis by inducing endothelial and epithelial cell injury, which activates the immune system and recruits fibroblasts to the lung tissue. Similarly, ACAs are linked to limited cutaneous SSc (lcSSc) and a lower risk of severe ILD, but their titers do not necessarily correlate with pulmonary involvement [22]. In contrast, anti-Scl-70 antibodies correlate with dcSSc, and there is a higher likelihood of ILD, which is a major complication affecting the lungs [24].

Although some studies have shown that the presence of these antibodies can help predict the course and severity of the disease [22,24], understanding these correlations is crucial for an early diagnosis and targeted treatment, potentially improving patient outcomes by helping to provide a more personalized medical approach. This knowledge shows the importance of antibody testing in the management of SSc, particularly for monitoring lung involvement and guiding therapeutic decisions.

Furthermore, Bhattacharyya et al. [17] highlight the importance of biomarkers as therapeutic targets, with the potential for research-led advancements in patient care. A distinguishing feature of autoantibodies is their accuracy regarding the diagnosis of particular subsets of SSc, with titer measurements relating to disease severity and reproducibility of laboratory measurements. Furthermore, patients with SSc-ILD may present with unique autoantibodies not often associated with other autoimmune diseases [17]. In line with these, autoantibodies, such as anti-Scl-70, ACAs, and anti-RNA polymerase III (ARA), serve as key diagnostic and prognostic biomarkers in SSc [18].

The autoimmune nature of SSc is further evidenced by Bhattacharyya et al. through the presence of anti-fibroblast antibodies in up to 40% of patients, which stimulate IL-6 production and pro-fibrotic chemokines, enhancing fibroblast activation and collagen synthesis [17]. Similarly, antibodies against fibrillin 1 and platelet-derived growth factor receptors (PDGFRs) have been shown to promote collagen gene expression and myofibroblast differentiation via endogenous TGF-β signaling pathways. The involvement of these autoantibodies in the fibrotic process underscores their role in perpetuating the chronic inflammation and fibrosis seen in SSc-ILD. The simultaneous presence of different SSc-specific autoantibodies is rare but highlights the complexity of the autoimmune response in SSc [20]. Cytokines play a pivotal role in the pathogenesis of lung fibrosis in SSc, particularly in the development of ILD, which is a significant cause of morbidity and mortality in SSc patients [18].

As Murguganandam et al. pointed out, transforming growth factor-beta (TGF-β) is central to the fibrotic process in SSc, driving the excessive deposition of extracellular matrix (ECM) proteins, particularly collagen, which increases lung tissue stiffness and reduces lung compliance [20]. Additionally, cytokines such as interleukins (IL-1, IL-4, IL-6, IL-8, IL-10 IL-13, IL-16, IL-17, IL-18, IL-22, IL-32, and IL-35); the chemokines CCL, C-X-C motif (CXC), and C-X3-C motif chemokine ligand 1 (CX3CL1) (fractalkine); and growth differentiation factor 15 (GDF15) are implicated in the recruitment and activation of fibroblasts, further contributing to fibrosis. The involvement of cytokines and autoantibodies suggests the complex immune dysregulation in SSc and highlights potential therapeutic targets for mitigating lung fibrosis and improving patient outcomes [20].

The complex pathogenesis of lung involvement in SSc is presented in Figure 2.

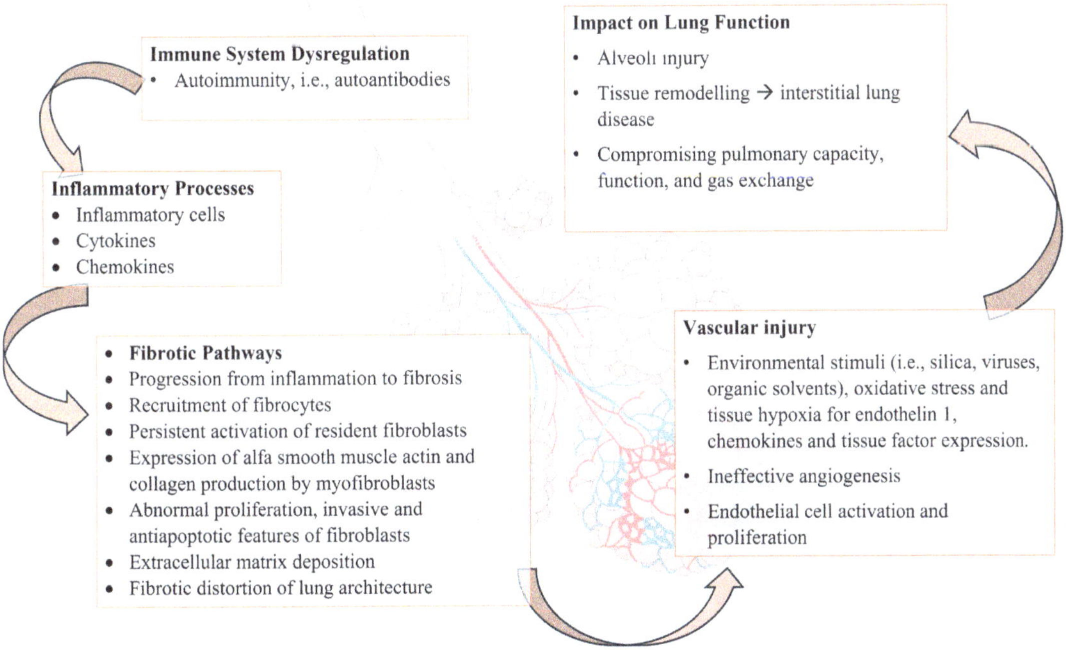

Figure 2. Pathogenesis of lung involvement in SSc is linked to the migration, activation, and proliferation of fibroblasts and differentiation into myofibroblasts. Autoreactive immune cells and produced antibodies and mediators (i.e., cytokines) further perpetuate the inflammation. When fibroblasts and myofibroblasts are persistently activated, they invade pulmonary tissue and produce collagen and extracellular matrix protein. Eventually, the excessive extracellular matrix protein remodels and distorts the lung architecture, leading to compromised lung function. Parts of the figure were drawn by using pictures from Servier Medical Art. Servier Medical Art by Servier is licensed under a Creative Commons BY 4.0 (https://creativecommons.org/licenses/by/4.0/; last accessed on 3 August 2024).

3. Clinical Manifestations and Diagnosis

3.1. Symptoms of Lung Involvement in SSc

When a patient with SSc presents with signs and symptoms referring to the chest, a variety of potential disorders should be considered. They include direct pulmonary involvement, indirect pulmonary complications, or a combination of both. Direct lung involvement can be subdivided into two common types: ILD and PAH [25]. Together, they account for around 60% of SSc-related deaths, with ILD being the leading cause of morbidity and mortality in SSc patients. SSc-induced PAH is most common in the lcSSc variant of the disease, while dcSSc is common in patients with ILD [19,26].

A considerable number of patients with SSc-ILD present with no specific symptoms, significantly when extrapulmonary manifestations of the disease limit their mobility. When symptoms are present, dyspnea, in exertion at first and eventually at rest; non-productive cough; and fatigue are most commonly reported. Patients with PAH can also present with hemoptysis, syncope, and symptoms of fluid retention. Perelas et al. note that the longer duration of the disease is associated with pulmonary involvement, specifically SSc-ILD [27].

3.2. Diagnostic Tools and Techniques

According to Solomon et al., up to 90% of patients will have interstitial abnormalities on high-resolution computed tomography (HRCT), while 40–70% will have pulmonary function test (PFT) changes [28]. HRCT is the standard modality for the non-invasive diagnosis of SSc-ILD. NSIP is the most common pattern detected in the scans of more than 80% of patients with SSc-ILD. This is characterized by peripheral ground-glass opacities, with an apical to basal gradient and possibly with subpleural spacing. The modality does have limitations, including the possibility of being normal in patients with PFT abnormalities or in patients with an abnormal chest auscultation (crackles) [28]. Despite the limitations, a normal HRCT at baseline can predict a low chance for the development of SSc-ILD, with around 85% of these patients having a normal scan at a mean follow-up of 5 years. PFTs are an essential non-invasive method for detecting pulmonary complications in the early stages.

Forced vital capacity and lung diffusing capacity for carbon monoxide (DLco) have been traditionally used to assess lung involvement in SSc. Spirometry and lung volumes show reasonable specificity but poor sensitivity to pulmonary fibrosis in SSc [29]. PFTs show a reduction in FVC in 40–75% of patients, with 15% having a severe reduction. Patients with minimal to no restriction had a 10-year survival rate of 87%, while patients with moderate and severe restriction had 75% and 58% 10-year survival rates, respectively. Functional vital capacity and DLco have been identified as adverse prognostic markers in SSc-related pulmonary injury. Almost all patients with pulmonary function test abnormalities will have a reduced DLco, with that being the most significant marker for poor outcomes and having a correlation with the extent of lung disease. Studies have indicated that DLco is preferable to spirometry in detecting lung involvement [29].

In the case of PAH, transthoracic echocardiography is the most widely used tool for screening. A plain CXR is the least sensitive test for evaluating PAH [30]. Still, it shows high specificity (up to 100% in one study), with findings including right pulmonary artery enlargement and loss of peripheral vasculature. Another valuable modality for the evaluation of patients with SSc is the use of biomarkers. ANAs are present in more than 90% of SSc patients and could be reliable biomarkers for diagnosis [30]. Additionally, several studies have suggested that TGF-β plays an essential role in the fibrotic process; therefore, it could be a potential biomarker for fibrosis development. Interleukin receptor-associated kinase-1 (IRAK-1), interferon regulatory factor (IRF5), connective tissue growth factor (CTGF), transducer and activator of transcription signal 4 (STAT4), and nucleotide-binding oligomerization domain (NOD)-like receptor containing a Pyrin domain 1 (NLRP1) have been reported to be implicated in SSc damage [21]. Genetic factors, including DRB1 alleles, have also been implicated. Several interleukins and chemokines like CCL18, CX3CL1, and CXCL4 can be elevated and have been associated with SSc-ILD [21].

3.3. Differential Diagnosis

Depending on the HRCT pattern, various differential diagnoses can be considered. That includes other CT diseases, drug-associated NSIP, interstitial pneumonia with autoimmune features, hypersensitivity pneumonitis, and idiopathic NSIP [31]. That is mainly in the early stage. The late fibrotic stage differential can include CT diseases, drug toxicity, chronic hypertensive pneumonitis, asbestosis, and idiopathic pulmonary fibrosis. SSc-ILD shares similarities with IPF, but differences can be observed. Under histological examination, a nonspecific interstitial pneumonia pattern is seen in SSc-ILD, while IPF is defined by usual interstitial pneumonia. A definite interstitial pneumonia honeycomb pattern is present in fewer than 10% of patients with SSc-ILD [31].

Figure 3 presents an overview of lung involvement in SSc, including clinical manifestations, diagnosis, prognosis, and follow-up.

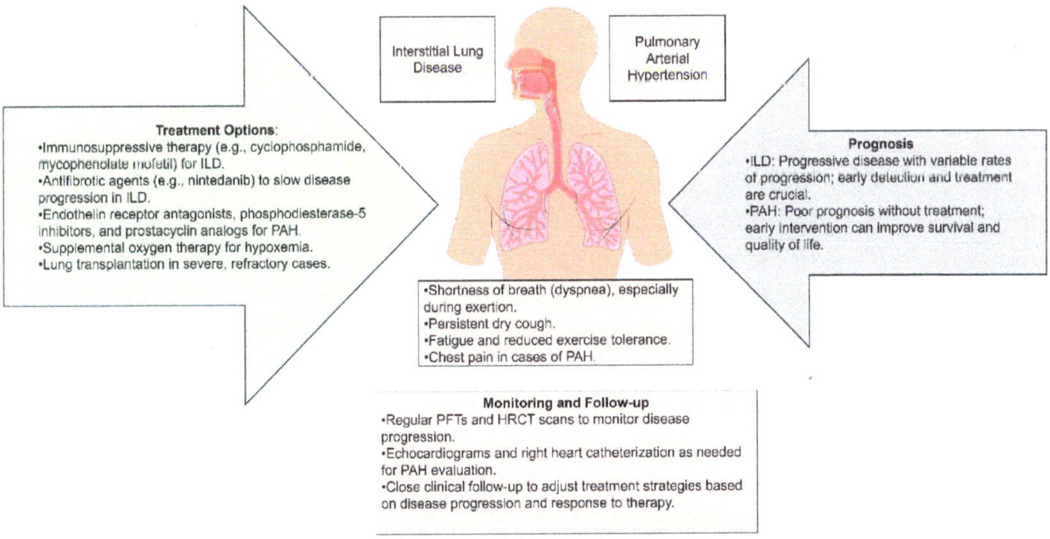

Figure 3. Interstitial lung disease and pulmonary arterial hypertension as lung involvement in SSc. Parts of the figure were drawn by using pictures from Servier Medical Art. Servier Medical Art by Servier is licensed under a Creative Commons Attribution 3.0 Unported License (https://creativecommons.org/licenses/by/3.0/; last accessed on 3 August 2024).

4. Prediction and Monitoring of Lung Involvement

4.1. Risk Factors and Predictive Models: Genetic Predisposition and Environmental and Lifestyle Factors

Lung involvement in the case of SSc typically affects the lung interstitium, in the context of ILD. The most common histopathological presentation of SSc-ILD is NSIP, which corresponds to the typical ground-glass pattern observed on lung CT [32]. Interestingly the UIP pattern, despite being consistent with "fibrotic" chest CT features of honeycombing and traction bronchiectasis, is less commonly seen in SSc-ILD. The highly variable course of SSc-ILD requires the use of strong prognostic predictors of severe and progressive disease with the aim of timely and precise clinical management. Genetic predictors in this context can act as discriminating factors for patients at higher risk for developing ILD while also offering predictive value to disease progression at the time of the initial disease diagnosis. Additionally, they can aid in risk stratification of the subgroup not included in the Goh staging system that does not meet the criterion of antecedent presence of ILD on HRCT [32].

The prevalence of ILD increases exponentially in individuals of Choctaw Native American, African, and Japanese descent when compared with a cohort of European descent. Simultaneously, the aforementioned ethnic groups exhibit an accelerated decline in lung function and worse overall survival rates when compared with European individuals [33].

Multiple HLA region associations have been made, with the HLA-DRB1 region playing a predominant role in the disease incidence among UK Caucasians, Spanish, and Black South African individuals. Conversely, the HLA-DQB1*0501 allele seems to be associated with the disease occurrence in Han Chinese [33].

Other genes implicated in SSc are shown to affect multiple aspects of innate immunity, as well as B- and T-lymphocyte activation processes. Some notable examples are single nucleotide polymorphisms (SNPs) in the genes of interferon regulatory factor 5 (IRF5), signal transducer and activator of transcription 4 (STAT4), and cell receptor CD3ζ (CD247) [33].

STAT4 is the transcription factor associated with the expression of type 1 interferons, IL-12 and IL-23. SNPs in the gene of IRF5 affect the transcription of interferon A and B, as well as other pro-inflammatory cytokines, and can thus alter the disease severity or even impact a protective effect. At the same time, specific polymorphisms can have a synergistic effect, e.g., the cumulative effect of IRF5 SNP with specific STAT4 SNP, leading to increased ILD severity. Another possible genetic association is with gene CD226, which codes for DNAX accessory molecule 1 and is implicated in cell-mediated cytotoxicity of T and NK cells [33].

NLRP1 provides a platform for the assembly of the inflammasome forming that has been found to have an additive effect with specific SNPs of STAT4 and ILR5 genes [30], leading to promoting the processing and maturation of pro-IL-1β. Additionally, single nucleotide polymorphisms are present in NLRP1 (i.e., rs8182352 variant) with both anti-topoisomerase-positive and SSc-related fibrosing alveolitis [34].

The IRAK1 gene, located on the X chromosome, encodes a protein kinase whose function results in enhanced NFκ-B activity. Connective tissue growth factor (CTGF) drives the differentiation of myofibroblasts, therefore contributing to extracellular matrix deposition in tissues. Sato et al. have successfully demonstrated that serum levels of CTGF can predict the extent of pulmonary fibrosis in SSc-ILD [35]. The CD247 gene codes for the T-cell receptor T3 ζ chain that forms the T-cell receptor (TCR)/CD3 complex [36].

Activating mutations in the MUC5B (mucin 5B) gene and overexpression of the components involved in the Wnt pathway (e.g., β-catenin and MMP7) have been known to contribute to the pathogenesis of IPF. Still, they do not appear to play a role in ILD [4].

A posttranscriptional mechanism of gene expression regulation through targeting the messenger RNAs (mRNAs) includes the synthesis of microRNAs (miRNAs). miRNAs comprise a class of endogenous short noncoding RNA molecules that serve as negative regulators of the gene expression [16]. Functional studies have shown that miRNAs regulate critical fibrosis-related signaling pathways and molecules related to fibroblast hyperactivity and abnormal synthesis of ECM proteins, as well as SSc-related genes, thus playing an important role in the pathogenesis of fibrosis [16,37]. miRNAs have been shown to directly or indirectly participate in the fibrotic process by targeting the transforming growth factor (TGF)/Smad3 canonical signaling pathway and the connective tissue growth factor (CTGF), by affecting the epithelial-to-mesenchymal transition and inducing myofibroblast proliferation and resistance to apoptosis [16,38].

Environmental and lifestyle risk factors associated with SSc are presented in Table 1.

Table 1. Risk factors associated with SSc.

Group of Factors	Examples
Genetic	IRF5, STAT4, CD247, CD226, NLRP1, IRAK1, CTGF, HLA DRB1, HLA-DQB1
Environmental and lifestyle	Silica, silicone breast implants Vinyl chloride, trichloroethylene, benzene, toluene Bleomycin, L-5-hydroxytryptophan Rapeseed oil Epoxy resins Infectious: CMV, EBV, parvovirus B19, retroviruses Neoplastic: lung cancer, breast cancer, esophageal cancer, hematological malignancies

Environmental factors can be attributable to occupational exposures (e.g., silica and organic solvents); infectious agents (bacterial and viral); and non-occupational/non-infectious exposure to drugs, pesticides, and silicones. The pathogenetic mechanisms implicated in SSc include (1) immune tolerance interference, e.g., epigenetic modification by drugs; (2) immune system activation, e.g., vinyl chloride-mediated activation of CD8+ subsets and enhanced immunogenicity; and (3) molecular mimicry shared by many infectious triggers [39].

Some infectious agents studied for their contributions to SSc are parvovirus B19, cytomegalovirus (CMV), Epstein–Barr virus (EBV), and retroviruses. Neoplastic and/or paraneoplastic associations have been made with lung and breast cancer. As Maria et al. concluded, lung cancer appears to be linked with SSc-ILD in the presence of anti-Scl-70 Ab. On the other hand, the most commonly encountered cancers involve the breast, which in turn seems to be dependent on the presence of anti-RNA-PolIII Ab [40].

The sex predisposition of SSc for females follows the classic trend of most autoimmune diseases. This, subsequently, culminates in men preferentially presenting with an active and diffuse disease with an increased incidence of lung involvement, which may have a negative predictive value on survival. Truchetet et al. have also proposed that the failure of the physiological silencing of one of the two X-chromosomal copies in females can enhance autoantibody production. Another suggestion that focuses on the SNP of genes found on the X chromosome, such as IL13RA2, IRAK1, and FOXP3, may further elucidate the pathogenesis of SSc and explain the female-predominant nature of the disease [41].

4.2. Biomarkers for Early Detection: Emerging Biomarkers and Role of Autoantibodies in Prediction

The prediction of early pulmonary involvement in patients with SSc is a crucial aspect of the treatment strategy. Recent advances have been made in searching for serological or proteomic biomarkers for early detection of lung involvement in this subset of patients [42].

PAH is a severe complication in about 7–12% of SSc patients. A bare minimum for detecting PAH in SSc patients includes PFT with measurement of diffusion capacity of the lung for carbon monoxide (DLCO) and the systolic pulmonary arterial pressure on echocardiography. According to the DETECT protocol, a clinical examination, PFTs, cardiac examination, and serum biomarkers can be used with high sensitivity but relatively low specificity for PAH [42]. Biomarker research focuses on identifying several circulating or tissue-specific biomarkers whose concentrations could be used to predict PAH.

Natriuretic peptides are molecules released by the cardiac myocytes in response to ischemia, hypoxia, and ventricular wall stress. Atrial natriuretic peptide (ANP) and the more stable brain (B-type) natriuretic peptide are secreted in response to atrial or ventricular stretching, aiming for vasodilation and increased diuresis and natriuresis. In recent years, the N-terminal Pro-Brain natriuretic peptide (NT-proBNP) has been proven to be a preferable biomarker due to its longer half-life and higher stability and accuracy than BNP. NT-proBNP levels have been higher in SSc patients with PAH than those without PAH [43]. The change in NT-proBNP levels has shown a prognostic prediction in PAH at baseline and in the follow-up of the patients [44]. Of note is that levels of NT-proBNP could be elevated in SSc patients without PAH as a result of primary cardiac involvement.

Vascular Endothelial Growth Factor-A (VEGF-A) is an essential regulator of angiogenesis, promoting new angiogenesis, vascular permeability, and endothelial cell migration. Circulating levels of VEGF-A have been described in SSc patients, as well as in SSc-PAH patients, in correlation with the systemic pulmonary arterial pressure, DLCO, and MRC dyspnea score [45].

Growth Differentiation Factor-15 (GDF-15) plays a vital role in cell growth and differentiation. It is a cytokine member of the TGF-β superfamily, and its levels are higher in SSc-PAH patients compared with SSc patients without PAH and healthy volunteers with high diagnostic accuracy [46]. Serum levels of type I, II, and III interferon (IFN) are elevated in SSc-PAH, and an association exists between SSc-PAH and serum levels of interferon γ inducible protein 10 (IP10) [47,48].

Regarding the role of SSc-specific autoantibodies, there is no clear association between ANAs in PAH SSc patients. According to the literature, patients with anticentromere (ACA), CENP-A, and/or CENP-B are more prone to develop PAH but not ILD [49]. The frequency of ILD has been reported to be higher in SSc patients with anti-Th/To-positivity [50]. Antibodies against ET-1 receptor type A and angiotensin receptor type 1 have been found to be higher in PAH associated with connective tissue disease, and in particular, SSc, as well as with the development of digital ulceration in SSc [51].

4.3. Monitoring Disease Progression

Monitoring disease progression in SSc is crucial for preventing disease complications and reducing mortality rates. Inflammatory serum markers like C-reactive protein are helpful for the prediction of disease progression. Elevated serum levels of CRP have been identified as an independent predictor of PAH with a poor prognosis [52]. Monitoring serum uric acid is recommended for the detection of scleroderma-renal crisis, as well as being a predictor of PAH-related ventricular dysfunction [53].

According to the recommendations for evaluating and monitoring patients with PAH and CTD, asymptomatic SSc patients should undergo resting echocardiography as a screening, followed by annual screening with echocardiography, DLCO, and biomarkers. Right heart catheterization is recommended in all cases of suspected PAH associated with CTD [54]. According to the DETECT algorithm, patients with SSc and an increased risk of developing PAH should undergo a two-step screening (Figure 4).

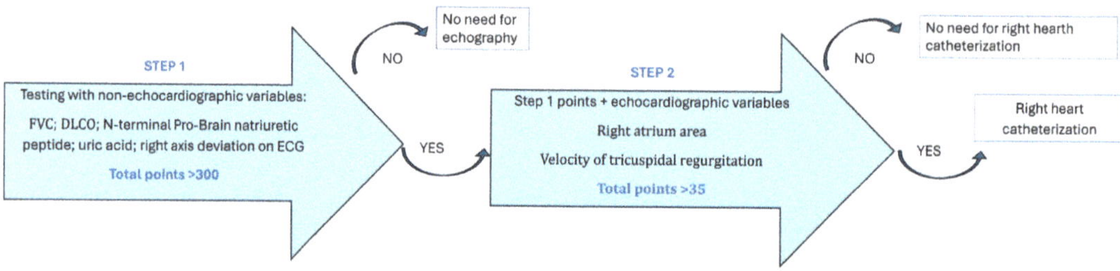

Figure 4. Algorithm for SSc management when the risk of PAH is high. FVC, forced vital capacity; DLCO, diffusing capacity for carbon monoxide; ACA, anticentromere antibodies.

5. Current and Emerging Therapies for SSc

5.1. Pharmacological Treatment

The approach to treating SSc and its effects on the lung is aimed at suppressing the three pathogenetically relevant processes inherent to disease progression: immune-mediated inflammation, fibrosis, and vasculopathy. Immunosuppressants receive the most attention given that they are, at a group level, indicated in virtually all patients from the time of the diagnosis [55].

In patients with predominantly skin disease, methotrexate is still considered the first treatment of choice, showing its moderately beneficial effect on inhibiting further skin thickening. Due to its anti-inflammatory and immunosuppressive effects, methotrexate has been used to manage mainly skin, joint, and muscle involvement in SSc. So far methotrexate is recommended for treating skin changes in patients with early diffuse SSc demonstrating efficacy in reducing skin fibrosis and improving skin scores [56]. However, its use in patients without lung involvement requires careful consideration. There is a concern that methotrexate could contribute to the development of lung fibrosis due to allergic, cytotoxic, or immunologic reactions, particularly in patients with pre-existing pulmonary symptoms or those at risk for pulmonary complications. The risk of methotrexate-induced lung fibrosis, although relatively low, needs to be weighed against its potential benefits. Clinical practice recommendations, based on current evidence, state that methotrexate may be used in early-stage SSc with skin involvement, provided that patients are closely monitored for any signs of lung involvement. Regular pulmonary assessments and imaging may be warranted to detect any early signs of lung fibrosis [56].

Cyclophosphamide and mycophenolate mofetil (MMF) serve as the following line of immunosuppressants, indicated either when the skin is pronouncedly affected or in the case of significantly affected internal organs, primarily the lung interstitium and the gastrointestinal tract [55].

The effect of these two immunosuppressants on progressive ILD was assessed in two randomized controlled trials: the Scleroderma Lung Studies (SLSs) 1 and 2. In the SLS1 study, oral cyclophosphamide was shown to be superior to a placebo in preventing decline in lung function tests [57].

In SLS2, MMF was shown to be non-inferior to cyclophosphamide in terms of efficacy, but it had a better tolerability profile. It is worth noting that the effect size of the treatment in both studies was modest at best, with a forced vital capacity (FVC) improvement of less than 3% predicted value in both the SLS1 and SLS2. This difference is in line with those observed in other studies. It indicates the expected benefits from the treatment: immunosuppression is intended to hamper further ILD progression rather than lead to a clinically meaningful improvement [58].

In the current therapeutic armamentarium, both cyclophosphamide and MMF are employed, and there is an increasing trend toward the use of MMF. The advantage of MMF is its more acceptable toxicity profile, making it suitable not only as an induction treatment option but also as a longer-term maintenance agent. On the other hand, cyclophosphamide is usually administered intravenously, circumventing the issue of adherence to treatment associated with oral MMF. Even though oral cyclophosphamide was employed in SLS1 and SLS2, the intravenous use of pulse cyclophosphamide (which has become a standard in most centers) is associated with a lower cumulative dose and, consequently, less toxicity [59].

Although azathioprine is not among the first immunosuppressive agents of choice, it can still be considered a maintenance option if MMF is not tolerated, is unavailable, or is contraindicated (such as in pregnancy) [60].

Among the biological treatment options for SSc, rituximab (RTX, an anti-CD20 monoclonal antibody) and tocilizumab (TCZ, a monoclonal antibody inhibiting the interleukin 6 receptor) have demonstrated their effects in clinical trials, primarily on the ILD component. They are used as a later treatment line after an inadequate response to a conventional immunosuppressive agent. The possibility of combining RTX and TCZ with MMF may be beneficial in selected patients, as well as a further addition of an antifibrotic agent [61]. In this recent meta-analysis of 20 studies, RTX has been shown to improve FVC by 4.49% at six months and by 7.03% at 12 months [61]. Even though these improvements seem numerically superior compared with other immunosuppressants, RTX was not superior to cyclophosphamide in its effect on FVC in the recently published RECITAL study conducted on patients with CTD-ILD [62].

Tocilizumab (TCZ) is a humanized anti-human IL-6 receptor antibody that binds to soluble and membrane-bound IL-6 receptors, and at detectable levels in the blood, TCZ is capable of almost completely blocking the transmembrane signaling of IL-6 [63]. TCZ is approved for use in the treatment of various immune-mediated diseases including rheumatoid arthritis (RA) and giant cell arteritis (GCA) [64]. The phase II faSScinate and phase III focuSSced trials evaluated the safety and efficacy of TCZ in patients with early active dcSSc. While the improvements in skin fibrosis were not statistically significant between the TCZ group and the placebo group, it was indicated that it might preserve lung function in patients with early SSc-ILD and elevated acute phase reactants. In 2021, it was approved by the FDA for use in patients with SSc-ILD based on the results of the focuSSced trial. More specifically, in the faSScinate trial, the difference in FVC between the placebo group and the TCZ group was 120 mL with a difference of 167 mL overall in the focuSSced one [65,66]. Collectively, the data from Khanna D et al. showed that the stabilization of lung function in patients receiving TCZ was consistent across all severity groups with SSc-ILD, showing that the effects of TCZ were observed in all subgroups.

Regarding safety, during the phase III study, 82 patients in the placebo groups had at least one adverse event, with the number in the TCZ group being 89 [66]. Only two of the TCZ group patients experienced cardiac disorders during the study compared with seven in the placebo group. Overall, no major differences in experienced adverse effects were observed between the two groups. Kuster S et al. [67] confirm the previously mentioned adverse effects and do not reveal significant new potential threats of TCZ during treatment.

Tocilizumab was approved for SSc-associated ILD based on the results of a randomized controlled trial, which did not meet its primary skin endpoint. The trial did show a numerical improvement in the modified Rodnan skin score at week 48 in the tocilizumab group compared with the placebo (−6.1 vs. −4.4, respectively). Interestingly, the change in FVC at week 48 was only −0.4% in the tocilizumab group compared with −4.6% in the placebo group ($p = 0.002$). However, this finding was a priori not taken into account as significant due to the hierarchical structure of the study disregarding any results of secondary endpoint analyses in the context of the study not meeting the primary endpoint [66].

The role of glucocorticoids is not as prominent in SSc compared with other connective tissue diseases due to an increased risk of renal crisis associated with their use. However, glucocorticoids are still used in patients exhibiting features overlapping with other inflammatory rheumatic conditions, such as arthritis, myositis, and serositis [68]. Antifibrotic drugs are promising therapeutic options available for SSc. Nintedanib is the first and currently only antifibrotic agent approved for the treatment of SSc, used in the treatment of ILD. At the same time, it does not affect the skin. In the current treatment paradigm, it is being used in cases of progressive pulmonary fibrosis, usually as an add-on option following an inadequate effect of immunosuppressive treatment. Its approval is based on its rather modest efficacy demonstrated in the SENCSIS trial: an absolute difference in the FVC predicted value of 1.2% (equaling 46.4 mL) between the nintendanib add-on group and the standard of care group. On the other hand, 75.7% of patients on nintendanib experienced diarrhea even in the trial (compared with 31.6% in the control group) [68]. Pirfenidone is another antifibrotic agent already being used for the treatment of idiopathic pulmonary fibrosis. There is growing evidence that its use may also be of benefit to patients with progressive pulmonary fibrosis in the context of SSc [68].

Current treatment options for PAH include endothelin receptor antagonists, phosphodiesterase 5 (PDE5) inhibitors, prostaglandin analogs, and soluble guanylate cyclase agonists. Endothelin receptor blockade, PDE5 inhibitors, and iloprost have also been shown to control the symptoms of secondary Raynaud's phenomenon and digital ulcers associated with vasculopathy inherent to the disease. The therapeutic approach to PAH in patients with SSc is analogous to treating idiopathic PAH. The initialization of therapy with a single agent is reserved only for a low-risk patient profile. In contrast, most patients should be concomitantly started on dual treatment (usually an endothelin receptor antagonist and a PDE5 inhibitor) [69].

It is worth noting that the recent change in the definition of the cutoff value of increased pulmonary artery pressure from 25 mmHg to 20 mmHg (and 3 Wood units to 2 Wood units) should allow for better control of patients under risk of development of PAH-related complications and poor outcomes [70].

5.2. Non-Pharmacological Approaches

Oxygen therapy is used in patients with evidence of partial or global respiratory insufficiency in an acute setting of an ILD exacerbation or respiratory infection or the setting of severe later-stage ILD and/or SSc-associated PAH despite treatment with pharmacological agents. Oxygen treatment aims to prevent further deterioration of the patient's condition, mainly to prevent secondary (especially right-sided) heart failure, as well as to improve quality of life and mortality. Given the lack of direct evidence of using supplementary oxygen in patients with SSc, data on the expected benefits are derived from other more frequent conditions [71].

Although there are some recommendations regarding nutrition for preventing pulmonary fibrosis, such as low sodium (salt) intake and avoiding added sugars and saturated and trans fat, no specific nutrition and diet could really prevent lung involvement in SSc patients [72].

The use of hyperbaric oxygen has been described as an adjunctive add-on treatment of intractable ulcers due to severe vascular insufficiency in patients with SSc. Despite some authorities favoring such a treatment modality, its efficacy and potential safety issues have not been assessed in well-designed clinical trials [73].

Pulmonary rehabilitation is an important adjunctive treatment option that increases the patient's quality of life and improves exertional capacity. Despite the relatively well-documented role of pulmonary rehabilitation in patients with other lung diseases, the role of pulmonary rehabilitation in SSc still needs to be fully appreciated in well-designed clinical studies. An interesting aspect may be speech therapy, which has been shown to decrease the incidence of aspiration episodes associated with exacerbations of ILD [74].

A systematic review by Murphy et al. (2022), which included 15 randomized controlled trials and one prospective quasi-experimental study, revealed within-group improvements in intervention groups (most focused on hands/upper extremities, followed by multicomponent, orofacial, and directed self-management). However, the study's heterogenicity, interventions that focus on hand and upper extremity outcomes or are multicomponent, provides some support for rehabilitation in SSc [75].

5.3. Future Directions and Research for SSc Lung Complications

Various molecular targets have been explored through preclinical studies and clinical trials. These include the blockade of the costimulatory CD28-CD80/86 T-cell signal with abatacept and the blockade of CD19 and CD20 on cells of B lineage, as well as the inhibition of CCL24 (Chemokine C-C motif ligand 24), tumor necrosis factor-alpha, transforming growth factor–beta, B-cell activating factor (BAFF), LPA1 receptor (lysophosphatidic acid receptor 1), sGC (soluble guanylate cyclase), Janus kinases, interleukins 6 and 17, endothelin receptor, and autotaxin [76].

Despite the high number of potential therapeutic targets, the biology of SSc as a predominantly pro-fibrotic condition is the main limiting feature toward achieving improved outcomes. A modest therapeutic effect of immunosuppressive agents has illustrated that the disease is recognized at a late stage or that active inflammation should not be the primary therapeutic target. On the other hand, nintendanib has not demonstrated its antifibrotic property beyond the lung interstitium. The fact that there are several immunosuppressive agents and several agents targeting PAH but only one available agent targeting fibrosis reveals a highly unmet need for the control of fibrosis in SSc.

6. Conclusions

In conclusion, the complexity and high patient burden of SSc-related lung disease calls for a more thorough understanding of the underlying pathophysiological mechanisms, the standardization of biomarker evaluation, and their integration into clinical practice. Predictive models and biomarkers for lung involvement in SSc can significantly enhance early diagnosis, enable more personalized treatment strategies, and improve patient outcomes. Many SSc patients are stable over time; however, predicting the progression of the disease, based on different markers, etc., would be of utmost importance. By identifying high-risk individuals and monitoring disease progression more effectively, these predictive tools can guide clinical decision-making, potentially reducing lung damage and improving overall prognosis. We believe these advancements will contribute to more targeted and proactive approaches in managing SSc-related lung complications.

Overcoming the challenges around lung involvement in SSc would denote a new era of refined diagnostic and personalized treatment options, offering hope for improved outcomes in SSc patients with lung involvement. Collaboration between multidisciplinary teams, technological advances, and meticulous research endeavors are all prerequisites for the future improvement of patient care.

Author Contributions: Conceptualization, I.E.K. and K.B.; methodology, I.P.; software, V.L.; validation, I.E.K., R.S. and T.V.; formal analysis, K.B.; investigation, I.P. and P.P.S.; resources, V.L.; data curation, P.P.S.; writing—original draft preparation, I.E.K., K.B., I.P., V.L. and P.P.S.; writing—review and editing, R.S. and T.V.; visualization, I.E.K., R.S. and T.V.; supervision, R.S.; project administration, T.V.; funding acquisition, T.V. All authors have read and agreed to the published version of the manuscript.

Funding: This study is financed by the European Union-NextGenerationEU, through the National Recovery and Resilience Plan of the Republic of Bulgaria, project no. BG-RRP-2.004-0008.

Acknowledgments: Parts of Figures 2 and 3 were drawn by using pictures from Servier Medical Art. Servier Medical Art by Servier is licensed under a Creative Commons BY 4.0 (https://creativecommons.org/licenses/by/4.0/; last accessed on 3 August 2024).

Conflicts of Interest: The authors declare no conflicts of interest.

References

1. Denton, C.P.; Khanna, D. Systemic sclerosis. *Lancet* **2017**, *390*, 1685–1699. [CrossRef] [PubMed]
2. Tian, J.; Kang, S.; Zhang, D.; Huang, Y.; Zhao, M.; Gui, X.; Yao, X.; Lu, Q. Global, regional, and national incidence and prevalence of systemic sclerosis. *Clin. Immunol.* **2023**, *248*, 109267. [CrossRef] [PubMed]
3. Perelas, A.; Silver, R.M.; Arrossi, A.V.; Highland, K.B. Systemic sclerosis-associated interstitial lung disease. *Lancet Respir. Med.* **2020**, *8*, 304–320. [CrossRef] [PubMed]
4. Khanna, D.; Tashkin, D.P.; Denton, C.P.; Renzoni, E.A.; Desai, S.R.; Varga, J. Etiology, Risk Factors, and Biomarkers in Systemic Sclerosis with Interstitial Lung Disease. *Am. J. Respir. Crit. Care Med.* **2020**, *201*, 650–660. [CrossRef] [PubMed] [PubMed Central]
5. Hoffmann-Vold, A.-M.; Allanore, Y.; Alves, M.; Brunborg, C.; Airó, P.; Ananieva, L.P.; Czirják, L.; Guiducci, S.; Hachulla, E.; Li, M.; et al. Progressive interstitial lung disease in patients with systemic sclerosis-associated interstitial lung disease in the EUSTAR database. *Ann. Rheum. Dis.* **2021**, *80*, 219–227. [CrossRef] [PubMed] [PubMed Central]
6. Gladue, H.; Altorok, N.; Townsend, W.; McLaughlin, V.; Khanna, D. Screening and diagnostic modalities for connective tissue disease-associated pulmonary arterial hypertension: A systematic review. *Semin. Arthritis Rheum.* **2014**, *43*, 536–541. [CrossRef] [PubMed] [PubMed Central]
7. Distler, O.; Highland, K.B.; Gahlemann, M.; Azuma, A.; Fischer, A.; Mayes, M.D.; Raghu, G.; Sauter, W.; Girard, M.; Alves, M.; et al. Nintedanib for Systemic Sclerosis–Associated Interstitial Lung Disease. *N. Engl. J. Med.* **2019**, *380*, 2518–2528. [CrossRef] [PubMed]
8. Parikh, R.; Konstantinidis, I.; O'Sullivan, D.M.; Farber, H.W. Pulmonary hypertension in patients with interstitial lung disease: A tool for early detection. *Pulm. Circ.* **2022**, *12*, e12141. [CrossRef]
9. Kacprzak, A.; Tomkowski, W.; Szturmowicz, M. Pulmonary Hypertension in the Course of Interstitial Lung Diseases—A Personalised Approach Is Needed to Identify a Dominant Cause and Provide an Effective Therapy. *Diagnostics* **2023**, *13*, 2354. [CrossRef]
10. Simonneau, G.; Montani, D.; Celermajer, D.S.; Denton, C.P.; Gatzoulis, M.A.; Krowka, M.; Williams, P.G.; Souza, R. Haemodynamic definitions and updated clinical classification of pulmonary hypertension. *Eur. Respir. J.* **2019**, *53*, 1801913. [CrossRef] [PubMed] [PubMed Central]
11. Dhont, S.; Zwaenepoel, B.; Vandecasteele, E.; Brusselle, G.; De Pauw, M. Pulmonary hypertension in interstitial lung disease: An area of unmet clinical need. *ERJ Open Res.* **2022**, *8*, 00272-2022. [CrossRef] [PubMed]
12. Arslan, A.; Smith, J.; Qureshi, M.R.; Uysal, A.; Patel, K.K.; Herazo-Maya, J.D.; Bandyopadhyay, D. Evolution of pulmonary hypertension in interstitial lung disease: A journey through past, present, and future. *Front. Med.* **2024**, *10*, 1306032. [CrossRef] [PubMed]
13. Haynes, Z.A.; Chandel, A.; King, C.S. Pulmonary Hypertension in Interstitial Lung Disease: Updates in Disease, Diagnosis, and Therapeutics. *Cells* **2023**, *12*, 2394. [CrossRef]
14. Denton, C.P.; Wells, A.U.; Coghlan, J.G. Major lung complications of systemic sclerosis. *Nat. Rev. Rheumatol.* **2018**, *14*, 511–527. [CrossRef] [PubMed]
15. Lafyatis, R. Transforming growth factor β—At the centre of systemic sclerosis. *Nat. Rev. Rheumatol.* **2014**, *10*, 706–719. [CrossRef] [PubMed]
16. Shumnalieva, R.; Kachakova, D.; Kaneva, R.; Kolarov, Z.; Monov, S. Serum miR-21 and miR-29a expression in systemic sclerosis patients. *Clin. Exp. Rheumatol.* **2023**, *41*, 1688–1694. [CrossRef] [PubMed]
17. Bhattacharyya, S.; Wei, J.; Varga, J. Understanding fibrosis in systemic sclerosis: Shifting paradigms, emerging opportunities. *Nat. Rev. Rheumatol.* **2011**, *8*, 42–54. [CrossRef] [PubMed] [PubMed Central]
18. Nihtyanova, S.I.; Denton, C.P. Scleroderma Lung Involvement, Autoantibodies, and Outcome Prediction: The Confounding Effect of Time. *J. Rheumatol.* **2017**, *44*, 404–406. [CrossRef] [PubMed]
19. Hassoun, P.M. Lung involvement in systemic sclerosis. *Presse Med.* **2011**, *40*, e25–e39. [CrossRef] [PubMed] [PubMed Central]
20. Muruganandam, M.; Ariza-Hutchinson, A.; Patel, R.A.; Sibbitt, W.L., Jr. Biomarkers in the Pathogenesis, Diagnosis, and Treatment of Systemic Sclerosis. *J. Inflamm. Res.* **2023**, *ume 16*, 4633–4660. [CrossRef] [PubMed] [PubMed Central]
21. Mulkoju, R.; Saka, V.K.; Rajaram, M.; Kumari, R.; Negi, V.S.; Mohapatra, M.M.; Govindaraj, V.; Dwivedi, D.P.; Babu, V.M. Pulmonary Manifestations in Systemic Sclerosis: Hospital-Based Descriptive Study. *Cureus* **2020**, *12*, e8649. [CrossRef] [PubMed] [PubMed Central]

22. Cavazzana, I.; Vojinovic, T.; Airo', P.; Fredi, M.; Ceribelli, A.; Pedretti, E.; Lazzaroni, M.G.; Garrafa, E.; Franceschini, F. Systemic Sclerosis-Specific Antibodies: Novel and Classical Biomarkers. *Clin. Rev. Allergy Immunol.* **2023**, *64*, 412–430. [CrossRef] [PubMed]
23. Doskaliuk, B.; Zaiats, L.; Yatsyshyn, R.; Gerych, P.; Cherniuk, N.; Zimba, O. Pulmonary involvement in systemic sclerosis: Exploring cellular, genetic and epigenetic mechanisms. *Rheumatol. Int.* **2020**, *40*, 1555–1569. [CrossRef] [PubMed]
24. Stochmal, A.; Czuwara, J.; Trojanowska, M.; Rudnicka, L. Antinuclear Antibodies in Systemic Sclerosis: An Update. *Clin. Rev. Allergy Immunol.* **2020**, *58*, 40–51. [CrossRef]
25. Khedoe, P.; Marges, E.; Hiemstra, P.; Ninaber, M.; Geelhoed, M. Interstitial Lung Disease in Patients with Systemic Sclerosis: Toward Personalized-Medicine-Based Prediction and Drug Screening Models of Systemic Sclerosis-Related Interstitial Lung Disease (SSc-ILD). *Front. Immunol.* **2020**, *11*, 1990. [CrossRef] [PubMed]
26. Deepa, A.; Rachel, R.P.; Ramchandran, P.; Devaraj, U.; Arnold, S.A.; Shobha, V.; D'Souza, G. Pulmonary involvement in systemic sclerosis: A clinical profile. *Lung India* **2016**, *33*, 144–147. [CrossRef] [PubMed] [PubMed Central]
27. Perelas, A.; Arrossi, A.V.; Highland, K.B. Pulmonary Manifestations of Systemic Sclerosis and Mixed Connective Tissue Disease. *Clin. Chest Med.* **2019**, *40*, 501–518. [CrossRef]
28. Solomon, J.J.; Olson, A.L.; Fischer, A.; Bull, T.; Brown, K.K.; Raghu, G. Scleroderma lung disease. *Eur. Respir. Rev.* **2013**, *22*, 6–19. [CrossRef] [PubMed] [PubMed Central]
29. Khanna, D.; Distler, O.; Cottin, V.; Brown, K.K.; Chung, L.; Goldin, J.G.; Matteson, E.L.; Kazerooni, E.A.; Walsh, S.L.; McNitt-Gray, M.; et al. Diagnosis and monitoring of systemic sclerosis-associated interstitial lung disease using high-resolution computed tomography. *J. Scleroderma Relat. Disord.* **2022**, *7*, 168–178. [CrossRef] [PubMed] [PubMed Central]
30. Di Maggio, G.; Confalonieri, P.; Salton, F.; Trotta, L.; Ruggero, L.; Kodric, M.; Geri, P.; Hughes, M.; Bellan, M.; Gilio, M.; et al. Biomarkers in Systemic Sclerosis: An Overview. *Curr. Issues Mol. Biol.* **2023**, *45*, 7775–7802. [CrossRef] [PubMed] [PubMed Central]
31. Wijsenbeek, M.; Suzuki, A.; Maher, T.M. Interstitial lung diseases. *Lancet* **2022**, *400*, 769–786. [CrossRef] [PubMed]
32. Ota, Y.; Kuwana, M. Updates on genetics in systemic sclerosis. *Inflamm. Regen.* **2021**, *41*, 17. [CrossRef]
33. Stock, C.J.W.; Renzoni, E.A. Genetic predictors of systemic sclerosis-associated interstitial lung disease: A review of recent literature. *Eur. J. Hum. Genet.* **2018**, *26*, 765–777. [CrossRef] [PubMed] [PubMed Central]
34. Dieudé, P.; Guedj, M.; Wipff, J.; Ruiz, B.; Riemekasten, G.; Airo, P.; Melchers, I.; Hachulla, E.; Cerinic, M.M.; Diot, E.; et al. *NLRP1* influences the systemic sclerosis phenotype: A new clue for the contribution of innate immunity in systemic sclerosis-related fibrosing alveolitis pathogenesis. *Ann. Rheum. Dis.* **2011**, *70*, 668–674. [CrossRef] [PubMed]
35. Sato, S.; Nagaoka, T.; Hasegawa, M.; Tamatani, T.; Nakanishi, T.; Takigawa, M.; Takehara, K. Serum levels of connective tissue growth factor are elevated in patients with systemic sclerosis: Association with extent of skin sclerosis and severity of pulmonary fibrosis. *J. Rheumatol.* **2000**, *27*, 149–154.
36. Dieudé, P.; Boileau, C.; Guedj, M.; Avouac, J.; Ruiz, B.; Hachulla, E.; Diot, E.; Cracowski, J.L.; Tiev, K.; Sibilia, J.; et al. Independent replication establishes the CD247 gene as a genetic systemic sclerosis susceptibility factor. *Ann. Rheum. Dis.* **2011**, *70*, 1695–1696. [CrossRef]
37. Wajda, A.; Walczyk, M.; Dudek, E.; Stypińska, B.; Lewandowska, A.; Romanowska-Próchnicka, K.; Chojnowski, M.; Olesińska, M.; Paradowska-Gorycka, A. Serum microRNAs in Systemic Sclerosis, Associations with Digital Vasculopathy and Lung Involvement. *Int. J. Mol. Sci.* **2022**, *23*, 10731. [CrossRef] [PubMed]
38. Li, Y.; Huang, J.; Hu, C.; Zhou, J.; Xu, D.; Hou, Y.; Wu, C.; Zhao, J.; Li, M.; Zeng, X.; et al. MicroRNA-320a: An important regulator in the fibrotic process in interstitial lung disease of systemic sclerosis. *Arthritis Res. Ther.* **2021**, *23*, 1–11. [CrossRef]
39. Mora, G.F. Systemic Sclerosis: Environmental Factors. *J. Rheumatol.* **2009**, *36*, 2383–2396. [CrossRef] [PubMed]
40. Maria, A.T.J.; Partouche, L.; Goulabchand, R.; Rivière, S.; Rozier, P.; Bourgier, C.; Le Quellec, A.; Morel, J.; Noël, D.; Guilpain, P. Intriguing Relationships Between Cancer and Systemic Sclerosis: Role of the Immune System and Other Contributors. *Front. Immunol.* **2019**, *9*, 3112. [CrossRef] [PubMed] [PubMed Central]
41. Truchetet, M.E.; Brembilla, N.C.; Chizzolini, C. Current Concepts on the Pathogenesis of Systemic Sclerosis. *Clin. Rev. Allergy Immunol.* **2023**, *64*, 262–283. [CrossRef] [PubMed] [PubMed Central]
42. Coghlan, J.G.; Denton, C.P.; Grünig, E.; Bonderman, D.; Distler, O.; Khanna, D.; Müller-Ladner, U.; Pope, J.E.; Vonk, M.C.; Doelberg, M.; et al. Evidence-based detection of pulmonary arterial hypertension in systemic sclerosis: The DETECT study. *Ann. Rheum. Dis.* **2014**, *73*, 1340–1349. [CrossRef] [PubMed] [PubMed Central]
43. Williams, M.H.; Handler, C.E.; Akram, R.; Smith, C.J.; Das, C.; Smee, J.; Nair, D.; Denton, C.P.; Black, C.M.; Coghlan, J.G. Role of N-terminal brain natriuretic peptide (N-TproBNP) in scleroderma-associated pulmonary arterial hypertension. *Eur. Heart J.* **2006**, *27*, 1485–1494. [CrossRef]
44. Nagaya, N.; Nishikimi, T.; Uematsu, M.; Satoh, T.; Kyotani, S.; Sakamaki, F.; Kakishita, M.; Fukushima, K.; Okano, Y.; Nakanishi, N.; et al. Plasma brain natriuretic peptide as a prognostic indicator in patients with primary pulmonary hypertension. *Circulation* **2000**, *102*, 865–870. [CrossRef]
45. Papaioannou, A.I.; Zakynthinos, E.; Kostikas, K.; Kiropoulos, T.; Koutsokera, A.; Ziogas, A.; Koutroumpas, A.; Sakkas, L.; Gourgoulianis, K.I.; Daniil, Z.D. Serum VEGF levels are related to the presence of pulmonary arterial hypertension in systemic sclerosis. *BMC Pulm. Med.* **2009**, *9*, 18. [CrossRef]

46. Meadows, C.A.; Risbano, M.G.; Zhang, L.; Geraci, M.W.; Tuder, R.M.; Collier, D.H.; Bull, T.M. Increased expression of growth differentiation factor-15 in systemic sclerosis-associated pulmonary arterial hypertension. *Chest* **2011**, *139*, 994–1002. [CrossRef] [PubMed]
47. George, P.M.; Oliver, E.; Dorfmuller, P.; Dubois, O.D.; Reed, D.M.; Kirkby, N.S.; Mohamed, N.A.; Perros, F.; Antigny, F.; Fadel, E.; et al. Evidence for the involvement of type I interferon in pulmonary arterial hypertension. *Circ. Res.* **2014**, *114*, 677–688. [CrossRef] [PubMed]
48. Eloranta, M.-L.; Franck-Larsson, K.; Lövgren, T.; Kalamajski, S.; Rönnblom, A.; Rubin, K.; Alm, G.V.; Rönnblom, L. Type I interferon system activation and association with disease manifestations in systemic sclerosis. *Ann. Rheum. Dis.* **2010**, *69*, 1396–1402. [CrossRef]
49. Hudson, M.; Mahler, M.; Pope, J.; You, D.; Tatibouet, S.; Steele, R.; Baron, M.; Canadian Scleroderma Research Group; Fritzler, M. Clinical correlates of CENP-A and CENP-B antibodies in a large cohort of patients with systemic sclerosis. *J. Rheumatol.* **2012**, *39*, 787–794. [CrossRef]
50. Mitri, G.M.; Lucas, M.; Fertig, N.; Steen, V.D.; Medsger, T.A. A comparison between anti-Th/To–and anticentromere antibody–positive systemic sclerosis patients with limited cutaneous involvement. *Arthritis Rheum.* **2003**, *48*, 203–209. [CrossRef]
51. Becker, M.O.; Kill, A.; Kutsche, M.; Guenther, J.; Rose, A.; Tabeling, C.; Witzenrath, M.; Kühl, A.A.; Heidecke, H.; Ghofrani, H.A.; et al. Vascular receptor autoantibodies in pulmonary arterial hypertension associated with systemic sclerosis. *Am. J. Respir. Crit. Care Med.* **2014**, *190*, 808–817. [CrossRef] [PubMed]
52. Launay, D.; Sitbon, O.; Cordier, J.-F.; Hachulla, E.; Mouthon, L.; Gressin, V.; Rottat, L.; Clerson, P.; Simonneau, G.; Humbert, M. Survival and prognostic factors in patients with incident systemic sclerosis-associated pulmonary arterial hypertension from the french registry. *Eur. Respir. J.* **2011**, *38*, 2338. [CrossRef]
53. Zhang, C.Y.; Ma, L.L.; Wang, L.X. Relationship between serum uric acid levels and ventricular function in patients with idiopathic pulmonary hypertension. *Exp. Clin. Cardiol.* **2013**, *18*, e37–e39. [PubMed]
54. Galiè, N.; Humbert, M.; Vachiery, J.L.; Gibbs, S.; Lang, I.; Torbicki, A.; Hoeper, M. 2015 ESC/ERS guidelines for the diagnosis and treatment of pulmonary hypertension: The Joint Task Force for the Diagnosis and Treatment of Pulmonary Hypertension of the European Society of Cardiology (ESC) and the European Respiratory Society (ERS): Endorsed by: Association for European Paediatric and Congenital Cardiology (AEPC), International Society for Heart and Lung Transplantation (ISHLT). *Eur. Heart J.* **2016**, *37*, 67–119. [CrossRef] [PubMed]
55. Kowal-Bielecka, O.; Fransen, J.; Avouac, J.; Becker, M.; Kulak, A.; Allanore, Y.; Distler, O.; Clements, P.; Cutolo, M.; Czirjak, L.; et al. Update of EULAR recommendations for the treatment of systemic sclerosis. *Ann. Rheum. Dis.* **2017**, *76*, 1327–1339. [CrossRef] [PubMed]
56. Dawson, J.K.; Quah, E.; Earnshaw, B.; Amoasii, C.; Mudawi, T.; Spencer, L.G. Does methotrexate cause progressive fibrotic interstitial lung disease? A systematic review. *Rheumatol. Int.* **2021**, *41*, 1055–1064. [CrossRef]
57. Tashkin, D.P.; Elashoff, R.; Clements, P.J.; Goldin, J.; Roth, M.D.; Furst, D.E.; Arriola, E.; Silver, R.; Strange, C.; Bolster, M.; et al. Cyclophosphamide versus Placebo in Scleroderma Lung Disease. *New Engl. J. Med.* **2006**, *354*, 2655–2666. [CrossRef]
58. Tashkin, D.P.; Roth, M.D.; Clements, P.J.; Furst, D.E.; Khanna, D.; Kleerup, E.C.; Goldin, J.; Arriola, E.; Volkmann, E.R.; Kafaja, S.; et al. Mycophenolate mofetil versus oral cyclophosphamide in scleroderma-related interstitial lung disease (SLS II): A randomised controlled, double-blind, parallel group trial. *Lancet Respir. Med.* **2016**, *4*, 708–719. [CrossRef]
59. Funatogawa, T.; Narita, Y.; Tamura, A.; Mii, K.; Sugitani, Y.; Uchida, T. Use of mycophenolate mofetil for systemic sclerosis and systemic sclerosis-associated interstitial lung disease: Information from a Japanese hospital claims database. *Mod. Rheumatol.* **2022**, *32*, 755–760. [CrossRef]
60. Hoyles, R.K.; Ellis, R.W.; Wellsbury, J.; Lees, B.; Newlands, P.; Goh, N.S.L.; Roberts, C.; Desai, S.; Herrick, A.L.; McHugh, N.J.; et al. A multicenter, prospective, randomized, double-blind, placebo-controlled trial of corticosteroids and intravenous cyclophosphamide followed by oral azathioprine for the treatment of pulmonary fibrosis in scleroderma. *Arthritis Rheum.* **2006**, *54*, 3962–3970. [CrossRef] [PubMed]
61. Goswami, R.P.; Ray, A.; Chatterjee, M.; Mukherjee, A.; Sircar, G.; Ghosh, P. Rituximab in the treatment of systemic sclerosis–related interstitial lung disease: A systematic review and meta-analysis. *Rheumatology* **2021**, *60*, 557–567. [CrossRef]
62. Maher, T.M.; Tudor, V.A.; Saunders, P.; Gibbons, M.A.; Fletcher, S.V.; Denton, C.P.; Hoyles, R.K.; Parfrey, H.; Renzoni, E.A.; Kokosi, M.; et al. Rituximab versus intravenous cyclophosphamide in patients with connective tissue disease-associated interstitial lung disease in the UK (RECITAL): A double-blind, double-dummy, randomised, controlled, phase 2b trial. *Lancet Respir. Med.* **2023**, *11*, 45–54. [CrossRef]
63. Okuda, Y. Review of tocilizumab in the treatment of rheumatoid arthritis. *Biol. Targets Ther.* **2008**, *2*, 75–82. [CrossRef] [PubMed] [PubMed Central]
64. Roofeh, D.; Lin, C.J.F.; Goldin, J.; Kim, G.H.; Furst, D.E.; Denton, C.P.; Huang, S.; Khanna, D.; focuSSced Investigators. Tocilizumab Prevents Progression of Early Systemic Sclerosis–Associated Interstitial Lung Disease. *Arthritis Rheumatol.* **2021**, *73*, 1301–1310. [CrossRef] [PubMed] [PubMed Central]
65. Khanna, D.; Denton, C.P.; Jahreis, A.; van Laar, J.M.; Frech, T.M.; Anderson, M.E.; Baron, M.; Chung, L.; Fierlbeck, G.; Lakshminarayanan, S.; et al. Safety and efficacy of subcutaneous tocilizumab in adults with systemic sclerosis (faSScinate): A phase 2, randomised, controlled trial. *Lancet* **2016**, *387*, 2630–2640. [CrossRef] [PubMed]

66. Khanna, D.; Lin, C.J.F.; Furst, D.E.; Goldin, J.; Kim, G.; Kuwana, M.; Allanore, Y.; Matucci-Cerinic, M.; Distler, O.; Shima, Y.; et al. Tocilizumab in systemic sclerosis: A randomised, double-blind, placebo-controlled, phase 3 trial. *Lancet Respir. Med.* **2020**, *8*, 963–974. [CrossRef]
67. Kuster, S.; Jordan, S.; Elhai, M.; Held, U.; Steigmiller, K.; Bruni, C., Cacciapaglia, F.; Vettori, S.; Siegert, E.; Rednic, S.; et al. Effectiveness and safety of tocilizumab in patients with systemic sclerosis: A propensity score matched controlled observational study of the EUSTAR cohort. *RMD Open* **2022**, *8*, e002477. [CrossRef] [PubMed] [PubMed Central]
68. Bolcto, G.; Avouac, J.; Allanore, Y. The role of antifibrotic therapies in the treatment of systemic sclerosis–associated interstitial lung disease. *Ther. Adv. Musculoskelet. Dis.* **2022**, *14*, 1759720X211066686. [CrossRef] [PubMed] [PubMed Central]
69. Pope, J.E.; Denton, C.P.; Johnson, S.R.; Fernandez-Codina, A.; Hudson, M.; Nevskaya, T. State-of-the-art evidence in the treatment of systemic sclerosis. *Nat. Rev. Rheumatol.* **2023**, *19*, 212–226. [CrossRef] [PubMed]
70. Maron, B.A. Revised Definition of Pulmonary Hypertension and Approach to Management: A Clinical Primer. *J. Am. Heart Assoc.* **2023**, *12*, e029024. [CrossRef] [PubMed]
71. Hardinge, M.; Annandale, J.; Bourne, S.; Cooper, B.; Evans, A.; Freeman, D.; Green, A.; Hippolyte, S.; Knowles, V.; MacNee, W.; et al. British Thoracic Society guidelines for home oxygen use in adults: Accredited by NICE. *Thorax* **2015**, *70*, i1–i43. [CrossRef] [PubMed]
72. Nutrition and Pulmonary Fibrosis. American Lung Association. Available online: https://www.lung.org/lung-health-diseases/lung-disease-lookup/pulmonary-fibrosis/patients/living-well-with-pulmonary-fibrosis/nutrition#:~:text=Eating%20a%20bland%20diet,%20made,BRAT%20diet),%20can%20help (accessed on 1 August 2024).
73. Biney, I.; Dudney, T.; Goldman, M.; Carder, L.; Schriver, E. Successful Use of Hyperbaric Oxygen as Adjunctive Therapy for a Nonhealing Venous Ulcer in a Patient with Systemic Sclerosis and Pulmonary Arterial Hypertension: A Case Report and Review of the Literature. *Case Rep. Pulmonol.* **2020**, *2020*, 4750375. [CrossRef] [PubMed]
74. Mugii, N.; Hamaguchi, Y.; Maddali-Bongi, S. Clinical significance and usefulness of rehabilitation for systemic sclerosis. *J. Scleroderma Relat. Disord.* **2018**, *3*, 71–80. [CrossRef] [PubMed]
75. Murphy, S.L.; Poole, J.L.; Chen, Y.T.; Lescoat, A.; Khanna, D. Rehabilitation Interventions in Systemic Sclerosis: A Systematic Review and Future Directions. *Arthritis Care Res.* **2022**, *74*, 59–69. [CrossRef] [PubMed]
76. Bohdziewicz, A.; Pawlik, K.K.; Maciejewska, M.; Sikora, M.; Alda-Malicka, R.; Czuwara, J.; Rudnicka, L. Future Treatment Options in Systemic Sclerosis—Potential Targets and Ongoing Clinical Trials. *J. Clin. Med.* **2022**, *11*, 1310. [CrossRef]

sclerosis

MDPI

Systematic Review

The Metabolomic View of Systemic Sclerosis—A Systematic Literature Review

Sebastian T. Jendrek [1,*], Franziska Schmelter [2], Christian Sina [2,3], Ulrich L. Günther [4] and Gabriela Riemekasten [1]

1 Clinic for Rheumatology and Clinical Immunology, University Hospital Schleswig-Holstein, Campus Lübeck, 23562 Lübeck, Germany; gabriela.riemekasten@uksh.de
2 Institute of Nutritional Medicine, University of Lübeck, 23562 Lübeck, Germany; franziska.schmelter@uksh.de (F.S.); christian.sina@uksh.de (C.S.)
3 Medical Department I, University Hospital Schleswig-Holstein, 23562 Lübeck, Germany
4 Institute of Chemistry and Metabolomics, University of Lübeck, 23562 Lübeck, Germany; ulrich.guenther@uni-luebeck.de
* Correspondence: sebastiantorben.jendrek@uksh.de

Abstract: The mortality risk in systemic sclerosis (SSc) is primarily determined by pulmonary involvement (interstitial lung disease (ILD), pulmonary fibrosis), pulmonary arterial hypertension (PAH), and cardiac involvement. With timely and intensive treatment, the disease can be halted or even improved. Therefore, early diagnosis remains crucial. Unfortunately, biomarkers currently available cannot meet this requirement. SSc is characterized by autoimmune inflammation, vasculopathy, and fibrosis. The immunometabolic characterization of autoimmune diseases contributes to a better understanding of the underlying inflammatory processes. In this narrative review, we included 13 studies on metabolomic patterns in SSc in accordance with the Preferred Reporting Items for Systematic Reviews and Meta-Analyses Guidelines (PRISMA). Current studies indicate an altered metabolome in SSc. All documented significant differences between patients with SSc and healthy controls, although the observed metabolomic patterns in SSc were inconsistent between studies. Metabolome alterations include, in particular, energy-related metabolic pathways such as glycolysis/gluconeogenesis, including the synthesis and degradation of ketones, fatty acid oxidation, amino acid-related metabolic pathways, lipid metabolism, and the tricarboxylic acid (TCA) cycle, including pyruvate metabolism. The most frequently examined organ complications with reported significant aberrations of the metabolome were skin involvement, ILD, and PAH. Conclusion: The detailed characterization of the SSc-specific metabolome promises a more comprehensive understanding of the pathogenic mechanisms of the disease. Furthermore, the detection of associations between specific metabolic aberrations and disease phenotypes bears hope for new biomarkers and an improved personalized approach to diagnostics, therapy, and follow-up in the management of SSc.

Keywords: metabolomics; metabolome; systemic sclerosis; biomarkers

1. Introduction

Systemic sclerosis (SSc) is a life-threatening rheumatic disease characterized by autoimmunity, vasculopathy, and inflammatory fibrosis, which represents an immense burden for patients due to its high morbidity and mortality [1–4]. In addition to a significant impairment in quality of life, the disease burden of SSc exceeds that of other rheumatic diseases [5,6]. A causal therapeutic approach does not exist. SSc is characterized by heterogeneous clinical symptoms, among which interstitial lung disease (ILD) with development of fibrosis, idiopathic and associated pulmonary arterial hypertension (PAH), and cardiac involvement are prognostically relevant [6]. Of note, these manifestations of systemic sclerosis are often clinically oligo or asymptomatic in the initial phase and develop slowly over time. Therefore, it is standard practice to use comprehensive clinical, radiological, and laboratory analyses to phenotype patients at initial presentation [7,8]. Early and accurate diagnosis of both the underlying disease and emerging organ involvement is crucial. The assessment of the individual disease course, particularly with regard to the prognostically pertinent risk of visceral organ involvement, represents an unsolved burden in daily clinical practice. Apart from the modified Rodnan Skin Score (mRSS), the autoantibody profile, and capillary microscopy [9–11], no biomarkers are routinely used, and individual prognosis remains difficult to estimate [6]. Consequently, there remains an unmet need for new biomarkers to determine disease activity and assess SSc-associated prognosis. With regard to pathogenesis, SSc is increasingly understood as a complex interplay between environmental factors and the development of autoantibodies. In the early active phase of the disease, inflammatory and vasculopathic mechanisms seem to predominate, whereas fibrosing processes become more dominant over time [12]. Furthermore, microvasculopathy with activation of endothelial cells, as well as surrounding perimyocytes and smooth muscle cells, has been observed. Humoral and cellular factors activate aberrant fibroblasts, leading to excessive extracellular matrix production and subsequent fibrosis of the skin and organs [13–17]. Environmental factors appear to modulate the risk of developing SSc [18]. For instance, individual case reports in the 1980s pointed to factors impairing tryptophan metabolism as possible modulators in the pathogenesis of scleroderma-like illness [19]. More recently, changes in the intestinal microbiome (dysbiosis) have been described in SSc [20,21]. Microbial communities play an essential role in host physiology and have profound effects on immune homeostasis and the host metabolome, either directly or via their metabolites and/or components. Thus, metabolomic analyses provide insights beyond metabolic and energy status. For example, metabolites and metabolic pathways influence post-translational modifications [22] of DNA and histones, thereby affecting gene expression [23,24]. Metabolic activities can also regulate apoptosis sensitivity [25,26] and serve as cellular or pathogen-derived RNA-binding proteins [27]. Finally, some metabolites act directly as pro- or anti-inflammatory signaling molecules [28–30]. Most SSc patients clinically show a body composition that differs significantly from healthy controls (HCs) (e.g., muscle function/bone density) [31].

Metabolomics is the comprehensive analytical characterization and large-scale scientific study of small molecules, commonly referred to as metabolites, within an organism, biofluids, cells, or tissues [32,33]. Despite variations in definition, Robert D. Hall defined the metabolome as the entirety of low-molecular-weight products within an organism, with a mass of less than 1500 Da [34]. These metabolites play critical roles in biological systems, acting as intermediates as well as end products of cellular processes, thereby reflecting the biochemical activity and physiological state of the organism. By profiling metabolites, metabolomics offers valuable insights into the underlying mechanisms of health, disease, and environmental interactions [32]. Two of the most powerful analytical techniques in metabolomics are mass spectrometry (MS) and nuclear magnetic resonance (NMR) spectroscopy. Mass spectrometry is characterized by its high sensitivity and selectivity. Furthermore, it can be coupled with various chromatographic separation systems, such as liquid chromatography (LC), gas chromatography (GC), and capillary electrophoresis (CE). These combinations reduce ion suppression, separate isobaric compounds, minimize the signal-to-noise ratio, and ultimately improve detection limits and spectrum complexity. Most commonly, LC and GC couplings with high-resolution mass spectrometry are used in metabolomic research. LC separates complex mixtures of metabolites based on their chemical properties, such as polarity and hydrophobicity, using a liquid mobile phase. Gas chromatography, by contrast, utilizes a gaseous mobile phase and is suited for volatile compounds. The mass spectrometer identifies and quantifies compounds by measuring their mass-to-charge (m/z) ratio. However, mass spectrometry has limitations, including the often extensive sample preparation, the complexity of processing large datasets, and notably, reduced reproducibility. NMR spectroscopy, on the other hand, offers a non-destructive approach to metabolomics by exploiting the magnetic properties of atomic nuclei. NMR provides highly reproducible and quantitative data, along with structural information about metabolites. Its ability to analyze complex mixtures without extensive sample preparation makes it a valuable tool in metabolomics. Nonetheless, the technique has disadvantages, such as lower sensitivity compared to MS. Signal overlap in complex NMR spectra, compounded by limited coupling possibilities, restricts the number of detectable and quantifiable metabolites [35,36]. In summary, the comprehensive analysis of the metabolome is challenged by its diversity and dynamic nature. MS and NMR are complementary techniques, each offering unique advantages for elucidating the intricate network of metabolites. Their integration is facilitating deeper biological insights and biomarker discovery [36].

Consequently, metabolomic analyses in SSc offer promising opportunities to expand our knowledge of pathogenesis, SSc-specific immunometabolism, phenotyping, prognostic characterization, and risk stratification.

2. Methods and Search Strategy

A systematic review of all papers published in English on the topic of metabolome analyses in systemic sclerosis was carried out using the databases PubMed, Scopus, and Web of Science in accordance with the Preferred Reporting Items for Systematic Reviews and Meta-Analyses Guidelines (PRISMA) [37] (Figure 1). The search terms/keywords used were ("metabolome") AND ("systemic sclerosis"), ("metabolome") AND ("scleroderma"), ("chromatography–mass spectrometry") AND ("systemic sclerosis"), ("chromatography–mass spectrometry") AND ("scleroderma"), ("NMR") AND ("systemic sclerosis"), ("NMR") AND ("scleroderma"). The time span of the publications was 2015–2025. The time of the systematic literature search was December 2024. Titles and abstracts were first reviewed for topical relevance, followed by a full-text review by the authors independently to ensure only articles that met the predefined inclusion and exclusion criteria were included. Our protocol is registered on the International Platform of Registered Systematic Review and Meta-analysis Protocols (INPLASY) under doi: 10.37766/inplasy2025.5.0077.

Inclusion criteria:

- Original research articles (cohort, case control studies), addressing the human, adult serum or plasma metabolome in SSc, published without restriction to a single metabolite and published in English within the last ten years.
- Use of HPLC/UPLC-MS or LC-MS or 1H-NMR.
- SSc diagnosis according to the 2013 American College of Rheumatology and European League Against Rheumatism ACR/EULAR classification criteria.

The exclusion criteria were defined as follows:

- Studies focusing on other biological samples, e.g., urine.
- In vitro studies.

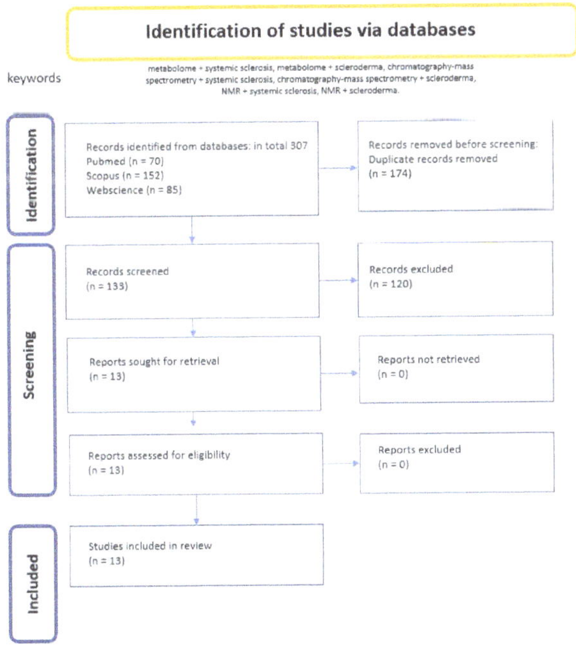

Figure 1. PRISMA 2020 flow diagram according to [37].

3. Results

A total of 307 papers were found. After applying the criteria described above, 13 papers were selected that met our criteria.

3.1. Serum or Plasma Metabolome in Systemic Sclerosis

A total of 17 studies on the serum or plasma metabolome in systemic sclerosis were identified that met the predefined inclusion criteria. Two of these studies did not primarily focus on SSc but either looked at connective tissue diseases in general [38] or analyzed the metabolome in systemic lupus erythematosus (SLE) and used SSc as a control group [39]. The number of SSc patients included in the individual studies varied between 19 and 206. The work of Xie et al. [40], which carried out a meta-analysis based on genome-wide association study (GWAS) data for plasma metabolites (taken from the GWAS catalog (GCST90199621-GCST90204603)) and included a total of 26,679 people (9095 SSc patients and 17,584 healthy controls), should be considered separately at this point. The individuals in this study came from 14 European–American SSc GWAS cohorts from a total of 10 countries. The plasma metabolite data included 1091 blood metabolites and 309 metabolite ratios. The majority of the studies report the serological status and clinical presentation, such as the limited and diffuse cutaneous form of SSc (lcSSc/dcSSc) of the patients. In our selected studies for review, nine studies used plasma and eight studies used serum for the analysis. Where healthy subjects were included as controls, significant differences between the metabolome of SSc and HCs were found. Eleven studies reported specific metabolomic fingerprints with respect to clinical subtype or organ involvement. One study postulated causal effects of specific gut microbiota and plasma metabolites on the development of SSc [40]. In the following, the study results on specific metabolome profiles or altered metabolome pathways will be presented from a clinical perspective, sorted according to the categories (I.) skin manifestations, (II.) interstitial lung disease/fibrosis, (III.) pulmonary arterial hypertension (PAH), and (IV.) disease prognosis or treatment response.

3.2. Skin Manifestation

Several metabolite changes were described in association with cutaneous manifestations in SSc, identifying both parameters with positive and negative correlation to skin fibrosis. Guo et al. [41] demonstrated a negative correlation between allysine and all-trans-retinoic acid (which also correlated with inflammatory parameters). Markers that correlated positively with mRSS in this study population were D-glucuronic acid and hexanoylcarnitine. Furthermore, sclerodactyly was negatively associated with thromboxane B2 and positively associated with phthalic acid.

In vitro background data support the role of amino acids in the immunometabolism of skin fibrosis in SSc, while increased collagen synthesis appears to be a concomitant symptom of cutaneous fibrosis. Interestingly, Ung et al. demonstrated an upregulation of amino acid metabolites such as glutamine, ornithine, proline, and citrulline, which are involved in collagen metabolism [42]. It is known that proline is required for collagen production and the synthesis of the extracellular matrix [43]. Proline is also present in increased amounts in fibroblasts stimulated with transforming growth factor beta (TGF-β) [44]. Glutamine, in turn, promotes proline synthesis and supports collagen production in fibroblasts [45]. With regard to glutamate metabolism, it has been shown that under the influence of TGF-β1, myofibroblasts have increased glutamate levels, while glutamine levels decrease, indicating accelerated glutaminolysis. Glutaminolysis is considered to be one of the main energy sources for effector T cells and facilitates the pro-inflammatory Th17 phenotype [46]. Smoleńska et al. [47] specifically investigated the amino acid metabolome in SSc, showing correlations between amino acids and their derivatives and clinical skin manifestations. In the diffuse cutaneous subtype (dcSSc), increased concentrations of sarcosine, β-alanine, methylnicotinamide (MNA), and L-NAME (N-nitroarginine methyl ester) were detectable. Calcinosis correlated positively with sarcosine, glutamate, proline, tyrosine, 3-methylhistidine, and ornithine levels. The extent of skin fibrosis measured by mRSS showed a negative correlation with sarcosine, proline, histidine, ornithine, asparagine, citrulline, and phenylalanine. L-NAME, glutamate, and lysine were associated with the increased occurrence of telangiectasias. This study revealed changes in amino acid metabolism, which could represent a link to SSc-associated vasculopathy. An increase in asymmetric dimethylarginine (ADMA) was detected. ADMA is an inhibitor of NO synthase, which supports the assumption of endothelial damage as the etiology of SSc.

However, besides alterations in amino acid pattern in the context of skin fibrosis in SSc, changes in lipid metabolism have also been observed. Recently, growing evidence suggests that changes in lipid metabolism could have a general influence on the modulation of fibrosis, immunity, and angiopathy in SSc [48]. Sphingomyelins were detected in reduced concentrations, which correlated with greater skin involvement [49]. Some metabolites of sphingomyelin, such as sphingosine 1-phosphate, regulate immune cell chemotaxis, vascular dilation, and angiogenesis via G protein-coupled receptors. Stimulation of lymphocytes, monocytes, and fibroblasts by sphingosine 1-phosphate has been described [50], which could establish a connection to inflammatory skin fibrosis. Furthermore, a correlation between specific lipoproteins and the severity of skin fibrosis was described in a study that simultaneously identified a specific lipoprotein pattern in SSc-ILD [51]. Jendrek et al. were able to retrace a negative correlation of high-density lipoprotein (HDL) and (apolipoprotein (Apo) A1/A2 levels with skin fibrosis measured by mRSS as a validated clinical endpoint in SSc [9].

3.3. Focus on Interstitial Lung Involvement (ILD) and Pulmonary Fibrosis

Visceral organ manifestations—especially interstitial lung disease with pulmonary fibrosis, cardiac involvement, and pulmonary arterial hypertension—significantly determine SSc-associated lethality [6]. Therefore, new prognostic and personalized biomarkers are urgently needed. Dyslipoproteinemia and alterations in the lipid profile are frequently present in SSc patients [52]. Lipids serve various functions, including acting as signaling substances for the immune system. Lipid subgroups such as short-chain fatty acids (SCFA) also appear to influence the differentiation of T lymphocytes by modulating histone deacetylase activity [53]. For example, supplementation of SCFA butyrate has demonstrated anti-inflammatory effects in chronic inflammatory bowel disease [54]. Comparable effects in SSc have not yet been investigated. However, butyrate levels are also found to be reduced in individuals with SSc [55,56].

With regard to ILD, the work of Guo et al. [41] provides a comprehensive metabolic fingerprint. This analysis included 127 non-treated (59.8% female) and 57 treated (59.6% female) individuals. Serum samples were analyzed using LC-MS. Parameters positively associated with ILD were γ-linolenic acid, dihydrothymine, etiocholanol glucuronide, L-pipecolic acid, carnosine, and L-cystathione. A negative association with the ILD diagnosis existed for the parameters proline, betaine, androsterone sulfate, phloretin-2′-O-glucuronide, 4-guanidinobutanoic acid, and NNAL-N-glucuronide (4-(methylnitrosamino)-1-(3-pyridyl)-1-butanol-N-glucuronide). Notably, the study also described a negative correlation between L-tryptophan and inflammatory markers.

However, studies focusing on the metabolic signature of SSc-ILD have yielded inconsistent results. For example, Belocchi et al. [57] were unable to demonstrate any metabolomic difference between patients with and without ILD. However, metabolic differences were detected between SSc and HC in this study. Diacylglycerol 38:5, phosphatidylcholine 36:4, 1-(9Z-pentadecenoyl)-glycero-3-phosphate, DL-2-aminooctanoic acid, 2,4-dinitrobenzenesulfonic acid, and α-N-phenylacetyl-L-glutamine differed significantly from HC. 59 SSc individuals (88.1% female, 17.1% dcSSc, 39% ACA positive, 39% anti-scl70 positive) were included and analyzed using LC-MS plasma analysis. Special attention was paid to intestinal involvement and microbiota disturbances. Therefore, the authors found that intestinal microbiota analysis could also distinguish SSc patients from HC (reduced prevalence of nine bacterial species from Firmicutes, Bacteroidetes, and Proteobacteria families). In general, it is accepted that this dysbiosis can lead to reduced butyrate production. Bögl et al. [58] provided metabolic evidence of intestinal microbiome dysregulation, although no significant association with ILD was observed. This work primarily identified amino acids (dimethylarginine, citrulline, ornithine, 1-methylhistidine, taurine, 3-methylhistidine, tryptophan, alanine, tyrosine, methionine, lysine, proline), their derivatives, and other metabolites (kynurenine, TMAO, trimethyllysine, hexanoylcarnitine, acetylcarnitine, choline, octanoylcarnitine, valerylcarnitine) as dysregulated in SSc.

However, another study by Meier et al. [59], which focused on SSc-ILD, was able to identify a distinct metabolomic profile in SSc-ILD. This study involved a smaller cohort of 36 SSc individuals (83.3% female, 25% dSSc, 33.3% ACA positive, 27.8% anti-Scl70 positive), analyzed using targeted LC-MS (110 molecules) from serum samples. Differences were shown between non-ILD-SSc, stable ILD-SSc, and progressive ILD-SSc. Remarkably, 85 distinct substances were identified, including various amino acid metabolites. Concentrations of L-threonine, xanthosine, 3-aminoisobutyric acid, leucine, isoleucine, and adenosine monophosphate were associated with ILD and correlated with a deterioration in lung function tests. L-tyrosine, leucine, isoleucine, and L-tryptophan were discussed as potential SSc-ILD biomarkers. Additional SSc-ILD biomarkers (L-glutamine and Ile-Ala) were identified by Sun et al. [60], performing untargeted LC-MS of serum in a cohort of 30 SSc individuals (80% female, 40% dcSSc). They found 38 compounds at different concentrations, 32 of which demonstrated good diagnostic value (including vitamin E, various lipid metabolites, and amino acids). In addition, different patterns were observed for cutaneous subtypes (dcSSc and lcSSc).

Our own group [51] showed that patients with SSc-ILD and lung fibrosis display reduced HDL levels. Furthermore, a reduction in ApoA1 + A2 and its HDL fractions reflected a distinct lipoprotein profile for SSc-ILD patients, independent of potential clinical confounders for dyslipidemia. Notably, SSc-ILD HDL levels correlate with FVC (forced vital capacity), DLCO (diffusion capacity of the lungs for carbon monoxide), and mRSS. These results suggest that HDL and its subfractions may be considered as potential new biomarkers for SSc-ILD. The correlation with severity of lung involvement, measured by FVC and DLCO, as well as the independent correlation with mRSS, underlined the relevance of HDL and lipoprotein profiling in SSc-ILD.

Further evidence of pathological lipid metabolism in SSc was provided by Ottria et al. [61]. This study included a discovery cohort with 20 SSc individuals (85% female, 35% dcSSc, 55% ACA positive, 25% anti-scl70 positive) and a validation cohort with 12 SSc individuals (92% female, 16.7% dcSSc, 25% ACA positive, 50% anti-scl70 positive). In the discovery group, LC-MS was used, and in the validation group, GC-MS (for carnitine) and a fatty acid analysis (via LC-MS) in plasma were performed. Using untargeted LC-MS analysis, 46 metabolites that differed from HC were initially detected, indicating impaired fatty acid oxidation and renal dysfunction in the SSc. The targeted analysis focusing on fatty acids and carnitine concentrations identified significant differences in the concentrations of lauric acid, myristic acid, arachidic acid, carnitine, isovalerylcarnitine, octanoylcarnitine, and palmitoylcarnitine. In addition, in a functional assay, inhibition of carnitine transporters in dendritic cells from patients with SSc suppressed pro-inflammatory reactions. Therefore, the authors discuss L-carnitine and acylcarnitines as potential biomarkers for SSc.

A different metabolome signature of SSc-ILD vs. SSc patients without ILD was also shown in the work of Fernández-Ochoa et al. [49]. The authors compared the lcSSc and dcSSc groups but found no significant plasma differences between SSc-ILD and SSc-nonILD. However, in urine samples, deregulated metabolites were acylcarnitines, acylglycines, and again metabolites derived from amino acids, especially proline, histidine, and glutamine, which could become biomarkers for SSc-ILD. 2-arachidonoylglycerol, which is upregulated in SSc compared to HC, was also discussed as a possible biomarker given its role in the endocannabinoid system and possible involvement in SSc-associated autoimmunity.

In a subsequent study [38], Fernández-Ochoa et al. presented that urine analysis can achieve greater accuracy in the differentiation of SSc from mixed connective tissue disease (MCTD) and undifferentiated connective tissue disease (UCTD), as well as rheumatoid arthritis or systemic lupus erythematosus. Unfortunately, the authors did not provide any information on specific deviations in SSc within this cohort.

3.4. Focus on Pulmonary Arterial Hypertension (SSc-PAH)

Pulmonary arterial hypertension (PAH) is characterized by damage to the smaller arteries in the precapillary circulation of the pulmonary vessels and occurs with an average frequency of about 9% (5–15%) in SSc. However, it is one of the main causes of death in SSc [62,63]. PAH can occur as a primary condition or develop as a consequence of SSc-ILD. Early diagnosis is important, as studies have shown that early therapeutic intervention can improve survival rates [64]. Since some PAH-specific therapeutics mediate their effect by modulating intracellular endothelial metabolism, investigating immunometabolic changes in SSc-PAH is relevant.

Two studies compared metabolomic patterns between SSc patients with PAH and SSc patients without PAH [56,65]. Another study [66] also included idiopathic pulmonary arterial hypertension (IPAH) as a disease control. Deidda et al. [56] initially reported that patients with SSc-PAH showed higher levels of carboxylic acids (e.g., lactate) and lipoproteins, while amino acid levels, especially L-arginine, were reduced compared to patients with SSc without PAH. The study used NMR spectroscopy, directly analyzing pulmonary artery blood. In detail, SSc-PAH patients had increased concentrations of acetoacetic ester, alanine, lactate, VLDL and LDL levels, and decreased γ-aminobutyric acid, arginine, betaine, choline, creatine/creatinine, glucose, glutamate/glutamine, glycine, histidine, phenylalanine, and tyrosine levels. In addition, significantly higher ADMA levels and reduced L-arginine levels were documented in SSc-PAH compared to non-PAH patients [65]. In this study, serum ADMA levels ≥ 0.7 μM were also discussed as a diagnostic biomarker with a sensitivity of 86.7% and a specificity of 90.0% for PAH [65]. The work of Alotaibi et al. [66], including a disease control group, analyzed plasma from SSc patients with and without PAH as well as from patients with IPAH. They found nine metabolites characteristic of SSc-PAH (lignoceric acid, nervonic acid, fatty acid esters of hydroxy fatty acids, nitrooleate, 11-testosterone, 17β-estradiol, new eicosanoid, prostaglandin F2α, leukotriene B4). Among these, several parameters seemed to correlate with the severity of SSc-PAH. In this study, it was also noted that lignoceric acid and leukotriene B4 are present in higher concentrations in SSc without pulmonary hypertension. Overall, the above observations support the hypothesis of a dysregulated metabolism of fatty acids, steroid hormones, and arachidonic acid. Another study [67] demonstrated that dysregulation of the kynurenine pathway could serve as a predictor for the development of SSc-PAH. However, a correlation with other manifestations of SSc-associated microvasculopathy, such as Raynaud's syndrome or the occurrence of telangiectasias, could not be established in this cohort.

3.5. Focus on Further Prognostic Metabolome Signatures Including Treatment Response:

The heterogeneous disease manifestations of SSc with their variable and unpredictable courses justify the urgent need for diagnostic, personalized, and prognostic biomarkers. However, only a few studies provide information on treatment response, primarily due to limitations in the study design and small cohort sizes. However, the analysis of the metabolome can offer, e.g., prognostic information about the cutaneous disease severity. The most important metabolic pathways that were altered in dcSSc compared to lcSSc included glycolysis and gluconeogenesis as well as glutamate-glutamine metabolism [55]. The previously mentioned study by Guo et al. [41] not only analyzed the correlation of metabolomic parameters with mRSS but also examined metabolic changes in response to therapy-induced regression of skin involvement. They found that some of the deviating metabolites (γ-carboxyethylhydroxychroman (γ-CEHC), paraxanthine, PS(18:0/18:1(9z)), 2,3-diaminosalicylic acid, MG(0:0/182(9Z,12Z)/0:0), and phloretin-2′-O-glucuronide) normalized during treatment in the SSc group, suggesting their potential as biomarkers for cutaneous treatment response. Additional parameters, such as mediagenic acid-3-O-β-D-glucuronide, 4′-O-methyl-(-)-epicatechin-3′-O-β-glucuronide, and valproic acid glucuronide, were identified, although no causal relationship was established. Prognostic factors for SSc-ILD were considered in the study by Meier et al. [59]. The colleagues were able to distinguish progressive SSc-ILD from stable SSc-ILD based on several metabolome changes. This study showed that the levels of L-leucine and L-isoleucine were highest in HC and gradually decreased from SSc patients without ILD to those with stable ILD. In addition, L-tryptophan, L-tyrosine, L-threonine, and adenosine monophosphate showed a similar decline, while 3-aminoisobutyric acid and 1-methyladenosine showed an inverse trend. Based on this study, the determination of branched chain amino acids (BCAA: L-leucine and L-isoleucine) was discussed as prognostic biomarkers for the course of SSc-ILD. BCAA levels also correlated significantly with disease activity. In a separate BCAA assay, a cut-off value of 250.3 μM was defined for the differentiation of stable ILD from progressive ILD [59]. These results were confirmed by analysis of a validation cohort.

Table 1 presents a summary, including the characteristics of the groups ex-amined in the studies, as well as the techniques used and selected key findings of the pa-pers.

Table 1. Overview of the original articles included in this review, with the methods used and a selection of the specific key findings. Abbreviations: IPAH (idiopathic pulmonary arterial hypertension); ACA (anti-centromere antibodies); dcSSc (diffuse systemic sclerosis); HC (healthy controls); ILD (interstitial lung disease); mRSS (modified Rodnan skin score); SLE (systemic lupus erythematosus); SSc (systemic sclerosis); L-NAME (N-nitroarginine methyl ester); FVC (forced vital capacity); DLCO (diffusion capacity of the lungs for carbon monoxide); pulmonary arterial hypertension (PAH).

Original Papers	Cohort/Control	Analytical Technique, Method	Result Selection
Fernández-Ochoa Á et al., 2020 [38]	N = 43 SSc (83.6% female)/HC	liquid chromatography–mass spectrometry (LC-MS), plasma and urine analysis	Differences in L-kynurenine and N-acetylaspartylglutamic acid compared to controls. No further characterization of SSc individuals. Focus on other autoimmune diseases. Urine metabolites can tendentially achieve better accuracy.
Bengtsson AA et al., 2016 [39]	N = 19 SSc (84% female, 52.6% dcSSc, 42.1% ACA positive, 21%, anti-Scl70 positive)	gas chromatography–mass spectroscopy (GC-MS)	Focus on SLE, SSc individuals served as control, e.g., increase in arginine and simultaneous decrease in 2-oxoglutaric acid for SSc compared to HC and SLE.
Guo M et al., 2023 [41]	N = 127 SSc non-treated (59.8% female, 57 treated (59.6% female)	high-performance liquid chromatography–quadrupole-time-of-flight mass spectrometry (HPLC-Q-TOFMS)/MS	Starch and sucrose metabolism, proline metabolism, androgen and estrogen metabolism, and tryptophan metabolism dysregulated in new-onset SSc, but restored upon treatment. Allysine and all-trans-retinoic acid negatively correlated, while D-glucuronic acid and hexanoyl carnitine positively correlated with mRSS. Proline betaine, phloretin 2′-Oglucuronide, gamma-linolenic acid, and L-cystathionine associated with SSc-ILD.
Smolenska Z et al., 2020 [47]	N = 42 SSc (83.3% female, 50% dcSSc)	liquid chromatography–mass spectrometry (LC-MS)	Increase in concentrations of NO synthase (NOS) inhibitor asymmetric dimethylarginine (ADMA) in SSc vs. HC. NOS inhibitor L-NAME elevated in patients with dcSSc or telangiectasia.
Fernández-Ochoa Á et al., 2019 [49]	N = 59 SSc (88.1% female, 16.9% dcSSc, 39% ACA positive, 39% anti-Scl70 positive)/HC	reversed-phase high-performance liquid chromatography coupled to electrospray ionization-quadrupole-time-of-flight mass spectrometry (RP-HPLC–ESI-Q-TOF-MS)	Main parameters in urine were acylcarnitines, acylglycines and metabolites derived from amino acids (proline, histidine, and glutamine). Main plasma biomarker was 2-arachidonoylglycerol (potential crosslink to endocannabinoid system).

Table 1. *Cont.*

Original Papers	Cohort/Control	Analytical Technique, Method	Result Selection
Jendrek ST et al., 2024 [51]	N = 100 SSc (75% female, 38% dcSSc, 62% lcSSc, 31% SSc-ILD)/HC	proton nuclear magnetic resonance spectroscopy (1H-NMR)	Reduced HDL levels are linked to SSc-ILD independently from clinical confounders. High-density lipoprotein (HDL) and (HDL) apolipoprotein (Apo) A1/A2 levels positively correlate with parameters of lung involvement in SSc-ILD such as FVC and DLCO. HDL and (HDL) ApoA1/A2 levels negatively correlate with skin fibrosis in SSc patients with and without ILD.
Bellocchi C et al., 2018 [57]	N = 59 SSc (88.1% female, 17.1% dcSSc, 39% ACA-positive, 39% anti-scl70 positive)/HC	high-performance liquid chromatography–mass spectrometry (HPLC-MS); 16S rRNA gene amplification and sequencing (fecal microbiota)	Metabolomic alterations in glycerophospholipidmetabolites and benzene derivatives. Microbial and metabolic data showed significant interactions between Desulfovibrio and alpha-N-phenylacetyl-l-glutamine and 2,4-dinitrobenzenesulfonic acid.
Bögl T et al., 2022 [58]	N = 52 SSc (84.6% female, 21.2% dcSSc, 34.6% ACA positive, 32.7 anti-Scl70 positive)/HC [Exclusion criteria for control group: acute infections, liver and/or kidney diseases and diabetes]	high-performance liquid chromatography–mass spectrometry (HPLC-MS)	SSc-specific alterations, inter alia, in the kynurenine pathway, the urea cycle, lipid metabolism.
Meier C et al., 2020 [59]	N = 36 SSc (83.3% female, 25% dSSc, 33.3% ACA positive, 27.8% anti-Scl70 positive)/HC	targeted liquid chromatography–mass spectrometry (LC-MS)	SSc/HC-discriminating profile consisting of 4 amino acids and 3 purine metabolites (L-tyrosine, L-tryptophan, and 1-methyl-adenosine). Differentiation between progressing and stable SSc-ILD through L-leucine, L-isoleucine, xanthosine, and adenosine monophosphate. L-leucine and xanthosine negatively correlated with changes in FVC% and xanthosine negatively correlated with changes in DLCO%.
Sun C et al., 2023 [60]	N = 30 SSc (80% female, 40% dcSSc)	ultra-high-pressure liquid chromatography–quadrupole-time-of-fight mass spectrometry (UPLC-Q-TOF)	Fatty acids, amino acids, and glycerophospholipids, primarily altered in SSc patients. Glutamine metabolism primarily altered in SSc-ILD, whereas amino acid metabolism and steroid hormone biosynthesis primarily altered in leading skin fibrosis.

Table 1. *Cont.*

Original Papers	Cohort/Control	Analytical Technique, Method	Result Selection
Thakkar V et al., 2016 [65]	Case–Control study: 15 consecutive treatment naive patients with newly diagnosed SSc-PAH and compared with 30 SSc-controls without PAH.	high-performance liquid chromatography–mass spectrometry (HPLC-MS);	Asymmetric dimethylarginine (ADMA) levels higher in SSc-PAH.
Alotaibi M et al., 2023 [66]	N = 400 SSc-PAH. Controls: N = 1.082 IPAH. Validation Cohort of 100 patients with SSc without PAH	liquid chromatography–high-resolution mass spectrometry (LC-MS)	Lignoceric acid and nervonic acid, eicosanoids/oxylipins and sex hormone metabolites distinguishing between SSc-PAH and IPAH.
Simpson CE et al., 2023 [67]	N = 62 SSc-PAH, N = 19 SSc comparators without PAH, N = 85 HC	liquid chromatography–mass spectrometry (LC-MS)	Kynurenine and its ratio to tryptophan (kyn/trp) increased over the surveillance period in patients with SSc who developed PAH.

4. Discussion

According to our defined inclusion and exclusion criteria, we identified 13 articles in this review focusing on serum or plasma metabolites in SSc patients and summarized the key findings on dysregulated metabolic pathways in SSc (Table 1).

Only two studies included cohorts of more than 100 individuals [41,51]. Almost all studies compared SSc-associated metabolome changes with healthy controls (HC). Exceptions included one study that focused on SSc-PAH and also included idiopathic pulmonary arterial hypertension (IPAH) as a control [66] and another study that considered other inflammatory rheumatic diseases, using SSc only as a control [38]. In this latter study, SSc individuals were phenotyped in a more restricted manner. Thus, metabolome-phenotype associations must be evaluated with caution in this study. The most frequently examined organ complications with reported significant aberrations of the metabolome were skin involvement, ILD, and PAH. Regarding other organ involvements, no consistent or significant associations with metabolome alterations have been identified in the studies to date. This lack of findings may be attributed to the heterogeneity of SSc manifestations and the often small cohort sizes. One study even found no significant changes in metabolome parameters comparing SSc patients with and without ILD. Furthermore, it remains unclear whether the observed metabolome aberrations are causal or a consequence of SSc.

It should also be noted that the studies that focused on the metabolome pattern in SSc-PAH examined blood from the pulmonary arteries. Consequently, comparability with other studies using peripheral blood as a sample source is limited.

Although the metabolome parameters associated with specific organ manifestations differed between studies, all authors consistently identified significant differences between SSc and HC. However, common disturbed metabolic pathways emerged across studies, particularly including energy-related metabolic pathways such as glycolysis/gluconeogenesis, the synthesis and degradation of ketones, fatty acid oxidation, amino acid-related metabolic pathways, lipid metabolism, and the TCA cycle with pyruvate metabolism. Given the complexity of metabolic profiles, we would like to present selected patterns below and discuss possible implications for SSc pathology. Interestingly, in individual cases [41], previously identified metabolomic abnormalities normalized during treatment, thus warranting further investigation into metabolome–immune phenotype associations. This also implies that, in addition to SSc organ involvement, treatment status and inflammatory activity should always be documented during sample collection in future metabolomic studies and that prospective approaches remain complementary.

Alterations in amino acid metabolism [41,42,56,58,59,65] have been frequently observed in SSc patients, possibly related to protein synthesis and catabolism. In addition to the aforementioned discussed role of specific amino acid metabolites in collagen metabolism and fibrosis development [42–45] and the potential pro-inflammatory Th17 shift through dominant glutaminolysis [46], further metabolome changes in SSc should be discussed in light of the energy metabolism of respective immune effector cells or target cells of autoimmune inflammation, SSc-associated vasculopathy and fibrosis. Referring to the observations of Murgia et al., differentiating cutaneous disease severity based on metabolic changes within glycolysis/gluconeogenesis and glutamate-glutamine metabolism, the respective energy source of immune effector cells may even be a contributing factor. In addition to glucose, amino acids play an important role for T cells as a primary energy source and as a substrate for protein and nucleic acid biosynthesis [68]. Notably, T cells possess a functional GABAergic system that is involved in modulating immune response [69]. Glutamate, a precursor of γ-aminobutyric acid (GABA), acts as an antioxidant through its immediate precursor glutathione [70,71]. Interestingly, glutamine, but not glutamate, uptake is enhanced during T cell activation [72,73], which could explain the observed relative increase in glutamate and decrease in glutamine in patients with dcSSc compared to lcSSc patients. Glutamine is not only important for protein synthesis but also contributes to other processes, which are important for T cell proliferation, including fatty acid synthesis and the synthesis of purine and pyrimidine nucleotides.

On the other hand, certain amino acid metabolites can facilitate a pro-inflammatory and pro-fibrotic environment, reinforcing the potential causal role of metabolomic changes. For example, BCAAs, particularly leucine and isoleucine, demonstrated prognostic value for the course of SSc-ILD and lung function parameters. Furthermore, especially L-leucine, stimulates protein synthesis and reduces protein degradation through the phosphorylation of mTOR [74]. mTOR plays an important role in anabolic processes by inducing cells to switch from oxidative phosphorylation to aerobic glycolysis [75], while its activity is increased in SSc and pulmonary fibrosis [76]. Another consistent finding across multiple studies is the tendency of SSc patients to lower tryptophan levels [41,58,59]. Possible explanations include enhanced metabolism of this essential amino acid, especially under inflammatory conditions, via the kynurenine-, serotonin-, and indole-3-pyruvate pathways [77]. The majority of tryptophan is metabolized via the kynurenine pathway, which is stimulated by pro-inflammatory substances such as lipopolysaccharides, tumor necrosis factor α, and interleukin 1 and 2 [78]. The resulting kynurenine stimulates CD4 and CD8 double-negative T lymphocytes and thus maintains the inflammatory process [79]. As already mentioned, disturbances in the kynurenine pathway appear to represent a common metabolomic marker for ILD and PAH [58,59,67]. These findings could point towards new avenues for treatment.

In addition to amino acids, several studies have identified a dyslipidemia in patients with SSc, correlating with specific organ manifestations and disease activity. Lipids fulfill multiple physiological functions, for example, acting as structural components of cellular membranes and as an energy source. Furthermore, lipids such as short-chain, medium-chain, and long-chain fatty acids influence immune response, particularly through T-lymphocyte differentiation [53]. Medium-chain fatty acids promote a Th1 and Th17 shift and inhibit Treg cells [80], while (long-chain) fatty acids represent the basis for the production of pro- and anti-inflammatory cytokines [81]. The importance of eicosanoids and other fatty acid derivatives in SSc has already been extensively investigated [48]. However, a detailed discussion is beyond the scope of this article.

Nevertheless, recent findings on changes in lipoprotein subfractions in SSc should be discussed in more detail [51]. A large study with more than 100 SSc patients demonstrated that SSc-ILD is characterized by a dyslipidemic profile. In this study, reduced HDL levels (measured by 1H NMR spectroscopy) were not only associated with SSc-ILD, but additionally, HDL and ApoA1/A2 levels were positively correlated with established parameters of disease severity in SSc-ILD, such as FVC and DLCO. Furthermore, a negative correlation between HDL and its apolipoproteins and skin fibrosis (measured by mRSS) and thus, another validated biomarker was observed [51]. Since these results persisted even after adjustment and multivariate analysis for typical confounding factors of HDL/LDL-dyslipidemia, the often neglected immunological effects of HDL may be discussed as a cause and link to SSc-microvasculopathy. Various immunomodulatory HDL effects have been described: inter alia, anti-apoptotic, anti-inflammatory, endothelial cell repair, and proliferation-enhancing effects. These effects are partly explained by downregulation of the expression of cell adhesion molecules, namely VCAM-1 and ICAM-1, and reduced expression of MCP-1 [82–86]. In this context, the distinct metabolomic profile of endothelial cells in SSc patients with PAH described by Deidda et al. [56], as well as the association of reduced HDL levels in SSc-PAH patients described by Borba et al. [87], should also be discussed. In addition, another group demonstrated a correlation between cholesterol efflux capacity and skin fibrosis [88].

Conclusively, it is reasonable to speculate that high-resolution metabolomic determination of the lipoprotein profile is suitable for a more individualized assessment of SSc-ILD. Nevertheless, several inherent limitations remain to be considered when applying and interpreting metabolomic analyses. For example, the comparability of studies using different analytical techniques is challenging. In this instance, MS and NMR profiling are widely used techniques for metabolome analysis, each with its own advantages and disadvantages. NMR spectroscopy is robust and reproducible. The sample preparation is relatively simple, and the measurement is non-destructive. However, compared to mass spectrometry, the detection limit is significantly lower. Mass spectrometry is sensitive and can simultaneously analyze a wide range of components. The complexity of the data makes the evaluation process intricate. Despite the promising potential of metabolomics to uncover novel biomarkers and pathophysiological mechanisms in SSc, some further methodological challenges could limit the robustness and reproducibility of current findings. A critical issue is the frequent mismatch between small sample sizes and the high dimensionality of metabolomic data, which increases the risk of overfitting and compromises the stability of feature selection [89]. In this context, it is important to note that of the 13 studies included in this review, 10 included fewer than 100 SSc individuals. Among the studies with fewer than 100 SSc individuals, six studies examined cohorts under 50 individuals (Table 1). Balanced and representative patient stratification with regard to disease activity/stage, (clinical/serological) phenotypes, and demographic characteristics such as age, gender, and ethnicity is, therefore, often lacking. However, since all of these factors can influence metabolite activities, future studies on potential metabolomic biomarkers should include careful patient characterization based on, inter alia, a combination of clinical, biochemical, and radiological profiling. In addition, stratification according to prevalent comorbidities such as sarcopenia, pulmonary cachexia, or chronic kidney disease is also desirable to exclude further metabolomic confounders.

With regard to biomarker studies, it remains necessary to conduct further longitudinal and comparative analyses on different disease phenotypes during disease progression using the same analytical techniques, since different clinical presentations manifest at the onset and during disease progression. In addition to considering age- and sex-matched healthy controls, the inclusion of disease controls in multicenter cohorts in future studies must be postulated in order to be able to specify potential biomarkers.

Furthermore, batch effects introduced during sample processing and data acquisition can confound biological signals if not adequately controlled [90]. Biological variability, stemming from disease heterogeneity, comorbidities, medication use, and lifestyle factors, adds another layer of complexity, often obscuring disease-specific metabolic signatures [91,92]. Compounding these issues is the limited availability of external validation cohorts, which limits the generalizability of proposed biomarkers.

Addressing these challenges requires rigorous study design, standardized protocols, appropriate statistical frameworks, and multicenter collaborations to enable robust validation in future large-scale cohort studies on SSc-associated metabolomics. Characteristic and clinically challenging features of SSc remain the great heterogeneity of clinical manifestations and the high variability of disease progression in individual patients. In this regard, disease-specific biomarkers can have different functions. They may be used for diagnosis, monitoring of therapy, or for prognosis.

In terms of (early) diagnostic utility, again, the work of Guo et al. should be mentioned, since this work reported some metabolites to be associated with the presence of abnormalities in capillaroscopy. Capillaroscopy is a non-invasive and easy-to-perform examination with high diagnostic value in the assessment of secondary Raynaud's phenomenon and the diagnostic differentiation of SSc. Furthermore, there is evidence that specific nailfold videocapillaroscopy patterns have an association with SSc-ILD and SSc-PAH independent of the SSc-autoantibodies [93], so that the question arises whether the presence of a simultaneous metabolic fingerprint can be delineated. Guo et al. [41] identified LysoPC(16:1(9Z)/0:0), Thromboxane A2, and 4-Vinylphenol sulfate upregulated in the presence of an abnormal capillaroscopy. However, only a dichotomous distinction was made between normal and abnormal nailfold capillaries. A detailed description of the capillaroscopic pattern, for example, early versus late or active pattern, was not provided. Nevertheless, a connection to (micro)vasculopathy seems conceivable due to the identified metabolites, since in the case of thromboxane, the contraction of smooth muscles in blood vessels and airways is mediated via the thromboxane receptors. The precise pathophysiological functions represented by the other two metabolites in different states remain to be specified. Finally, it should be mentioned that Caramaschi et al. [94] exclusively examined plasma homocysteine (Hcy) levels using a high-performance liquid chromatography method with fluorescent detection [94] and found a significant correlation between plasma Hcy concentration and the nailfold videocapillaroscopic pattern in SSc, with a progressive increase from the early to the active and, above all, the late pattern. This study is not included in our review because it focused exclusively on homocysteine. Also, not included in our review is the study by Volpe et al. [95] since this study investigated the urine metabolome.

Taken together, due to the aforementioned inherent limitations of metabolomic studies in general and the design of the studies conducted so far, no reliable statement can be made regarding the diagnostic utility of metabolomic profiling with regard to early diagnosis of SSc. If used for (early) diagnosis, more elaborate study designs would have been necessary in order to show that metabolic signatures are not associated with other—and in terms of pathophysiology similar—diseases. On the other hand, some studies demonstrated correlations between specific metabolites and disease activity, thus providing the groundwork for a potential prognostic utility of metabolomic profiling with regard to visceral organ manifestations. Therefore, further studies with prospective study designs remain mandatory to better evaluate individual metabolomic parameters not only with regard to their prognostic utility but also in terms of treatment response.

5. Conclusions

The challenge of metabolic characterization of SSc lies in its rarity and the highly variable disease course. However, this is precisely why the need for integrated studies on non-invasive, prognostic, and early diagnostic biomarkers remains urgent, with the intention to improve treatment and intervene in the progression of the disease through a personalized approach. As demonstrated, metabolic characterization in SSc offers promising perspectives with regard to diagnosis, disease endotyping, and the detection of additional biomarkers. Although the metabolome can be influenced by various factors, and the studies to date only allow speculation about a causal relationship between the observed metabolic disturbances and SSc-specific inflammation, the data at least indicate the existence of common metabolome patterns within the disease. Currently, the interpretation of these metabolic patterns or associations should be undertaken with great caution, as the results are based on the use of various analytical metabolomic techniques and the cohorts were partly small and can only be compared to a limited extent or not at all with regard to aspects such as disease duration, phenotype, and specific therapies.

However, some of the reported metabolic fingerprints not only correlate with disease activity, but also in vitro data suggest the modulation of autoimmunity, vasculopathy, fibrosis, and intestinal dysbiosis by the respective metabolic pathways. Consequently, further studies remain mandatory to characterize the role of these alterations in the pathophysiology of the disease. Based on the studies conducted to date, mainly, but not exclusively, amino acid and lipid metabolism, as well as dysregulation of the TCA cycle, appear to have great potential to define metabolomic networks as treatment targets or as biomarkers not only for diagnosis, but also for prognosis and response to treatment.

Author Contributions: Conceptualization: S.T.J. and F.S.; methodology: S.T.J., F.S., C.S. and U.L.G.; investigation: S.T.J., F.S. and G.R.; data curation: S.T.J., U.L.G., C.S. and G.R.; writing—original draft preparation: S.T.J. and F.S.; writing—review and editing: C.S., U.L.G. and G.R.; supervision: U.L.G., G.R. and C.S.; project administration: S.T.J. All authors have read and agreed to the published version of the manuscript.

Funding: This research received no external funding.

Institutional Review Board Statement: Not applicable.

Informed Consent Statement: Not applicable.

Data Availability Statement: Data based on the literature review are available on reasonable request. Researchers interested in performing additional analysis are invited to submit proposals: For approved projects, after review by our institution summary tables will be provided as requested. Proposals should be directed to Sebastian. Jendrek@uksh.de. Raw data is not available to other researchers, since no new data were created.

Acknowledgments: The authors would like to thank all working groups and patients involved in the cited studies for their dedicated work and cooperation.

Conflicts of Interest: The authors declare no conflicts of interest.

References

1. Gabrielli, A.; Avvedimento, E.V.; Krieg, T. Scleroderma. *N. Engl. J. Med.* **2009**, *360*, 1989–2003. [CrossRef] [PubMed]
2. Steen, V.D. Autoantibodies in systemic sclerosis. *Semin. Arthritis Rheum.* **2005**, *35*, 35–42. [CrossRef] [PubMed]
3. Moinzadeh, P.; Aberer, E.; Ahmadi-Simab, K.; Blank, N.; Distler, J.H.W.; Fierlbeck, G.; Genth, E.; Guenther, C.; Hein, R.; Henes, J.; et al. Disease progression in systemic sclerosis-overlap syndrome is significantly different from limited and diffuse cutaneous systemic sclerosis. *Ann. Rheum. Dis.* **2015**, *74*, 730–737. [CrossRef]
4. Mok, C.C.; Kwok, C.L.; Ho, L.Y.; Chan, P.T.; Yip, S.F. Life expectancy, standardized mortality ratios, and causes of death in six rheumatic diseases in Hong Kong, China. *Arthritis Rheum.* **2011**, *63*, 1182–1189. [CrossRef]
5. Steen, V.D.; Medsger, T.A. Changes in causes of death in systemic sclerosis, 1972–2002. *Ann. Rheum. Dis.* **2007**, *66*, 940–944. [CrossRef]
6. Elhai, M.; Meune, C.; Boubaya, M.; Avouac, J.; Hachulla, E.; Balbir-Gurman, A.; Riemekasten, G.; Airò, P.; Joven, B.; Vettori, S.; et al. Mapping and predicting mortality from systemic sclerosis. *Ann. Rheum. Dis.* **2017**, *76*, 1897–1905. [CrossRef] [PubMed]
7. Smith, V.; Scirè, C.A.; Talarico, R.; Airo, P.; Alexander, T.; Allanore, Y.; Bruni, C.; Codullo, V.; Dalm, V.; De Vries-Bouwstra, J.; et al. Systemic sclerosis: State of the art on clinical practice guidelines. *RMD Open* **2018**, *4*, e000782. [CrossRef]
8. Hachulla, E.; Agard, C.; Allanore, Y.; Avouac, J.; Bader-Meunier, B.; Belot, A.; Berezne, A.; Bouthors, A.-S.; Condette-Wojtasik, G.; Constans, J.; et al. French recommendations for the management of systemic sclerosis. *Orphanet J. Rare Dis.* **2021**, *16*, 322. [CrossRef]
9. Furst, D.; Khanna, D.; Matucci-Cerinic, M.; Clements, P.; Steen, V.; Pope, J.; Merkel, P.; Foeldvari, I.; Seibold, J.; Pittrow, D.; et al. Systemic sclerosis—Continuing progress in developing clinical measures of response. *J. Rheumatol.* **2007**, *34*, 1194–1200.
10. Caramaschi, P.; Canestrini, S.; Martinelli, N.; Volpe, A.; Pieropan, S.; Ferrari, M.; Bambara, L.M.; Carletto, A.; Biasi, D. Scleroderma patients nailfold videocapillaroscopic patterns are associated with disease subset and disease severity. *Rheumtology* **2007**, *46*, 1566–1569. [CrossRef]
11. Domsic, R.T. Scleroderma: The role of serum autoantibodies in defining specific clinical phenotypes and organ system involvement. *Curr. Opin. Rheumatol.* **2014**, *26*, 646–652. [CrossRef]
12. Hachulla, E.; Czirjak, L. *EULAR Textbook on Systemic Sclerosis*, 1st ed.; BMJ Publishing Group Ltd.: London, UK, 2013.
13. van Laar, J.M.; Farge, D.; Sont, J.K.; Naraghi, K.; Marjanovic, Z.; Larghero, J.; Schuerwegh, A.J.; Marijt, E.W.A.; Vonk, M.C.; Schattenberg, A.V.; et al. Autologous hematopoietic stem cell transplantation vs intravenous pulse cyclophosphamide in diffuse cutaneous systemic sclerosis:a randomizedclinical trial. *JAMA* **2014**, *311*, 2490–2498. [CrossRef] [PubMed]

14. Scleroderma Lung Study Research Group; Tashkin, D.P.; Elashoff, R.; Clements, P.J.; Goldin, J.; Roth, M.D.; Furst, D.E.; Arriola, E.; Silver, R.; Strange, C.; et al. Cyclophosphamide versus placebo in scleroderma lung disease. *N. Engl. J. Med.* **2006**, *354*, 2655–2666. [CrossRef] [PubMed]
15. Iudici, M.; Cuomo, G.; Vettori, S.; Bocchino, M.; Zamparelli, A.S.; Cappabianca, S.; Valentini, G. Low-dose pulse cyclophosphamide in interstitial lung disease associated with systemic sclerosis (SSc-ILD): Efficacy of maintenance immunosuppression in responders and non-responders. *Semin. Arthritis Rheum.* **2015**, *44*, 437–444. [CrossRef]
16. Assassi, S.; Mayes, M.D. What does global gene expression profiling tell us about the pathogenesis of systemic sclerosis? *Curr. Opin. Rheumatol.* **2013**, *25*, 686–691. [CrossRef]
17. Becker, M.O.; Brückner, C.; Scherer, H.U.; Wassermann, N.; Humrich, J.Y.; Hanitsch, L.G.; Schneider, U.; Kawald, A.; Hanke, K.; Burmester, G.R.; et al. The monoclonal anti-CD25 antibody basiliximab for the treatment of progressive systemic sclerosis: An open-label study. *Ann. Rheum. Dis.* **2011**, *70*, 1340–1341. [CrossRef]
18. Mora, G.F. Systemic sclerosis: Environmental factors. *J. Rheumatol.* **2009**, *36*, 2383–2396. [CrossRef] [PubMed]
19. Sternberg, E.M.; Van Woert, M.H.; Young, S.N.; Magnussen, I.; Baker, H.; Gauthier, S.; Osterland, C.K. Development of a scleroderma-like illness during therapy with L15-Hydroxytryptophan and carbidopa. *N. Engl. J. Med.* **1980**, *303*, 782–787. [CrossRef]
20. Volkmann, E.R.; Hoffmann-Vold, A.-M.; Chang, Y.-L.; Jacobs, J.P.; Tillisch, K.; Mayer, E.A.; Clements, P.J.; Hov, J.R.; Kummen, M.; Midtvedt, Ø.; et al. Systemic sclerosis is associated with specific alterations in gastrointestinal microbiota in two independent cohorts. *BMJ Open Gastroenterol.* **2017**, *4*, e000134. [CrossRef]
21. Patrone, V.; Puglisi, E.; Cardinali, M.; Schnitzler, T.S.; Svegliati, S.; Festa, A.; Gabrielli, A.; Morelli, L. Gut microbiota profile in systemic sclerosis patients with and without clinical evidence of gastrointestinal involvement. *Sci. Rep.* **2017**, *7*, 14874. [CrossRef]
22. Murphy, M.P.; O'Neill, L.A.J. Krebs cycle reimagined: The emerging roles of succinate and itaconate as signal transducers. *Cell* **2018**, *174*, 780–784. [CrossRef] [PubMed]
23. Fan, J.; Krautkramer, K.A.; Feldman, J.L.; Denu, J.M. Metabolic regulation of histone post-translational modifications. *ACS Chem. Biol.* **2015**, *10*, 95–108. [CrossRef]
24. Cameron, A.M.; Lawless, S.J.; Pearce, E.J. Metabolism and acetylation in innate immune cell function and fate. *Semin. Immunol.* **2016**, *28*, 408–416. [CrossRef] [PubMed]
25. Mason, E.F.; Rathmell, J.C. Cell metabolism: An essential link between cell growth and apoptosis. *Biochem. Biophys. Acta* **2011**, *1813*, 645–654. [CrossRef]
26. Voss, K.; Larsen, S.E.; Snow, A.L. Metabolic reprogramming and apoptosis sensitivity: Defining the contours of a T cell response. *Cancer Lett.* **2017**, *408*, 190–196. [CrossRef] [PubMed]
27. Kim, B.; Arcos, S.; Rothamel, K.; Jian, J.; Rose, K.L.; McDonald, W.H.; Bian, Y.; Reasoner, S.; Barrows, N.J.; Bradrick, S.; et al. Discovery of widespread host protein interactions with the pre-replicated genome of CHIKV Using VIR-CLASP. *Mol. Cell* **2020**, *78*, 624–640. [CrossRef]
28. Pollizzi, K.N.; Powell, J.D. Integrating canonical and metabolic signalling programmes in the regulation of T cell responses. *Nat. Rev. Immunol.* **2014**, *14*, 435–446. [CrossRef]
29. Jellusova, J. Cross-talk between signal transduction and metabolism in B cells. *Immunol. Lett.* **2018**, *201*, 1–13. [CrossRef]
30. Zasfona, Z.; O'Neill, L.A.J. Cytokine-like roles for metabolites in immunity. *Mol. Cell* **2020**, *78*, 814–823. [CrossRef]
31. Krause, L.; Becker, M.O.; Brueckner, C.S.; Bellinghausen, C.-J.; Becker, C.; Schneider, U.; Haeupl, T.; Hanke, K.; Hensel-Wiegel, K.; Ebert, H.; et al. Nutritional status as marker for disease activity and severity predicting mortality in patients with systemic sclerosis. *Ann. Rheum. Dis.* **2010**, *69*, 1951–1957. [CrossRef]
32. Villas-Bas, S.G.; Roessner-Tunali, U.; Hansen, M.A.E.; Smedsgaard, J.; Nielsen, J. *Metabolome Analysis: An Introduction*, 1st ed.; John Wiley & Sons, Inc.: Hoboken, NJ, USA, 2007.
33. Fiehn, O. Combining Genomics, Metabolome Analysis, and Biochemical Modelling to Understand Metabolic Networks. *Comp. Funct. Genom.* **2001**, *2*, 155–168. [CrossRef] [PubMed]
34. Hall, R.D. Plant Metabolomics: From Holistic Hope, to Hype, to Hot Topic. *N. Phytol.* **2006**, *169*, 453–468. [CrossRef]
35. Karu, N.; Deng, L.; Slae, M.; Guo, A.C.; Sajed, T.; Huynh, H.; Wine, E.; Wishart, D.S. A Review on Human Fecal Metabolomics: Methods, Applications and the Human Fecal Metabolome Database. *Anal. Chim. Acta* **2018**, *1030*, 1–24. [CrossRef]
36. Dettmer, K.; Aronov, P.A.; Hammock, B.D. Mass Spectrometry-Based Metabolomics. *Mass Spectrom. Rev.* **2007**, *26*, 51–78. [CrossRef]
37. Page, M.J.; McKenzie, J.E.; Bossuyt, P.M.; Boutron, I.; Hoffmann, T.C.; Mulrow, C.D.; Shamseer, L.; Tetzlaff, J.M.; Akl, E.A.; Brennan, S.E.; et al. The PRISMA 2020 statement: An updated guideline for reporting systematic reviews. *BMJ* **2021**, *372*, n71. [CrossRef]
38. Fernández-Ochoa, Á.; Brunius, C.; Borrás-Linares, I.; Quirantes-Piné, R.; Cádiz-Gurrea, M.d.l.L.; PRECISESADS Clinical Consortium; Riquelme, M.E.A.; Segura-Carretero, A. Metabolic disturbances in urinary and plasma samples from seven different systemic autoimmune diseases detected by HPLCESI-QTOF-MS. *J. Proteome Res.* **2020**, *19*, 3220–3229. [CrossRef]

39. Bengtsson, A.A.; Trygg, J.; Wuttge, D.M.; Sturfelt, G.; Theander, E.; Donten, M.; Moritz, T.; Sennbro, C.-J.; Torell, F.; Lood, C.; et al. Metabolic profiling of systemic lupus erythematosus and comparison with primary Sjögren's syndrome and systemic sclerosis. *PLoS ONE* **2016**, *11*, e0159384. [CrossRef] [PubMed]
40. Xie, S.; Meng, Q.; Wang, L. The effect of gut microbiome and plasma metabolome on systemic sclerosis: A bidirectional two-sample Mendelian randomization study. *Front. Microbiol.* **2024**, *15*, 1427195. [CrossRef] [PubMed]
41. Guo, M.; Liu, D.; Jiang, Y.; Chen, W.; Zhao, L.; Bao, D.; Li, Y.; Distler, J.H.; Zhu, H. Serum metabolomic profiling reveals potential biomarkers in systemic sclerosis. *Metabolism* **2023**, *144*, 155587. [CrossRef]
42. Ung, C.Y.; Onoufriadis, A.; Parsons, M.; McGrath, J.A.; Shaw, T.J. Metabolic perturbations in fibrosis disease. *Int. J. Biochem. Cell Biol.* **2021**, *139*, 106073. [CrossRef]
43. Karna, E.; Szoka, L.; Huynh, T.Y.L.; Palka, J.A. Proline-dependentregulation of collagen metabolism. *Cell Mol. Life Sci.* **2020**, *77*, 1911–1918. [CrossRef] [PubMed]
44. Schwörer, S.; Berisa, M.; Violante, S.; Qin, W.; Zhu, J.; Hendrickson, R.C.; Cross, J.R.; Thompson, C.B. Proline biosynthesis is a vent for TGFβ-induced mitochondrial redox stress. *EMBO J.* **2020**, *39*, e103334. [CrossRef] [PubMed]
45. Kay, E.J.; Koulouras, G.; Zanivan, S. Regulation of extracellular matrix production in activated fibroblasts: Roles of amino acid metabolism in collagen synthesis. *Front. Oncol.* **2021**, *11*, 719922. [CrossRef]
46. Cruzat, V.; Macedo Rogero, M.; Keane, K.N.; Curi, R.; Newsholme, P. Glutamine: Metabolism and immune function, supplementation and clinical translation. *Nutrients* **2018**, *10*, 1564. [CrossRef] [PubMed]
47. Smolenska, Z.; Zabielska-Kaczorowska, M.; Wojteczek, A.; Kutryb-Zajac, B.; Zdrojewski, Z. Metabolic Pattern of Systemic Sclerosis: Association of Changes in Plasma Concentrations of Amino Acid-Related Compounds With Disease Presentation. *Front. Mol. Biosci.* **2020**, *7*, 585161. [CrossRef] [PubMed]
48. Gogulska, Z.; Smolenska, Z.; Turyn, J.; Mika, A.; Zdrojewski, Z. Lipid alterations in systemic sclerosis. *Front. Mol. Biosci.* **2021**, *8*, 761721. [CrossRef]
49. Fernández-Ochoa, Á.; Quirantes-Piné, R.; Borrás-Linares, I.; Gemperline, D.; Riquelme, M.E.A.; Beretta, L.; Segura-Carretero, A. Urinary and plasma metabolite differences detected by HPLC-ESI-QTOF-MS in systemic sclerosis patients. *J. Pharm. Biomed. Anal.* **2019**, *162*, 82–90. [CrossRef]
50. Cartier, A.; Hla, T. Sphingosine 1-phosphate: Lipid signaling in pathology and therapy. *Science* **2019**, *366*, eaar5551. [CrossRef]
51. Jendrek, S.T.; Schmelter, F.; Schinke, S.; Hackel, A.; Graßhoff, H.; Lamprecht, P.; Humrich, J.Y.; Sina, C.; Müller, A.; Günther, U.; et al. Metabolomic signature identifies HDL and apolipoproteins as potential biomarker for systemic sclerosis with interstitial lung disease. *Respir. Med.* **2024**, *234*, 107825. [CrossRef]
52. Hettema, M.E.; Zhang, D.; de Leeuw, K.; Stienstra, Y.; Smit, A.J.; Kallenberg, C.G.; Bootsma, H. Early atherosclerosis in systemic sclerosis and its relation to disease or traditional risk factors. *Arthritis Res. Ther.* **2008**, *10*, R49. [CrossRef]
53. Park, J.; Kim, M.; Kang, S.G.; Jannasch, A.H.; Cooper, B.; Patterson, J.; Kim, C.H. Short-chain fatty acids induce both effector and regulatory T cells by suppression of histone deacetylases and regulation of the mTOR-S6K pathway. *Mucosal Immunol.* **2015**, *8*, 80–93. [CrossRef]
54. Cleophas, M.C.P.; Ratter, J.M.; Bekkering, S.; Quintin, J.; Schraa, K.; Stroes, E.S.; Netea, M.G.; Joosten, L.A.B. Effects of oral butyrate supplementation on inflammatory potential of circulating peripheral blood mononuclear cells in healthy and obese males. *Sci. Rep.* **2019**, *9*, 775. [CrossRef] [PubMed]
55. Murgia, F.; Svegliati, S.; Poddighe, S.; Lussu, M.; Manzin, A.; Spadoni, T.; Fischetti, C.; Gabrielli, A.; Atzori, L. Metabolomic profile of systemic sclerosis patients. *Sci. Rep.* **2018**, *8*, 7627. [CrossRef] [PubMed]
56. Deidda, M.; Piras, C.; Dessalvi, C.C.; Locci, E.; Barberini, L.; Orofino, S.; Musu, M.; Mura, M.N.; Manconi, P.E.; Finco, G.; et al. Distinctive metabolomic fingerprint in scleroderma patients with pulmonary arterial hypertension. *Int. J. Cardiol.* **2017**, *241*, 401–406. [CrossRef]
57. Bellocchi, C.; Fernández-Ochoa, Á.; Montanelli, G.; Vigone, B.; Santaniello, A.; Milani, C.; Quirantes-Piné, R.; Borrás-Linares, I.; Ventura, M.; Segura-Carrettero, A.; et al. Microbial and metabolic multi-omic correlations in systemic sclerosis patients. *Ann. N. Y. Acad. Sci.* **2018**, *1421*, 97–109. [CrossRef]
58. Bögl, T.; Mlynek, F.; Himmelsbach, M.; Sepp, N.; Buchberger, W.; Geroldinger-Simić, M. Plasma metabolomic profiling reveals four possibly disrupted mechanisms in systemic sclerosis. *Biomedicines* **2022**, *10*, 607. [CrossRef] [PubMed]
59. Meier, C.; Freiburghaus, K.; Bovet, C.; Schniering, J.; Allanore, Y.; Distler, O.; Nakas, C.; Maurer, B. Serum metabolites as biomarkers in systemic sclerosis-associated interstitial lung disease. *Sci. Rep.* **2020**, *10*, 21912. [CrossRef]
60. Sun, C.; Zhu, H.; Wang, Y.; Han, Y.; Zhang, D.; Cao, X.; Alip, M.; Nie, M.; Xu, X.; Lv, L.; et al. Serum metabolite differences detected by HILIC UHPLC-Q-TOF MS in systemic sclerosis. *Clin. Rheumatol.* **2023**, *42*, 125–134. [CrossRef]
61. Ottria, A.; Hoekstra, A.T.; Zimmermann, M.; van der Kroef, M.; Vazirpanah, N.; Cossu, M.; Chouri, E.; Rossato, M.; Beretta, L.; Tieland, R.G.; et al. Fatty acid and carnitine metabolism are dysregulated in systemic sclerosis patients. *Front. Immunol.* **2020**, *11*, 822. [CrossRef]

62. Avouac, J.; Airo, P.; Meune, C.; Beretta, L.; Dieude, P.; Caramaschi, P.; Tiev, K.; Cappelli, S.; Diot, E.; Vacca, A.; et al. Prevalence of pulmonary hypertension in systemic sclerosis in European Caucasians and metaanalysis of 5 studies. *J. Rheumatol.* **2010**, *37*, 2290–2298. [CrossRef]
63. Naranjo, M.; Hassoun, P.M. Systemic sclerosis-associated pulmonary hypertension: Spectrum and impact. *Diagnostics* **2021**, *11*, 911. [CrossRef] [PubMed]
64. Humbert, M.; Yaici, A.; de Groote, P.; Montani, D.; Sitbon, O.; Launay, D.; Gressin, V.; Guillevin, L.; Clerson, P.; Simonneau, G.; et al. Screening for pulmonary arterial hypertension in patients with systemic sclerosis: Clinical characteristics at diagnosis and long-term survival. *ArthritisRheum* **2011**, *63*, 3522–3530. [CrossRef] [PubMed]
65. Thakkar, V.; Stevens, W.; Prior, D.; Rabusa, C.; Sahhar, J.; Walker, J.G.; Roddy, J.; Lester, S.; Rischmueller, M.; Zochling, J.; et al. The role of asymmetric dimethylarginine alone and in combination with N-terminal pro-B-type natriuretic peptide as a screening biomarker for systemic sclerosis-related pulmonary arterial hypertension: A case control study. *Clin. Exp. Rheumatol.* **2016**, *1*, 129–136.
66. Alotaibi, M.; Shao, J.; Pauciulo, M.W.; Nichols, W.C.; Hemnes, A.R.; Malhotra, A.; Kim, N.H.; Yuan, J.X.-J.; Fernandes, T.; Kerr, K.M.; et al. Metabolomic pro files differentiate Scleroderma PAH from idiopathic PAH and correspond with worsened functional capacity. *Chest* **2023**, *163*, 204–215. [CrossRef]
67. Simpson, C.E.; Ambade, A.S.; Harlan, R.; Roux, A.; Aja, S.; Graham, D.; Shah, A.A.; Hummers, L.K.; Hemnes, A.R.; Leopold, J.A.; et al. Kynurenine pathway metabolism evolves with development of preclinical and scleroderma-associated pulmonary arterial hypertension. *Am. J. Physiol. Cell. Mol. Physiol.* **2023**, *325*, L617–L627. [CrossRef] [PubMed]
68. Yang, Z.; Matteson, E.L.; Goronzy, J.J.; Weyand, C. T-cell metabolism in autoimmune disease. *Arthritis Res. Ther.* **2015**, *17*, 29. [CrossRef]
69. Peng, Y.; Wu, C.; Qin, X.; Du, H.; Li, N.; Ren, W. The immunological function of GABAergic system. *Front. Biosci.* **2017**, *22*, 1162–1172. [CrossRef]
70. Wu, G.; Fang, Y.; Yang, S.; Lupton, J.R.; Turner, N.D. Glutathione metabolism and its implications for health. *J. Nutr.* **2004**, *134*, 489–492. [CrossRef]
71. Newsholme, P.; Curi, R.; Curi, T.P.; Murphy, C.; Garcia, C.; de Melo, M.P. Glutamine metabolism by lymphocytes, macrophages, and neutrophils: Its importance in health and disease. *J. Nutr. Biochem.* **1999**, *10*, 316–324. [CrossRef]
72. Carr, E.L.; Kelman, A.; Wu, G.S.; Gopaul, R.; Senkevitch, E.; Aghvanyan, A.; Turay, A.M.; Frauwirth, K.A. Glutamine uptake and metabolism are coordinately regulated by ERK/MAPK during T lymphocyte activation. *J. Immunol.* **2010**, *185*, 1037–1044. [CrossRef]
73. Ardawi, M.S.M. Glutamine and glucose metabolism in human peripheral lymphocytes. *Metabolism* **1988**, *37*, 99–103. [CrossRef] [PubMed]
74. Wilkinson, D.J.; Hossain, T.; Hill, D.S.; Phillips, B.E.; Crossland, H.; Williams, J.; Loughna, P.; Churchward-Venne, T.A.; Breen, L.; Phillips, S.M.; et al. Effects of leucine and its metabolite beta-hydroxy-beta-methylbutyrate on human skeletal muscle protein metabolism. *J. Physiol.* **2013**, *591*, 2911–2923. [CrossRef] [PubMed]
75. Suto, T.; Karonitsch, T. The immunobiology of mTOR in autoimmunity. *J. Autoimmun.* **2019**, *110*, 102373. [CrossRef] [PubMed]
76. Lawrence, J.; Nho, R. The role of the mammalian target of rapamycin (mTOR) in pulmonary fibrosis. *Int. J. Mol. Sci.* **2018**, *19*, 778. [CrossRef]
77. Badawy, A.A.B. Tryptophan metabolism and disposition in cancer biology and immunotherapy. *Biosci. Rep.* **2022**, *42*, BSR20221682. [CrossRef]
78. Ramprasath, T.; Han, Y.-M.; Zhang, D.; Yu, C.-J.; Zou, M.-H. Tryptophan catabolism and inflammation: A Novel Therapeutic Target for aortic diseases. *Front. Immunol.* **2021**, *12*, 731701. [CrossRef]
79. Perl, A.; Hanczko, R.; Lai, Z.-W.; Oaks, Z.; Kelly, R.; Borsuk, R.; Asara, J.M.; Phillips, P.E. Comprehensive metabolome analyses reveal N-acetylcysteine-responsive accumulation of kynurenine in systemic lupus erythematosus: Implications for activation of the mechanistic target of rapamycin. *Metabolomics* **2015**, *11*, 1157–1174. [CrossRef]
80. Haghikia, A.; Jörg, S.; Duscha, A.; Berg, J.; Manzel, A.; Waschbisch, A.; Hammer, A.; Lee, D.-H.; May, C.; Wilck, N.; et al. Dietary fatty acids directly Impact Central Nervous System Autoimmunity via the small intestine. *Immunity* **2015**, *43*, 817–829. [CrossRef]
81. Ji, X.; Wu, L.; Marion, T.; Luo, Y. Lipid metabolism in regulation of B cell development and autoimmunity. *Cytokine Growth Factor Rev.* **2023**, *73*, 40–51. [CrossRef]
82. Nofer, J.-R.; van der Giet, M.; Tölle, M.; Wolinska, I.; Lipinski, K.V.W.; Baba, H.A.; Tietge, U.J.; Gödecke, A.; Ishii, I.; Kleuser, B.; et al. HDL induces NO-dependent vasorelaxation via the lysophospholipid receptor S1P3. *J. Clin. Investig.* **2004**, *113*, 569–581. [CrossRef]
83. Calabresi, L.; Gomaraschi, M.; Franceschini, G. Endothelial protection by high-density lipoproteins: From bench to bedside. *Arter. Thromb. Vasc. Biol.* **2003**, *23*, 1724–1731. [CrossRef]

84. Assanasen, C.; Mineo, C.; Seetharam, D.; Yuhanna, I.S.; Marcel, Y.L.; Connelly, M.A.; Williams, D.L.; de la Llera-Moya, M.; Shaul, P.W.; Silver, D.L. Cholesterol binding, efflux, and a PDZ-interacting domain of scavenger receptor-BI mediate HDL-initiated signaling. *J. Clin. Investig.* **2005**, *115*, 969–977. [CrossRef]
85. Gong, M.; Wilson, M.; Kelly, T.; Su, W.; Dressman, J.; Kincer, J.; Matveev, S.V.; Guo, L.; Guerin, T.; Li, X.-A.; et al. HDL-associated estradiol stimulates endothelial NO synthase and vasodilation in an SR-BI-dependent manner. *J. Clin. Investig.* **2003**, *111*, 1579–1587. [CrossRef]
86. Barter, P.J.; Nicholls, S.; Rye, K.-A.; Anantharamaiah, G.; Navab, M.; Fogelman, A.M. Antiinflammatory properties of HDL. *Circ. Res.* **2004**, *95*, 764–772. [CrossRef] [PubMed]
87. Borba, E.F.; Borges, C.T.L.; Bonfá, E. Lipoprotein profile in limited systemic sclerosis. *Rheumatol. Int.* **2005**, *25*, 379–383. [CrossRef] [PubMed]
88. Ferraz-Amaro, I.; Delgado-Frías, E.; Hernández-Hernández, V.; Sánchez-Pérez, H.; de Armas-Rillo, L.; Armas-González, E.; Machado, J.D.; Diaz-González, F. HDL cholesterol efflux capacity and lipid profile in patients with systemic sclerosis. *Arthritis Res. Ther.* **2021**, *23*, 62. [CrossRef] [PubMed]
89. Scalbert, A.; Brennan, L.; Fiehn, O.; Hankemeier, T.; Kristal, B.S.; van Ommen, B.; Pujos-Guillot, E.; Verheij, E.; Wishart, D.; Wopereis, S. Mass-spectrometry-based metabolomics: Limitations and recommendations for future progress with particular focus on nutrition research. *Metabolomics* **2009**, *5*, 435–458. [CrossRef]
90. Wachsmuth, C.; Oefner, P.; Dettmer, K. 1—Equipment and metabolite identification (ID) strategies for mass-based metabolomic analysis. In *Metabolomics in Food and Nutrition*; Woodhead Publishing Series in Food Science; Technology and Nutrition; Woodhead Publishing: Sawston, UK, 2013; pp. 3–28. [CrossRef]
91. Dunn, W.B.; Ellis, D.I. Metabolomics: Current analytical platforms and methodologies. *TrAC Trends Anal. Chem.* **2005**, *24*, 285–294.
92. Li, S.; Looby, N.; Chandran, V.; Kulasingam, V. Challenges in the Metabolomics-Based Biomarker Validation Pipeline. *Metabolites* **2024**, *14*, 200. [CrossRef]
93. Markusse, I.M.; Meijs, J.; de Boer, B.; Bakker, J.A.; Schippers, H.P.C.; Schouffoer, A.A.; Marsan, N.A.; Kroft, L.J.M.; Ninaber, M.K.; Huizinga, T.W.J.; et al. Predicting cardiopulmonary involvement in patients with systemic sclerosis: Complementary value of nailfold videocapillaroscopy patterns and disease-specificautoantibodies. *Rheumatology* **2017**, *56*, 1081–1088. [CrossRef]
94. Caramaschi, P.; Volpe, A.; Canestrini, S.; Bambara, L.M.; Faccini, G.; Carletto, A.; Biasi, D. Correlation between homocysteine plasma levels and nailfold videocapillaroscopic patterns in systemic sclerosis. *Clin. Rheumatol.* **2007**, *26*, 902–907. [CrossRef] [PubMed]
95. Volpe, A.; Biasi, D.; Caramaschi, P.; Mantovani, W.; Bambara, L.M.; Canestrini, S.; Ferrari, M.; Poli, G.; Degan, M.; Carletto, A.; et al. Levels of F2-isoprostanes in systemic sclerosis: Correlation with clinical features. *Rheumatology* **2006**, *45*, 314–320. [CrossRef] [PubMed]

MDPI AG
Grosspeteranlage 5
4052 Basel
Switzerland
Tel.: +41 61 683 77 34

Sclerosis Editorial Office
E-mail: sclerosis@mdpi.com
www.mdpi.com/journal/sclerosis

www.ingramcontent.com/pod-product-compliance
Lightning Source LLC
Chambersburg PA
CBHW041948260926
51850CB00018B/1964
9783725858033